G-quadruplex and Microorganisms

G-quadruplex and Microorganisms

Special Issue Editor

Sara N. Richter

MDPI • Basel • Beijing • Wuhan • Barcelona • Belgrade

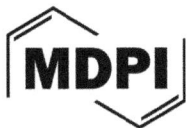

MDPI

Special Issue Editor
Sara N. Richter
University of Padua
Italy

Editorial Office
MDPI
St. Alban-Anlage 66
4052 Basel, Switzerland

This is a reprint of articles from the Special Issue published online in the open access journal *Molecules* (ISSN 1420-3049) from 2018 to 2019 (available at: https://www.mdpi.com/journal/molecules/special_issues/Gquadruplex_Microorganisms)

For citation purposes, cite each article independently as indicated on the article page online and as indicated below:

LastName, A.A.; LastName, B.B.; LastName, C.C. Article Title. *Journal Name* **Year**, *Article Number*, Page Range.

ISBN 978-3-03921-243-9 (Pbk)
ISBN 978-3-03921-244-6 (PDF)

Cover image courtesy of Sara N. Richter.

Contents

About the Special Issue Editor

Sara N. Richter is a Professor of Microbiology and Clinical Microbiology at the Department of Molecular Medicine, The University of Padua, Italy. Her research is focused on non-canonical nucleic acid structures and their presence in the genome of viruses, bacteria, and human cells in relation to infective and proliferative diseases. Together with her collaborators, she is investigating the function of non-canonical structures, their interaction with proteins, and the possibility to target them with small molecules to revert pathological traits. To date, Prof. Richter's research has generated more than 80 peer-reviewed publications. She has been awarded the European Research Council Starting and Consolidator grants, two Bill and Melinda Gates Foundation grants, and an AIRC-Italian Foundation for Cancer Research grant for her research on non-canonical nucleic acid structures and their targeting in viruses and tumors. Prof. Richter graduated in Pharmaceutical Chemistry and Technology and obtained two Ph.D. degrees in Drug Sciences and Virology at the University of Padua. She was a post-doctoral fellow at the Robert Wood Johnson Medical School, Rutgers University, Piscataway, NJ, USA.

Preface to "G-quadruplex and Microorganisms"

G-quadruplexes (G4s) are nucleic acid secondary structures that form in DNA or RNA guanine (G)-rich strands. Four G residues are connected through Hoogsteen-type hydrogen bonds, forming a G-tetrad, and two or more G-tetrads can stack on top of each other forming a G4, which is stabilized by coordinating monovalent cations, such as K^+.

G4s have been extensively described in the human genome, especially in telomeres and oncogene promoters, where their involvement in the regulation of different biological pathways such as replication, transcription, translation, and genome instability has been suggested. In addition to humans, putative G4-forming sequences have been found in other mammalian genomes, plants, yeasts, protozoa, bacteria, and viruses. In particular, in recent years, the presence of G4s in microorganisms has attracted increasing interest. In prokaryotes, G4 sequences have been found in several human pathogens and bacterial species present in the environment. Bacterial enzymes able to process G4s have also been identified. In viruses, G4s are involved in key steps of the viral life cycle: They have been associated with pathogenic mechanisms of the human immunodeficiency virus (HIV), herpes simplex virus 1 (HSV-1), human papilloma virus and have been detected in several other virus genomes. New evidence shows the presence of G4s in parasitic protozoa, such as *Plasmodium falciparum*. G4 binding proteins and mRNA G4s have been implicated in the regulation of microorganisms' genome replication and translation. G4 ligands have been developed and tested both as tools to study the complexity of G4-mediated mechanisms in the viral life cycle and as therapeutic agents. Moreover, new techniques to study G4 folding and their interactions with proteins have been developed. This Special Issue focuses on G4s present in microorganisms, addressing all the above aspects.

Sara N. Richter
Special Issue Editor

molecules

MDPI

Article

Conserved G-Quadruplexes Regulate the Immediate Early Promoters of Human *Alphaherpesviruses*

Ilaria Frasson, Matteo Nadai and Sara N. Richter *

Department of Molecular Medicine, University of Padua, via A. Gabelli 63, 35121 Padua, Italy
* Correspondence: sara.richter@unipd.it; Tel.: +39-0498272346

Received: 31 May 2019; Accepted: 26 June 2019; Published: 27 June 2019

Abstract: Human *Alphaherpesviruses* comprise three members, herpes simplex virus (HSV) 1 and 2 and varicella zoster virus (VZV). These viruses are characterized by a lytic cycle in epithelial cells and latency in the nervous system, with lifelong infections that may periodically reactivate and lead to serious complications, especially in immunocompromised patients. The mechanisms that regulate viral transcription have not been fully elucidated, but the master role of the immediate early (IE) genes has been established. G-quadruplexes are non-canonical nucleic-acid structures that control transcription, replication, and recombination in many organisms including viruses and that represent attractive antiviral targets. In this work, we investigate the presence, conservation, folding and activity of G-quadruplexes in the IE promoters of the *Alphaherpesviruses*. Our analysis shows that all IE promoters in the genome of HSV-1, HSV-2 and VZV contain fully conserved G-quadruplex forming sequences. These comprise sequences with long loops and bulges, and thus deviating from the classic G-quadruplex motifs. Moreover, their location is both on the leading and lagging strand and in some instances they contain exuberant G-tracts. Biophysical and biological analysis proved that all sequences actually fold into G-quadruplex under physiological conditions and can be further stabilized by the G-quadruplex ligand BRACO-19, with subsequent impairment of viral IE gene transcription in cells. These results help shed light on the control of viral transcription and indicate new viral targets to design drugs that impair the early steps of *Alphaherpesviruses*. In addition, they validate the significance of G-quadruplexes in the general regulation of viral cycles.

Keywords: G-quadruplex; immediate early promoters; *Alphaherpesvirinae*; Herpesvirus; virus

1. Introduction

In the last years the fact that the DNA can adopt complex secondary structures other than the double-stranded (ds) form wrapped around histones and packaged as chromatin [1] has become evident [2–4]. Guanine (G)-rich sequences in nucleic acids can assemble into G-quadruplex (G4) structures, comprising G-tetrads linked by loop nucleotides. Each G-tetrad is composed of four G residues connected through Hoogsteen-type hydrogen bonds. G4s are highly polymorphic structures, the topology of which depends on the strand stoichiometry and polarity, the nature and length of the loops and their location in the sequence [5]. The G4 parallel, antiparallel or mixed topology is directly correlated to the *syn* and *anti* conformational state of the glycosidic bond between the G base and the sugar [2]. The *anti* conformation characterizes a parallel folding, while antiparallel G4s can adopt both *syn* and *anti* orientations [6]. A number of different experimental techniques are used to study G-quadruplex formation, each examining different aspects of the structures, and hence reporting on different aspects of their formation. Circular Dichroism (CD) is a sensitive tool, widely used to investigate the conformations of nucleic acids. Based on the CD profile of maximum and minimum peaks at signature wavelengths (around 240, 260 and 290 nm), this technique allows identification of the G4 folding and characterization of the G4 topology [7]. UV absorption is an additional useful technique: G4s show both a hypochromic and a hyperchromic sigmoid transition at 295 and 240 nm, respectively [8]. The Thermal Difference Spectra (TDS) acquired by subtracting the UV absorbance spectra of the unfolded from the folded form of a given sample yield profiles that are characteristic of the G4 (i.e., a negative peak around 295 nm, and two positive peaks around 275 and 243 nm). Other useful techniques to highlight G4 formation are *Taq* polymerase stop assay [9] and mass spectrometry [10,11]. Finally, to acquire the structural details of G4 folding at the atomic level, NMR and X-ray crystallography are the ideal techniques, recently reported also in cells [6,12,13].

G4s have been shown to regulate key cellular processes, including gene expression and mRNA translation, many of which are in turn linked to significant human disorders [14–16]. The most recent literature has broadened the G4 spectrum of influence also to pathogens [17–23]. In the last years many viruses have been reported to have putative G4 sequences (PQS) in their genome, and in most cases the biological role of these structures and the potential administration of G4-ligands as active and selective antiviral agents have been described [24]. Interestingly, G4s and PQS that are significant from a functional standpoint have been repeatedly identified in members of the *Herpesviridae* virus family both at the genomic and mRNA level [17–19,25–27]. This family contains over 100 ds-DNA viruses that infect humans and a wide range of eukaryotic organisms, with eight members that are exclusively human pathogens [28]. These viruses differ significantly with respect to base composition and sequence arrangement of their DNA, but share many biologic properties including the ability to remain latent in their host. On the basis of these, the human non-zoonotic *Herpesviruses* have been classified into three subfamilies, i.e., *Alphaherpesvirinae*, *Betaherpesvirinae* and *Gammaherpesvirinae*. The members of the *Alphaherpesvirinae* subfamily are characterized by a short reproductive cycle, rapid spread in culture, efficient killing of infected cells, and capacity to establish latent infections primarily but not exclusively in sensory ganglia. This subfamily contains the genera *Simplexvirus* (HSV-1, HSV-2) and *Varicellovirus* (VZV). The life cycle of these genera is characterized by a coordinated and sequential cascade of expression of three temporal classes of viral genes [29,30]: the viral tegument protein VP16 binds to the TAATGARAT signal sequence and activates transcription of the immediate early (IE) viral genes [31], the products of which in turn activate transcription of the early and late viral genes; transcription of the late viral genes is also coupled to viral DNA replication. IE gene products include regulatory proteins, while early and late gene products comprise the viral replication machinery and the structural components of the virus, respectively.

We have recently demonstrated and visualized the presence of G4s in the HSV-1 genome [27] and their targeting by two classes of G4-ligands, which efficiently inhibited viral replication [17,32]. In addition, we evidenced that several members of the *Herpesviridae* family, i.e., HSV-1, HSV-2, VZV, HHV-4 and HHV-8, are statistically significantly enriched in G4 patterns [33]. These data suggest a conserved and essential role of G4s in *Herpesviruses*.

Here we show that conserved and stable G4s are present in crucial points of the *Alphaherpesvirinae* (i.e., HSV-1, HSV-2 and VZV) genome, in particular in promoters of IE genes, the major regulators of the life cycle of these viruses. The IE promoters contain multiple G4s on both leading and lagging strands; these viral G4s are in general stable and can be further stabilized by G4-ligands. Their folding results in inhibition of transcription. A significant parallelism in conserved G4s in key genomic regulatory regions within members of the same viral subfamily becomes apparent. Our results point for the first time to a G4-mediated regulation of the initial viral steps of this important class of human pathogens and may pave the way to a deeper understanding of *Alphaherpesvirinae* infection regulation.

2. Results

2.1. Detection of PQS in Herpesviridae Immediate Early (IE) Promoters

G4s have been reported to regulate transcription, both at the cellular and viral level, when embedded in promoter regions [15,24]. The HSV-1 infective cycle is predominately driven by the five immediate early (IE) genes, namely *ICP0*, *ICP4*, *ICP27* (UL54), *ICP22* and *ICP47* (US12) [34]. Our previous investigation showed that the GGG-island type PQS in HSV-1 were distributed along four defined genomic features, i.e., coding sequences (CDS), repeat regions (RR), 5'- and 3'-untranslated (UTR), and promoter regions, with a particularly high concentration in the RR and 5'–regulatory region [33]. However, while CDS and RR are explicitly described in RefSeq and GenBank databases, the annotation for promoters in viruses is generally inconsistent. To check whether G4s were reliably present in the promoters of HSV-1 IE genes, we first selected the region up to 1 kb upstream of the Transcription Start Site (TSS) of any unambiguous IE transcripts in the HSV-1 reference genome (NC_001806.2) [35]. The selected regions were examined for the presence of specific genomic features, such as the TAATGARAT signals, TATA boxes, replication origins, polyA signals or CDSs on the opposite strand, in order to restrict our analysis to sequences that most likely contained promoters. This analysis yielded five prominent sequences.

To corroborate our findings, we looked for any reported biological evidence: interestingly, all five regions were indicated to exert promoter activity in IE genes [36–40], with the peculiarity that the same sequence repeated in two different genomic regions constitutes the promoter of the *ICP22* and *ICP47* genes [37]. We thus checked these four promoter regions for PQS by running an initial algorithm-driven analysis to search for [G(2)L(1–7)]4, [G(3)L(1–12)]4 and [G(4)L(1–12)]4-type G4s, followed by a manual sequence revision to highlight the possible presence of "non-canonical" G4s (i.e., G(3)L(0-12)) or bulged PQS [41]. Subsequently the degree of conservation of each sequence was retrieved from the G4 virus website (http://www.medcomp.medicina.unipd.it/main_site/doku.php?id=g4virus#data_download) in order to discard non-conserved regions. Interestingly, all identified PQS were fully conserved, both in terms of G-tracts and loop-length and -composition, in the entire set of fully sequenced genomes present in the National Center for Biotechnology Information (NCBI) databank. The HSV-1 IE promoters contained multiple PQS (Table 1), embedded both in the leading and lagging strand.

Table 1. Putative Quadruplex Sequences (PQS) in the Herpes Simplex Virus 1 (HSV-1) Immediate Early (IE) promoter sequences. Each PQS is indicated by the 5' nucleotide (nt) position on the viral reference genome (NC_001806.2). The leading and the lagging strands are indicated with respect to the Transcription Start Site (TSS) position. The conservation ratio (C (%)) of the entire sequence (G tracts and loops) among all the strains available in the National Center for Biotechnology Information (NCBI) databank is also indicated.

HSV-1	Leading Strand	Lagging Strand	C (%)
ICP0			
1875	GCGGGAGGGGCATGCTA ATGGGGTTCTTTGGGG		100
1881	GGGGCATGCTAATGGGGT TCTTTGGGGGACACCGGG		100
1966	GGGGGCGCCGGGTTG GTCCCCGGGGACGGGG		100
2009	GGGCCTGCCTCCCCTGGG ACGCGCGGCCATTGGGGG		100
2066	GGGGAGGGGAAAGGCGTGGGG		100
ICP4			
R146532		GGGCGGGGCGCG AGGGCGGGTGGG	100
146574	GGGCGGGGCCGGG GGTTCGACCAACGGG		100
146578	GGGGCCGGGGGTTCGAC CAACGGGCCGCGGCCACGGG		100
146666	GGGGTGGGCCCGCC GGGGGGGCGGGGGG		100
146947	GGGGCCGGGGGTTCGACCA ACGGGCCGCGGCCACGGG		100

Table 1. *Cont.*

HSV-1	Leading Strand	Lagging Strand	C (%)
ICP22/ICP47			
131746	GGGCAGGGGGC GGGGCCCGGG		100
R131803		GGGCGGGACCGGGGGGCCCGGG GACGGCCAACGGGCGCGCGGGG	100
131857	GGGACCAACGGGACG GCGGGCGGCCCAAGGG		100
132059	GGGGGCGGGCCCGGGCGGC GGGGGGCGGGTCTCTCCGGCG		100
132065	GGGCCCGGGCG GCGGGGGGCGGG		100
132070	GGGCGGCGGGGGG CGGGTCTCTCCGGCG		100
R132290		GGGTGGGGTGGGCGGG	100
132411	GGGGGCGGAGGAGGGGGGAC GCGGGGGCGGAGGAGGGGG		100
132424	GGGGGGACGCGGGGGCGGAG GAGGGGGGACGCGGGGG		100
ICP27			
113501	GGGGCGGGGGCCCC GCCCGGGGGGCGG		100
113519	GGGGGGCGGAACGA GGAGGGGTTTGGG		100

ICP0 displayed five PQSs, two preceding the TAATGARAT signal, and three upstream the TATA box, all on the leading strand (Figure 1A); *ICP4* promoter contained five PQSs, four embedded in the region encompassing the TAATGARAT signal and the TATA box, the most distal G4 being on the lagging strand, and one close to the TSS (Figure 1B); *ICP22/ICP47* promoter included 9 PQSs, 6 upstream of the TATA box signal, both on the leading and lagging strand and the remaining 3 between the TATA box and the TSS (Figure 1C); *ICP27* promoter displayed two partially overlapped PQSs embedded between the TAATGARAT signal and the TATA box (Figure 1D). Notably, *ICP0* and *ICP22/ICP47* promoters contained bulged PQS. Moreover, the majority of the predicted PQS had at least one region possibly forming GC stem loops.

To check whether the G4 pattern identified in the HSV-1 IE promoters was also present and conserved in all members of the *Alphaherpesviruses*, we extended our analysis to HSV-2 and VZV IE gene promoters. First of all, we identified the homologues genes in the three viruses (Table 2) [42,43] and then performed the same algorithm and manual predictive analysis described for HSV-1.

Table 2. IE genes/proteins (they maintain the same name) in the three *Alphaherpesviruses*. The proteins of each single virus can complement the relative homologue of the other two classes. The only exception is Varicella Zoster Virus-Open Reading Frame 4 (VZV-ORF4), which cannot entirely substitute for HSV-1/HSV-2 ICP27 protein.

	HSV-1	HSV-2	VZV
	ICP0	ICP0	ORF61
	ICP4	ICP4	ORF62
IE genes/proteins	ICP27	ICP27	ORF4
	ICP47	ICP47	n.p.
	ICP22	ICP22	ORF63

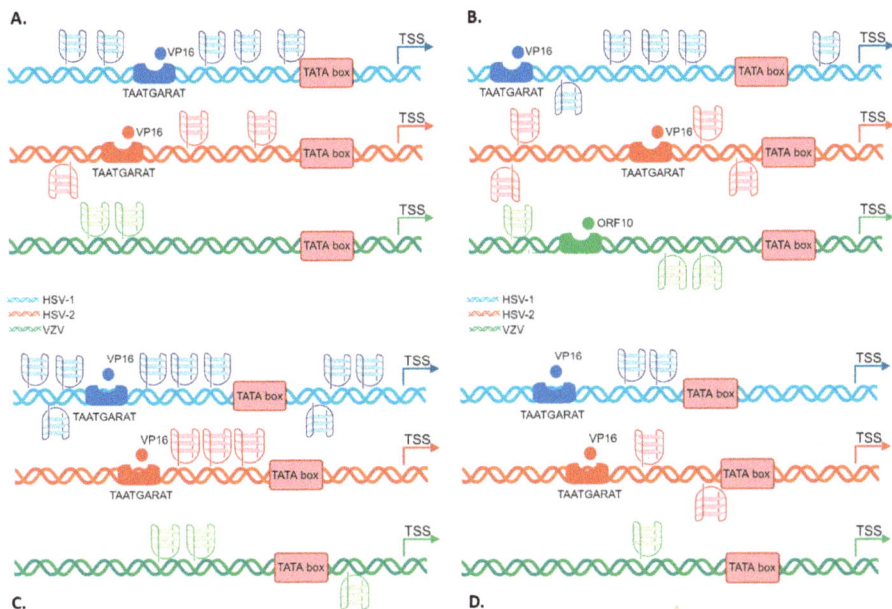

Figure 1. Schematic comparative representation of G4s in *Alphaherpesvirus* IE promoters. The four IE promoters (**A**. *ICP0*; **B**. *ICP4* or *ORF62*; **C**. *ICP22/ICP47* or *ORF63* and **D**. *ICP27*) are reported. HSV-1, HSV-2 and VZV promoter schemes are shown in blue, red and green, respectively. The TAATGARAT region is shown as a blue/red box with the VP16 protein nearby (or as a green box with *ORF10* protein in the case of VZV); the TATA box is represented as a red box; the arrow indicates the position of the Transcriptional Start Site (TSS). The position of each of these features on the double helix with respect to the TSS is on scale. In each promoter, the predicted G4s are shown above and below the DNA strand for G4s present in the leading and lagging strand, respectively.

Notably, also HSV-2 and VZV presented fully conserved PQS within the IE promoters, as reported in Table 3.

HSV-2, has always been considered a close homologue of HSV-1, but recent research highlighted that the two viruses are less related than initially believed [44]. Our analysis retrieved fewer PQS in the HSV-2 IE promoter regions with respect to HSV-1, but all of them were conserved in all sequenced circulating strains. VZV, despite sharing a similar biology with HSV-1 and HSV-2, including latency in sensory neurons, has a different genome organization and gene expression regulation [45,46]. The number of PQS predicted for VZV promoters was the smallest among the three viruses (*n* = 6); however, all of them retained the highest degree of conservation. PQS were retrieved on both strands: similarly to HSV-1 *ICP22* and *ICP47*, *ORF62* and *ORF63* of VZV are transcribed in opposite directions from a 1.5-kb intergenic region that acts as a bidirectional promoter [44] and also contains the VZV origin of replication [47]. *ORF62* and *ORF63* TSSs lie on opposite strands, thus PQS on the leading strand with respect to *ORF63*, on the lagging strand may act as regulators of *ORF62*, and vice versa. VZV is also the only virus with a predicted GG-island type PQS (*ORF4* 4278). Even if the TAATGARAT sequence is not present in VZV promoters, a TAATGARAT-VP16-like transcriptional enhancement can be mimicked by the ORF10 protein [48]. The ORF10 protein has been shown to influence the transcription of the VZV immediate-early (IE) gene, *ORF62*, but not of *ORF61*, *ORF4* or *ORF63* [49,50]. The relative comparison of PQS position on each *Alphaherpesviruses* IE promoter is reported in Figure 2.

Table 3. PQS in the HSV-2 and VZV IE promoter sequences. Each PQS is indicated by the 5′ nt position on the viral reference genome (NC_001798.2 and NC_001348.1). The leading and the lagging strands are indicated with respect to the TSS position. The conservation ratio (C (%)) of the entire sequence (G tracts and loops) among all the strains available in the NCBI databank is also indicated.

HSV-2	Leading Strand	Lagging Strand	C (%)
ICP0			
1571		GGGAAGCCGGCGCGGGGCG GTCGCCGGGGCGGAGTCCGGG	100
1913	GGGGGCGGGCACCACTCAGGGCC GCGCCGGCGGGGCGCCGGGGGG		100
2027	GGGGACGGGGCCGC CCCGAGAGGGGGGG		100
ICP4			
149044		GGGGCGCGCGGGGCGGGGGG	100
149088	GGGGCCGGCGGGGG CCAACGGGAGCGCGGGG		100
149287	GCGGACGCGCGGG CGTCGGGGCGGGG		100
149570		GGGGCGGCAGTG GGGGGGGGTGG	100
ICP22/ICP47			
132299	GGGGGGCCGGGC CGGGGGGACGGG		100
132325	GGGGGGACGGGC CGGGGGGACGGG		100
132988	GGGCCCGGACG GGGGGCGGG		100
ICP27			
114386	GGGGACGGCGGGGGCGGGGG CGGTGACGCCCGACGGGGAGGG		100
114579		GGGGCTGGGATGGCGG GTGTCCTCCGAGGGGG	100
VZV	**Leading Strand**	**Lagging Strand**	**C (%)**
ORF61			
104021		GGGGTCCGCCGGGCGCCCAGAAACC GGGGGGGGGTTATTTTCGGGGGGGGG	100
105081	GGGCGGGCGACGGGCGGG		100
ORF62/ORF63			
109246	GGGGAGGAAATATGCG GTCGAGGGGGGGG		99
109703	GCGGTTTTATGGGGT GTGGGCGGG		100
110410		GGGTAAAATGGCAATGGGGGATT CCGGGGCGGGAGACCTTCGATTGGG	100
ORF4			
4278	GGGTGCAGGTAA GCTTGTTTGGGG		100

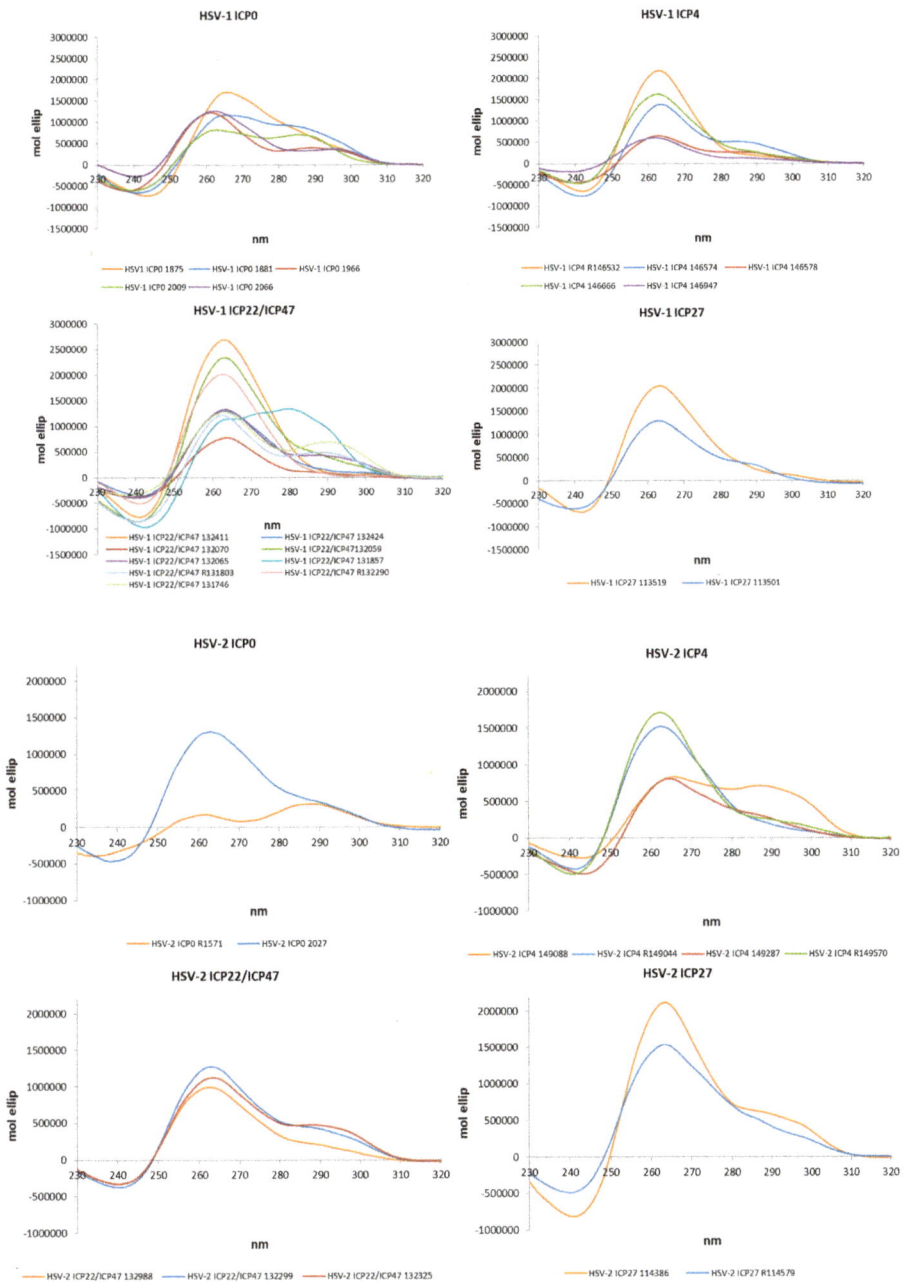

Figure 2. *Cont.*

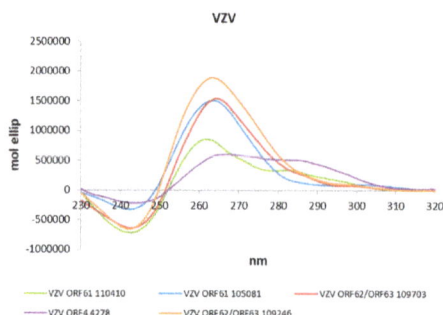

Figure 2. Circular Dichroism (CD) spectra of the PQS embedded in the *Alphaherpesvirus* IE promoters in PB 20 mM and KCl 70 mM.

These data indicate the possibility that IE gene expression of *Alphaherpesviruses* is regulated by G4s.

2.2. The Identified PQSs Fold into G4 Structures

The actual ability of *Alphaherpesvirus* IE promoter PQSs to form G4 structures was initially assessed by Circular Dichroism (CD), as this technique is considered a reliable tool to study nucleic acids conformation [51]. All sequences were analysed in the presence of K^+ to establish G4 folding, topology and thermal stability. Table 4 and in Figure 2 show that all predicted PQS did actually fold into G4 structures. The large majority (77%) of G4s displayed a parallel topology, with a maximum positive peak at ~260 nm and a minimum at ~240 nm. Some G4s were also characterized by a modest shoulder at 295 nm, without wavelength shift of the minimum peak at 240 nm and were considered parallel G4s (Table 4). The remaining sequences (18%) showed two maxima at 265 and 295 nm and a minimum at 245 nm and were thus classified as hybrid structures.

Table 4. CD and Thermal Difference Spectra (TDS) analysis of PQS embedded in the *Alphaherpesvirus* IE promoters. Both analyses were performed at 100 mM KCl. Topology and T_m values in the presence and absence of B19 are reported. For mixed structures, T_m values were calculated at both 260 and 290 nm. n.a.: oligonucleotide not available due to its too high G content.

HSV-1	Topology	T_m	T_m (B19)	ΔT_m	TDS
ICP0					
1875	parallel	60.9 ± 0.1	73.3 ± 0.2	12.4	+
1881	hybrid	51.9 ± 0.3/45.9 ± 0.2	80.7 ± 1.2/66.3 ± 0.5	28.8/20.4	+ *
1966	parallel	68.6 ± 0.1	>90	>21.4	+
2009	hybrid	54.9 ± 0.6/65.0 ± 0.4	69.2 ± 0.6/>90	14.3/>25	+/−
2066	parallel	>90			+
ICP4					
R146532	parallel	79.5 ± 0.1	>90	>10.5	+
146574	parallel	63.4 ± 0.2	>90	>26.6	+
146578	parallel	66.2 ± 0.1	80.3 ± 0.4	14.1	+/−
146666	parallel	>90			+
146947	parallel	69.2 ± 0.2	>90	>20.8	+
ICP22/ICP47					
131746	hybrid	>90/71.4 ± 0.8			+
R131803	hybrid	73.7 ± 0.8/76.7 ± 0.9	>90/85.1 ± 0.8	>16.3/8.4	+ *
131857	hybrid	62.4 ± 0.5/65.3 ± 0.2	69.6 ± 0.9/67.6 ± 0.4	7.2/2.3	+ *
132059	parallel	>90			+
132065	hybrid	>90/78.8 ± 0.7			+

Table 4. *Cont.*

HSV-1	Topology	T_m	T_m (B19)	ΔT_m	TDS
132070	parallel	74.2 ± 0.1	>90	>15.8	+ *
R132290	parallel	>90			+ **
132411	parallel	>90			+
132424	parallel	>90			+ **
ICP27					
113501	parallel	>90			+/−
113519	parallel	>90			+
HSV-2					
ICP0					
1571	hybrid	77.7 ± 0.8/79.0 ± 0.7	>90/71.2 ± 1.1	>12.3/−7.8	+/−
1913	n.a.				
2027	parallel	>90			+
ICP4					
149044	parallel	>90			+
149088	hybrid	67.2 ± 0.7/72.6 ± 0.7	64.5 ± 0.9/>90	−2.7/>17.4	+
149287	parallel	67.2 ± 0.7	84.1 ± 2.2	16.9	+
149570	parallel	81.8 ± 0.8	>90	>8.2	+
ICP22/ICP47					
132299	parallel	>90			+
132988	parallel	>90			+
132325	parallel	>90			+
ICP27					
114386	parallel	75.9 ± 0.4	>90	>14.1	+ *
114579	parallel	66.8 ± 0.9	83.4 ± 0.7	16.6	+
VZV					
ORF61					
104021	n.a.				
105081	parallel	75.9 ± 0.4	>90	>14.1	+
ORF62/ORF63					
109246	parallel	>90			+
109703	parallel	57.7 ± 0.2	84.7 ± 0.5	27.0	+
110410	parallel	56.5 ± 0.4	85.2 ± 0.8	28.7	+/−
ORF4					
4278	hybrid	57.5 ± 0.3/53.2 ± 0.5	79.2 ± 0.9/82.0 ± 0.9	21.7/28.8	+

+/− G4 TDS lacking negative peak at 295 nm; * 150 mM KCl; ** 50 mM KCl.

The stability of all G4s was assessed by melting experiments monitored by CD. The melting temperatures (T_m) were calculated according to the van 't Hoff equation (Table 4 and Figure S1). In half of the analysed sequences (58%) the CD signal decreased over temperature, leading to discrete T_m values. Notably, the remaining sequences (42%) maintained their G4 folding up to the maximum tested temperature (90 °C). For hybrid structures, where two transitions were visible, T_m values were calculated at both wavelengths.

We next investigated the *Alphaherpesvirus* IE promoter sequences in the presence of the commercially available G4-ligand, BRACO-19 (B19), which has been reported to specifically recognize and stabilize G4 structures over double- and single-stranded nucleic acids [52]. The effect of B19 was assessed by CD thermal unfolding analysis. B19 was able to further stabilize all G4s, with an increase in T_m higher than 10 °C (Table 4). In cases where several transitions were observed, T_m values for each transition were annotated. The results obtained with B19 further confirm the ability of all the predicted sequences to fold into G4 structures.

TDS spectra analysis was next employed to corroborate G4 folding. Mergny and others [8,53] established that G4 structures exhibit a TDS negative peak at 295 nm, and two positive peaks at 275 and 243 nm, respectively. The vast majority (86%) of analysed sequences displayed the G4 distinctive TDS spectrum (Table 4 and Figure S1). Bulged sequences, sequences containing more than four G-islands and sequences retaining the ability to form stem-loops displayed the characteristic TDS at higher cation concentration (KCl 150 mM), which allowed increased stabilization of the G4 over possible competitor structures. Five sequences displayed only the two positive peaks, and thus reported a non-definite TDS spectrum (indicated as +/−). It is possible that "non canonical" G4 structures cannot confidently be distinguished by TDS analysis.

For these reasons, two non-canonical G4s were additionally explored by *Taq* polymerase stop assay. These corresponded to the HSV-1 *ICP0* and *ICP27* promoter sequences (*ICP0* 2066 and *ICP27* 113501+113519): the first one was a putative bulged G4 that displayed G4-representative CD and TDS profiles, the second with long G-tracts and the possibility to form GC stem loops, had showed an ambiguous TDS profile. The *Taq* polymerase stop assay indicates the ability of a G4 to block or pause the enzyme activity and allows evaluation of G4 structures within an extended DNA environment. Samples were incubated in the absence and presence of increasing concentrations of KCl (Figure 3), and 1 µM B19. Stop sites resulted specific and located mainly at, or just before, the most 3′ G-tract involved in G4 formation (Figure 3, * symbol). Additional stop sites (Figure 3, ¤, §, #, ¥ and & symbols) corresponding to other G-tracts indicated the "breathing" of the G4 structure and possibly the ability of the tested oligonucleotides to fold into multiple G4 structures, preferentially stabilized at different K^+ concentrations. The G4-ligand B19 blocked enzyme processing mainly in correspondence of the most 3′ tract involved in G4 formation, suggesting that the structure with the longest sequence is likely the most stable and thus the one preferentially bound by B19 (Figure 3, * symbol). These data indicate that both the tested non-canonical G4s are able to fold into G4, and thus provide evidence that the TDS assay may lack the negative peak at 295 nm while still depicting a non-canonical G4.

Taken together these data indicate that IE PQS can fold into dynamic G4 structures, which are induced and stabilized by increasing concentrations of K^+ and a G4-ligand.

2.3. G4s Tune IE Promoter Activity at the Cellular Level

The biological role of G4s at the promoter level is still matter of debate since little is known on how G4 structures and their interaction with transcription factors and other proteins may contribute to regulate viral promoters. Here, we decided to study the activity of two representative promoters, i.e., HSV-1 *ICP0* and *ICP27* in cells. These two promoters were chosen both for their peculiar G4 content and for their unique roles during HSV-1 infection. ICP0 is the viral ubiquitin ligase that has been described to act as a powerful viral transactivator—both during productive infection and in reactivation from latency [54]. In contrast, at the nuclear level ICP27 induces the expression of a restricted number of early and late genes, such as UL42 (polymerase processivity factor) and UL44 (glycoprotein C) but it remains highly expressed during the whole viral life cycle [55]. The two sequences, *ICP0* and *ICP27* (NC_001806.2 nts 1551-2261 and nts 113451-113734, respectively) were cloned upstream of the firefly luciferase gene in a promoterless plasmid. The two promoters were studied in U-2 OS cells, a human osteosarcoma cell line that withstands HSV-1 infection [56], in the absence and presence of increasing concentrations of B19. The assay was performed monitoring also cell viability in the presence of B19 ($CC_{50\ U2\text{-}OS}$ > 100 µM) to avoid luciferase signal variation due to cytotoxicity. As shown in Figure 4, the activity of both promoters decreased in a dose dependent manner, up to ~65% of the untreated control in *ICP0* and up to ~55% in *ICP27*, proving that in this case G4s act as suppressors of transcription.

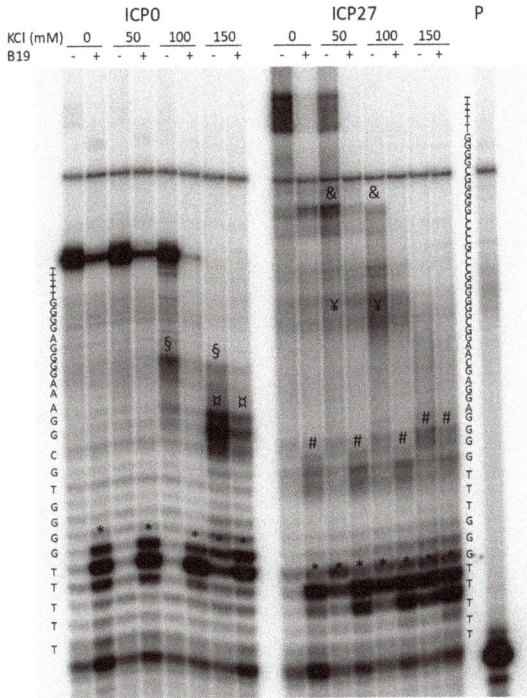

Figure 3. Sequencing PAGE of *Taq*-amplified *ICP0* and *ICP27* templates in the absence or presence of increasing concentrations of KCl and the G4-ligand B19. Symbols *, ¤, §, #, ¥ and & indicate pausing sites just before the G4 regions in the templates. P indicates the lane of the labeled primer.

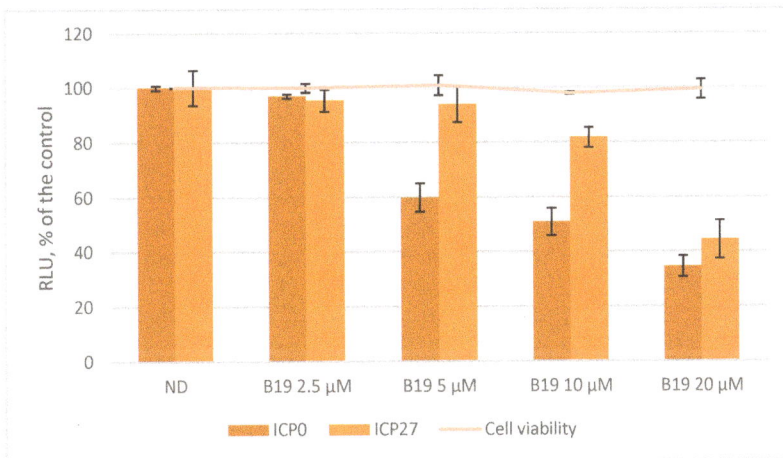

Figure 4. Luciferase assay on HSV-1 ICP0 and ICP27 promoters in U-2 OS (human osteosarcoma) cells in the presence of the G4 ligand B19 (2.5–20 μM). Cell viability, determined by MTT (3-(4,5-dimethylthiazolyl-2)-2,5-diphenyltetrazolium bromide) assay, in the presence of B19 is also indicated.

These findings support the hypothesis that G4s tune the activity of *Alphaherpesvirus* IE promoters, as indicated by the B19-mediated G4 stabilization, which down-regulates ICP0 and ICP27 transcription.

3. Discussion

In the past few years, interest in the characterization of G4 structures and their role within viral genomes has greatly increased, providing possibly innovative antiviral targets against many human pathogens. In this context, our group proved that HIV-1 transcription is modulated by the tuned folding/unfolding of G4s located in the U3 region of the LTR promoter [23,57]. We successively demonstrated that the HSV-1 genome contains an impressively high number of putative G4s that were visualized during infection in cells by means of an anti-G4 antibody [17,27]. In support of the presence and involvement of G4s in key viral processes, we found that two G4-ligands (B19 and a core extended naphthalene diimide) displayed remarkable antiviral activity in both viruses [17,32,58,59].

The HSV-1 cycle is strictly regulated by five IE proteins (namely ICP0, ICP4, ICP22, ICP27 and ICP47), that are also responsible in vivo for the establishment of latency at the neuronal level [34,60]. The five genes that encode for these proteins are immediately transcribed after infection and mutations altering their expression are strongly associated with a dysregulated viral cycle [60].

In this work, we investigated the presence of G4s within the promoter regions of IE genes of all members of the *Alphaherpesvirus* subfamily. The promoters were unambiguously identified based both on the presence of characterizing motifs, such as the TATA box and the TAATGARAT sequence and on previously reported biological evidence. In each promoter, we found several multiple and non-overlapping G4 folding motifs, interestingly located both on the leading and lagging strands. At the promoter level, G4 structures on the lagging strand have been shown so far only in few examples, in particular in the promoter region of the REarranged during Transfection (RET) proto-oncogene [61,62] and as regulators of DNA strand replication [63] in mammalian cells. In the human papillomavirus as well as in the human cytomegalovirus, G4s on the lagging strand were predicted only in non-coding regulatory regions, lacking experimentally proved promoter activity [18,64]. Promoters containing multiple G4s have been described in oncogenes [65–67], however, none of these features has been reported in viruses as yet. This work indicates the possibility that the large and strictly regulated genome of *Herpesviruses* controls gene transcription at the promoter level through G4-mediated mechanisms, as reported for the human genome. ICP4 is the major viral transcription factor, and its promoter presents 5 G4s. The G4 most distant from the TSS is embedded in the lagging strand close to the TAATGARAT sequence, which is a recognition signal for the viral protein VP16 [31]: it is possible that this G4 is involved in the transactivation activity of VP16. The *ICP22* and *ICP47* promoters, which share the same sequence albeit in two different locations along the genome, display a high number of G4s, also in this case located on both strands: we envisage the possibility of a control on both transcription and replication, since in the same region resides oriS, one of the origins of viral genome replication [68]. ICP0 plays a major role both on viral transactivation during the lytic cycle and in reactivation from latency: it contains five G4s nearby the TAATGARAT sequence and TATA box. ICP27 is an essential HSV-1 IE protein along with ICP4, but in contrast to the latter which is expressed only in the early stages and is involved in transcription initiation, ICP27 is a multifunctional protein and its expression remains high throughout the viral cycle, with post-translational modifications that regulate its activity [69–71]. The *ICP27* promoter is the one that contains fewer G4s. Four out of five *ICP0* G4s, displaying low Tm ($50 < Tm < 68\ °C$), were significantly stabilized by the G4-ligand, whereas *ICP27* G4s were very stable even in the absence of B19 and thus were less affected by the G4-ligand. These features are likely the reason why we observed a lower degree of response to the G4-ligand B19 in cells for *ICP27* compared to *ICP0*.

As HSV-1, HSV-2 and VZV are closely related viruses, all displaying a wide host-cell range, similar pathogenesis and analogous genome organization, we evaluated the presence of G4s also in HSV-2 and VZV IE promoters. The vast majority of the retrieved sequences, besides being fully conserved within all sequenced strains, were experimentally proven by at least two techniques to fold into G4 structures.

Finally, we found that many of the *Alphaherpesvirus* IE promoter G4-forming sequences described in this work formed "non-canonical" G4s: they were able to fold even in the absence of loops (i.e., HSV-1 *ICP4* 149570; VZV *ORF62/63* 109246) or in the presence of putative stem-forming sequences in the loop (i.e., HSV-1 *ICP0* 1966; HSV-1 *ICP4* 146666, 146578 and 146947; HSV-1 *ICP22/ICP47* R131803, 131857, 132059) or with bulges (i.e., HSV-1 *ICP0* 2009 and 2066; HSV-2 *ICP4* 149044, 149287). This fact indicates that the classic prediction methods based on motif recognition may overlook many non-canonical G4s that actually form. In this view, the newest machine learning models trained with sequences of experimentally validated G4 may yield more reliable results [72]. Moreover, several G4s (see HSV-1 *ICP4*, HSV-1 *ICP22/ICP47*, HSV-2 *ICP0*, HSV-2 *ICP27* and VZV *ORF62/ORF63*) presented 5 G-tracts; multiple G-tracts have been previously described for another strictly regulated viral promoter, the LTR sequence of HIV-1 virus [23]. These data may corroborate the recently proposed hypothesis by Burrows CJ and co-workers that the tracts exceeding four work as "spare tires" in promoters [73].

The described data provide a possible new direction for active antiviral design. Up to date, only polymerase inhibitors have been found active against HSV-1, HSV-2 and VZV. However, because of the emergence of resistant strains that may be extremely dangerous especially in transplant and immunocompromised patients [74], new antivirals with a different mechanism of action are highly wished for. We propose that selective anti-IE promoters G4-ligands could hinder the viral cycle at a much earlier stage, preventing the discomfort, the possible neuronal damage, the painful sequelae (specific to VZV) in normal human hosts and the possible life-threatening effects in immunocompromised patients caused by the *Alphaherpesviruses*.

4. Materials and Methods

4.1. PQS Detection and Evaluation of Conservation

The complete set of human *Alphaherpesvirus* genome sequences were downloaded from GenBank. The first analysis was performed with free G4 hunting software (QGRS http://bioinformatics.ramapo.edu/QGRS/index.php and Quadbase http://quadbase.igib.res.in/), using the standard parameters of the two programs (Minimum G-tetrad 2 and 3, Loop length1-7 for GG and 1–12 for GGG). Since *Herpesviridae* are dsDNA viruses, the presence of PQS was analysed on both genome strands.

4.2. Oligonucleotides and Cell Lines

Desalted oligonucleotides were purchased from Invitrogen and from Sigma-Aldrich, Milan, Italy (Table 1, Table 3). U2-OS (ECACC 92022711) were purchased from Sigma Aldrich and maintained in Dulbecco's Modified Eagle's medium (DMEM) (Gibco, Thermo Fisher Scientific, Waltham, MA, USA) supplemented with 10% heat-in- activated fetal bovine serum (FBS, Gibco, Thermo Fisher Scientific, Waltham, MA, USA). Cells were grown in a humidified incubator maintained at 37 °C with 5% CO_2.

4.3. Circular Dichroism Spectroscopy

DNA oligonucleotides were diluted to a final concentration (4 µM) in phosphate buffer (PB, 20 mM, pH 7.4) and KCl 70 mM. All samples were annealed at 95 °C for 5 min and gradually cooled to room temperature. The G4-ligand Braco-19 (B19, ENDOTHERM, Saarbruecken, Germany) was added from stock at final concentration of 16 µM. CD spectra were recorded on a Chirascan-Plus (Applied Photophysics, Leatherhead, UK) equipped with a Peltier temperature controller using a quartz cell of 5 mm optical path length, over a wavelength range of 230–320 nm. For the determination of T_m, spectra were recorded over a temperature range of 20–90 °C, with temperature increase of 5 °C. The reported spectra are baseline-corrected for signal contributions due to the buffer. Observed ellipticities were converted to mean residue ellipticity (θ) = deg $\times$ cm^2 $\times$ dmol^{-1} (mol ellip). T_m values were calculated according to the van't Hoff equation, applied for a two-state transition from a folded to unfolded state, assuming that the heat capacity of the folded and unfolded states are equal [75].

4.4. Taq Polymerase Stop Assay

Taq polymerase stop assay was carried out as previously described [23]. Briefly, the 5′-end labelled primer was annealed to its template (Table S1) in lithium cacodylate buffer in the presence or absence of KCl (50–150 mM) and by heating at 95 °C for 5 min and gradually cooling to room temperature. Where specified, samples were incubated with 1 μM B19 for 24 h after the annealing step. Primer extension was conducted with 2 U of AmpliTaq Gold DNA polymerase (Applied Biosystem, Carlsbad, California, USA) at 47 °C for 30 min. Reactions were stopped by ethanol precipitation, primer extension products were separated on a 16% denaturing gel, and finally visualized by phosphorimaging (Typhoon FLA 9000).

4.5. Plasmids Construction

The ICP0 and ICP27 promoter regions were amplified by PCR on the HSV-1 genome (GU734771.1) extracted from U2-OS infected cells. The promoter amplicons were subcloned into pGL4.10-Luc2 (Promega) within XhoI and *Hind*III sites. The resulting pGL4.10-ICP0 and pGL4.10-ICP27 vectors contained the sequenced regions corresponding to nts 1551-2261 (ICP0) and nts 113451-113734 (ICP27) in the HSV-1 reference genome (NC_001806.2), fused to the luciferase-coding region.

4.6. Reporter Assays

Vectors pGL4.10-ICP0 and pGL4.10-ICP27 (150 ng each) were transfected in 1.2×10^5 U2-OS cells per well onto 12-well plates, using *Lipo3000* transfection reagent (Invitrogen, Life Technologies Italia, Monza, Italy). B19 was added to the cell medium 1 h after transfection at increasing concentrations (5–20 μM), to avoid interference, if any, with transfection. Expression of firefly luciferase was determined 24 h after transfection using the Britelite plus Reporter Gene Assay System (PerkinElmer Inc., Milan, Italy) at a Victor X2 multilabel plate reader (PerkinElmer Inc., Milan, Italy), according to the manufacturer's instructions. Cells were lysed in 0.1% Triton-X100-PBS and protein concentration was determined by BCA assay (Thermo Scientific Pierce, Monza, Italy). Luciferase signals were subsequently normalized to total protein content, according to the manufacturer's protocol (http://ita.promega.com/~/pdf/resources/pubhub/cellnotes/normalizing-genetic-reporter-assays/). Each assay was performed in duplicate and each set of experiments was repeated at least three times.

4.7. Cellular Cytotoxicity

Cytotoxic effects were determined by MTT assay. U-2 OS cells were grown and maintained according to manufacturer's instructions (https://www.lgcstandards-atcc.org). Cells were plated into 96-microwell plates to a final volume of 100 μL and allowed an overnight period for attachment. The following day, the tested compound (B19) was added to each well and tested in triplicate. Control cells were treated in the exact same conditions. Cell survival was evaluated by MTT assay, 24 h after treatment: 10 μL of freshly dissolved solution of MTT (5 mg/mL in PBS) were added to each well, and after 4 h of incubation, MTT crystals were solubilized in solubilization solution (10% sodium dodecyl sulphate (SDS) and 0.01 M HCl). After overnight incubation at 37 °C, absorbance was read at 540 nm. Data were expressed as mean values of at least three individual experiments conducted in triplicate. The percentage of cell survival was calculated as follows: cell survival = (Awell − Ablank)/(Acontrol − Ablank) × 100, where blank denotes the medium without cells. Each experiment was repeated at least three times.

5. Conclusions

The work presented here provides for the first time a comprehensive analysis on the presence of G4s in the IE promoter regions of the three *Alphaherpesviruses* that infect humans. In these viruses, regulation of gene expression has been largely debated in the last decades but clear data are still lacking. Thus, the fact that in all *Alphaherpesviruses* the promoters of all genes involved in the first steps

Molecules **2019**, *24*, 2375

of infection and in the control of expression of the later genes contain 100% conserved G4 forming regions is a potent indication of their significance. Our data broaden the boosting recognition of G4s as molecular switches of gene expression at the viral level [24]. The in-depth understanding of the role of G4s at the viral promoter level will likely allow unravelling the mechanisms that regulate *Alphaherpesviruses* infection and latency in the human nervous system, with the subsequent possibility to design innovative drugs to manage the infection of some of the most widespread latency-associated human pathogens.

Supplementary Materials: The following are available online, Figure S1: CD thermal unfolding spectra, CD thermal unfolding fitting and TDS of *Alphaherpesvirus* IE promoter G4 sequences, Table S1: Oligonucleotides used in the *Taq* polymerase stop assay.

Author Contributions: Conceptualization, I.F. and S.N.R.; methodology, I.F. and M.N.; validation, I.F., M.N. and S.N.R.; formal analysis, I.F. and S.N.R.; investigation, I.F. and M.N.; data curation, I.F. and M.N.; funding acquisition, S.N.R.; writing—original draft preparation, I.F.; writing—review and editing, S.N.R.

Funding: This research was funded by the European Research Council grant number (ERC Consolidator 615879) and by the DMM, University of Padua (PRID RICH-SID18_01).

Conflicts of Interest: The authors declare no conflict of interest.

References

1. Cutter, A.R.; Hayes, J.J. A brief review of nucleosome structure. *FEBS Lett.* **2015**, *589*, 2914–2922. [CrossRef] [PubMed]
2. Burge, S.; Parkinson, G.N.; Hazel, P.; Todd, A.K.; Neidle, S. Quadruplex DNA: Sequence, topology and structure. *Nucleic Acids Res.* **2006**, *34*, 5402–5415. [CrossRef] [PubMed]
3. Bochman, M.L.; Paeschke, K.; Zakian, V.A. DNA secondary structures: Stability and function of G-quadruplex structures. *Nat. Rev. Genet.* **2012**, *13*, 770–780. [CrossRef] [PubMed]
4. Bacolla, A.; Wang, G.; Vasquez, K.M. New Perspectives on DNA and RNA Triplexes As Effectors of Biological Activity. *PLoS Genet.* **2015**, *11*, e1005696. [CrossRef] [PubMed]
5. Harkness, R.W.; Mittermaier, A.K. G-quadruplex dynamics. *Biochim. Biophys. Acta-Proteins Proteomics* **2017**, *1865*, 1544–1554. [CrossRef] [PubMed]
6. Huppert, J.L. Four-stranded nucleic acids: Structure, function and targeting of G-quadruplexes. *Chem. Soc. Rev.* **2008**, *37*, 1375–1384. [CrossRef] [PubMed]
7. del Villar-Guerra, R.; Trent, J.O.; Chaires, J.B. G-Quadruplex Secondary Structure Obtained from Circular Dichroism Spectroscopy. *Angew. Chemie Int. Ed.* **2018**, *57*, 7171–7175. [CrossRef]
8. Mergny, J.L.; Phan, A.T.; Lacroix, L. Following G-quartet formation by UV-spectroscopy. *FEBS Lett.* **1998**, *435*, 74–78. [CrossRef]
9. Han, H.; Hurley, L.H.; Salazar, M. A DNA polymerase stop assay for G-quadruplex-interactive compounds. *Nucleic Acids Res.* **1999**, *27*, 537–542. [CrossRef]
10. Scalabrin, M.; Palumbo, M.; Richter, S.N. Highly Improved Electrospray Ionization-Mass Spectrometry Detection of G-Quadruplex-Folded Oligonucleotides and Their Complexes with Small Molecules. *Anal. Chem.* **2017**, *89*, 8632–8637. [CrossRef]
11. Tretyakova, N.; Villalta, P.W.; Kotapati, S. Mass spectrometry of structurally modified DNA. *Chem. Rev.* **2013**, *113*, 2395–2436. [CrossRef] [PubMed]
12. Manna, S.; Sarkar, D.; Srivatsan, S.G. A Dual-App Nucleoside Probe Provides Structural Insights into the Human Telomeric Overhang in Live Cells. *J. Am. Chem. Soc.* **2018**, *140*, 12622–12633. [CrossRef] [PubMed]
13. Bao, H.-L.; Liu, H.; Xu, Y. Hybrid-type and two-tetrad antiparallel telomere DNA G-quadruplex structures in living human cells. *Nucleic Acids Res.* **2019**, *47*, 4940–4947. [CrossRef] [PubMed]
14. Fay, M.M.; Lyons, S.M.; Ivanov, P. RNA G-Quadruplexes in Biology: Principles and Molecular Mechanisms. *J. Mol. Biol.* **2017**, *429*, 2127–2147. [CrossRef] [PubMed]
15. Rhodes, D.; Lipps, H.J. G-quadruplexes and their regulatory roles in biology. *Nucleic Acids Res.* **2015**, *43*, 8627–8637. [CrossRef] [PubMed]
16. Cammas, A.; Millevoi, S. RNA G-quadruplexes: Emerging mechanisms in disease. *Nucleic Acids Res.* **2016**, *45*, gkw1280. [CrossRef] [PubMed]

17. Artusi, S.; Nadai, M.; Perrone, R.; Biasolo, M.A.; Palù, G.; Flamand, L.; Calistri, A.; Richter, S.N. The Herpes Simplex Virus-1 genome contains multiple clusters of repeated G-quadruplex: Implications for the antiviral activity of a G-quadruplex ligand. *Antiviral Res.* **2015**, *118*, 123–131. [CrossRef]
18. Ravichandran, S.; Kim, Y.-E.; Bansal, V.; Ghosh, A.; Hur, J.; Subramani, V.K.; Pradhan, S.; Lee, M.K.; Kim, K.K.; Ahn, J.-H. Genome-wide analysis of regulatory G-quadruplexes affecting gene expression in human cytomegalovirus. *PLoS Pathog.* **2018**, *14*, e1007334. [CrossRef]
19. Norseen, J.; Johnson, F.B.; Lieberman, P.M. Role for G-quadruplex RNA binding by Epstein-Barr virus nuclear antigen 1 in DNA replication and metaphase chromosome attachment. *J. Virol.* **2009**, *83*, 10336–10346. [CrossRef]
20. Harris, L.M.; Monsell, K.R.; Noulin, F.; Famodimu, M.T.; Smargiasso, N.; Damblon, C.; Horrocks, P.; Merrick, C.J. G-Quadruplex DNA Motifs in the Malaria Parasite Plasmodium falciparum and Their Potential as Novel Antimalarial Drug Targets. *Antimicrob. Agents Chemother.* **2018**, *62*, e01828-17. [CrossRef]
21. Fleming, A.M.; Ding, Y.; Alenko, A.; Burrows, C.J. Zika Virus Genomic RNA Possesses Conserved G-Quadruplexes Characteristic of the Flaviviridae Family. *ACS Infect. Dis.* **2016**, *2*, 674–681. [CrossRef] [PubMed]
22. Harris, L.M.; Merrick, C.J. G-quadruplexes in pathogens: A common route to virulence control? *PLoS Pathog.* **2015**, *11*, e1004562. [CrossRef] [PubMed]
23. Perrone, R.; Nadai, M.; Frasson, I.; Poe, J.A.; Butovskaya, E.; Smithgall, T.E.; Palumbo, M.; Palù, G.; Richter, S.N. A Dynamic G-Quadruplex Region Regulates the HIV-1 Long Terminal Repeat Promoter. *J. Med. Chem.* **2013**, *56*, 6521–6530. [CrossRef] [PubMed]
24. Ruggiero, E.; Richter, S.N. G-quadruplexes and G-quadruplex ligands: Targets and tools in antiviral therapy. *Nucleic Acids Res.* **2018**, *46*, 3270–3283. [CrossRef] [PubMed]
25. Bhartiya, D.; Chawla, V.; Ghosh, S.; Shankar, R.; Kumar, N. Genome-wide regulatory dynamics of G-quadruplexes in human malaria parasite Plasmodium falciparum. *Genomics* **2016**, *108*, 224–231. [CrossRef] [PubMed]
26. Madireddy, A.; Purushothaman, P.; Loosbroock, C.P.; Robertson, E.S.; Schildkraut, C.L.; Verma, S.C. G-quadruplex-interacting compounds alter latent DNA replication and episomal persistence of KSHV. *Nucleic Acids Res.* **2016**, *44*, 3675–3694. [CrossRef] [PubMed]
27. Artusi, S.; Perrone, R.; Lago, S.; Raffa, P.; Di Iorio, E.; Palù, G.; Richter, S.N. Visualization of DNA G-quadruplexes in herpes simplex virus 1-infected cells. *Nucleic Acids Res.* **2016**, *44*, 10343–10353. [CrossRef]
28. Roizman, B.; Baines, J. The diversity and unity of herpesviridae. *Comp. Immunol. Microbiol. Infect. Dis.* **1991**, *14*, 63–79. [CrossRef]
29. Honess, R.W.; Roizman, B. Regulation of herpesvirus macromolecular synthesis: Sequential transition of polypeptide synthesis requires functional viral polypeptides. *Proc. Natl. Acad. Sci. USA* **1975**, *72*, 1276–1280. [CrossRef]
30. Honess, R.W.; Roizman, B. Regulation of herpesvirus macromolecular synthesis. I. Cascade regulation of the synthesis of three groups of viral proteins. *J. Virol.* **1974**, *14*, 8–19.
31. Babb, R.; Huang, C.C.; Aufiero, D.J.; Herr, W. DNA recognition by the herpes simplex virus transactivator VP16: A novel DNA-binding structure. *Mol. Cell. Biol.* **2001**, *21*, 4700–4712. [CrossRef] [PubMed]
32. Callegaro, S.; Perrone, R.; Scalabrin, M.; Doria, F.; Palù, G.; Richter, S.N. A core extended naphtalene diimide G-quadruplex ligand potently inhibits herpes simplex virus 1 replication. *Sci. Rep.* **2017**, *7*, 2341. [CrossRef] [PubMed]
33. Lavezzo, E.; Berselli, M.; Frasson, I.; Perrone, R.; Palù, G.; Brazzale, A.R.; Richter, S.N.; Toppo, S. G-quadruplex forming sequences in the genome of all known human viruses: A comprehensive guide. *PLoS Comput. Biol.* **2018**, *14*, e1006675. [CrossRef] [PubMed]
34. Pesola, J.M.; Zhu, J.; Knipe, D.M.; Coen, D.M. Herpes simplex virus 1 immediate-early and early gene expression during reactivation from latency under conditions that prevent infectious virus production. *J. Virol.* **2005**, *79*, 14516–14525. [CrossRef] [PubMed]
35. Bedrat, A.; Lacroix, L.; Mergny, J.-L. Re-evaluation of G-quadruplex propensity with G4Hunter. *Nucleic Acids Res.* **2016**, *44*, 1746–1759. [CrossRef] [PubMed]
36. Rice, S.A.; Knipe, D.M. Gene-specific transactivation by herpes simplex virus type 1 alpha protein ICP27. *J. Virol.* **1988**, *62*, 3814–3823. [PubMed]

16

37. McGeoch, D.J.; Dolan, A.; Donald, S.; Rixon, F.J. Sequence determination and genetic content of the short unique region in the genome of herpes simplex virus type 1. *J. Mol. Biol.* **1985**, *181*, 1–13. [CrossRef]
38. Dauber, B.; Saffran, H.A.; Smiley, J.R. The herpes simplex virus 1 virion host shutoff protein enhances translation of viral late mRNAs by preventing mRNA overload. *J. Virol.* **2014**, *88*, 9624–9632. [CrossRef]
39. Lee, J.S.; Raja, P.; Knipe, D.M. Herpesviral ICP0 Protein Promotes Two Waves of Heterochromatin Removal on an Early Viral Promoter during Lytic Infection. *MBio* **2016**, *7*, e02007-15. [CrossRef]
40. Kuddus, R.; Gu, B.; DeLuca, N.A. Relationship between TATA-binding protein and herpes simplex virus type 1 ICP4 DNA-binding sites in complex formation and repression of transcription. *J. Virol.* **1995**, *69*, 5568–5575.
41. Chan, C.-Y.; Umar, M.I.; Kwok, C.K. Spectroscopic analysis reveals the effect of a single nucleotide bulge on G-quadruplex structures. *Chem. Commun. (Camb.)* **2019**, *55*, 2616–2619. [CrossRef] [PubMed]
42. Dolan, A.; Jamieson, F.E.; Cunningham, C.; Barnett, B.C.; McGeoch, D.J. The genome sequence of herpes simplex virus type 2. *J. Virol.* **1998**, *72*, 2010–2021. [PubMed]
43. Cohen, J.I. *The Varicella-Zoster Virus Genome*; Springer: Berlin/Heidelberg, Germany, 2010; pp. 1–14.
44. Jones, J.O.; Sommer, M.; Stamatis, S.; Arvin, A.M. Mutational Analysis of the Varicella-Zoster Virus ORF62/63 Intergenic Region. *J. Virol.* **2006**, *80*, 3116–3121. [CrossRef] [PubMed]
45. Norberg, P.; Tyler, S.; Severini, A.; Whitley, R.; Liljeqvist, J.-Å.; Bergström, T. A genome-wide comparative evolutionary analysis of herpes simplex virus type 1 and varicella zoster virus. *PLoS ONE* **2011**, *6*, e22527. [CrossRef] [PubMed]
46. Szpara, M.L.; Gatherer, D.; Ochoa, A.; Greenbaum, B.; Dolan, A.; Bowden, R.J.; Enquist, L.W.; Legendre, M.; Davison, A.J. Evolution and diversity in human herpes simplex virus genomes. *J. Virol.* **2014**, *88*, 1209–1227. [CrossRef] [PubMed]
47. Reinhold, W.C.; Straus, S.E.; Ostrove, J.M. Directionality and further mapping of varicella zoster virus transcripts. *Virus Res.* **1988**, *9*, 249–261. [CrossRef]
48. Che, X.; Zerboni, L.; Sommer, M.H.; Arvin, A.M. Varicella-zoster virus open reading frame 10 is a virulence determinant in skin cells but not in T cells in vivo. *J. Virol.* **2006**, *80*, 3238–3248. [CrossRef] [PubMed]
49. Moriuchi, M.; Moriuchi, H.; Straus, S.E.; Cohen, J.I. Varicella-Zoster Virus (VZV) Virion-Associated Transactivator Open Reading Frame 62 Protein Enhances the Infectivity of VZV DNA. *Virology* **1994**, *200*, 297–300. [CrossRef]
50. Moriuchi, H.; Moriuchi, M.; Straus, S.E.; Cohen, J.I. Varicella-zoster virus open reading frame 10 protein, the herpes simplex virus VP16 homolog, transactivates herpesvirus immediate-early gene promoters. *J. Virol.* **1993**, *67*, 2739–2746.
51. Zhou, J.; Rosu, F.; Amrane, S.; Korkut, D.N.; Gabelica, V.; Mergny, J.L. Assembly of chemically modified G-rich sequences into tetramolecular DNA G-quadruplexes and higher order structures. *Methods* **2014**, *67*, 159–168. [CrossRef]
52. Harrison, R.J.; Cuesta, J.; Chessari, G.; Martin, A.R.; Sanji, K.B.; Anthony, P.R.; Morrell, J.; Sharon, M.G.; Christopher, M.I.; Farial, A.T.; et al. Trisubstituted Acridine Derivatives as Potent and Selective Telomerase Inhibitors. *J. Med. Chem.* **2003**, *46*, 4463–4476. [CrossRef] [PubMed]
53. Mergny, J.-L. Thermal difference spectra: A specific signature for nucleic acid structures. *Nucleic Acids Res.* **2005**, *33*, e138. [CrossRef] [PubMed]
54. Smith, M.C.; Boutell, C.; Davido, D.J. HSV-1 ICP0: Paving the way for viral replication. *Future Virol.* **2011**, *6*, 421–429. [CrossRef] [PubMed]
55. Sedlackova, L.; Perkins, K.D.; Lengyel, J.; Strain, A.K.; van Santen, V.L.; Rice, S.A. Herpes simplex virus type 1 ICP27 regulates expression of a variant, secreted form of glycoprotein C by an intron retention mechanism. *J. Virol.* **2008**, *82*, 7443–7455. [CrossRef] [PubMed]
56. Suk, H.; Knipe, D.M. Proteomic analysis of the herpes simplex virus 1 virion protein 16 transactivator protein in infected cells. *Proteomics* **2015**, *15*, 1957–1967. [PubMed]
57. De Nicola, B.; Lech, C.J.; Heddi, B.; Regmi, S.; Frasson, I.; Perrone, R.; Richter, S.N.; Phan, A.T. Structure and possible function of a G-quadruplex in the long terminal repeat of the proviral HIV-1 genome. *Nucleic Acids Res.* **2016**, *44*, 6442–6451. [CrossRef]
58. Perrone, R.; Doria, F.; Butovskaya, E.; Frasson, I.; Botti, S.; Scalabrin, M.; Lago, S.; Grande, V.; Nadai, M.; Freccero, M.; et al. Synthesis, Binding and Antiviral Properties of Potent Core-Extended Naphthalene Diimides Targeting the HIV-1 Long Terminal Repeat Promoter G-Quadruplexes. *J. Med. Chem.* **2015**, *58*, 9639–9652. [CrossRef]

59. Perrone, R.; Butovskaya, E.; Daelemans, D.; Palu, G.; Pannecouque, C.; Richter, S.N. Anti-HIV-1 activity of the G-quadruplex ligand BRACO-19. *J. Antimicrob. Chemother.* **2014**, *69*, 3248–3258. [CrossRef]
60. Harkness, J.M.; Kader, M.; DeLuca, N.A. Transcription of the herpes simplex virus 1 genome during productive and quiescent infection of neuronal and nonneuronal cells. *J. Virol.* **2014**, *88*, 6847–6861. [CrossRef]
61. Lopergolo, A.; Perrone, R.; Tortoreto, M.; Doria, F.; Beretta, G.L.; Zuco, V.; Freccero, M.; Borrello, M.G.; Lanzi, C.; Richter, S.N.; et al. Targeting of RET oncogene by naphthalene diimide-mediated gene promoter G-quadruplex stabilization exerts anti-tumor activity in oncogene-addicted human medullary thyroid cancer. *Oncotarget* **2016**, *7*, 49649–49663. [CrossRef]
62. Tong, X.; Lan, W.; Zhang, X.; Wu, H.; Liu, M.; Cao, C. Solution structure of all parallel G-quadruplex formed by the oncogene RET promoter sequence. *Nucleic Acids Res.* **2011**, *39*, 6753–6763. [CrossRef] [PubMed]
63. Lerner, L.K.; Sale, J.E. Replication of G Quadruplex DNA. *Genes (Basel)* **2019**, *10*. [CrossRef] [PubMed]
64. Tlučková, K.; Marušič, M.; Tóthová, P.; Bauer, L.; Šket, P.; Plavec, J.; Viglasky, V. Human Papillomavirus G-Quadruplexes. *Biochemistry* **2013**, *52*, 7207–7216. [CrossRef] [PubMed]
65. Palumbo, S.L.; Ebbinghaus, S.W.; Hurley, L.H. Formation of a unique end-to-end stacked pair of G-quadruplexes in the hTERT core promoter with implications for inhibition of telomerase by G-quadruplex-interactive ligands. *J. Am. Chem. Soc.* **2009**, *131*, 10878–10891. [CrossRef] [PubMed]
66. Sun, D.; Liu, W.-J.; Guo, K.; Rusche, J.J.; Ebbinghaus, S.; Gokhale, V.; Hurley, L.H. The proximal promoter region of the human vascular endothelial growth factor gene has a G-quadruplex structure that can be targeted by G-quadruplex-interactive agents. *Mol. Cancer Ther.* **2008**, *7*, 880–889. [CrossRef] [PubMed]
67. Rigo, R.; Sissi, C. Characterization of G4–G4 Crosstalk in the *c-KIT* Promoter Region. *Biochemistry* **2017**, *56*, 4309–4312. [CrossRef] [PubMed]
68. Summers, B.C.; Leib, D.A. Herpes simplex virus type 1 origins of DNA replication play no role in the regulation of flanking promoters. *J. Virol.* **2002**, *76*, 7020–7029. [CrossRef]
69. Zhi, Y.; Sandri-Goldin, R.M. Analysis of the phosphorylation sites of herpes simplex virus type 1 regulatory protein ICP27. *J. Virol.* **1999**, *73*, 3246–3257.
70. Smith, I.L.; Hardwicke, M.A.; Sandri-Goldin, R.M. Evidence that the herpes simplex virus immediate early protein ICP27 acts post-transcriptionally during infection to regulate gene expression. *Virology* **1992**, *186*, 74–86. [CrossRef]
71. Sandri-Goldin, R.M. The many roles of the highly interactive HSV protein ICP27, a key regulator of infection. *Future Microbiol.* **2011**, *6*, 1261–1277. [CrossRef]
72. Sahakyan, A.B.; Chambers, V.S.; Marsico, G.; Santner, T.; Di Antonio, M.; Balasubramanian, S. Machine learning model for sequence-driven DNA G-quadruplex formation. *Sci. Rep.* **2017**, *7*, 14535. [CrossRef] [PubMed]
73. Omaga, C.A.; Fleming, A.M.; Burrows, C.J. The Fifth Domain in the G-Quadruplex-Forming Sequence of the Human *NEIL3* Promoter Locks DNA Folding in Response to Oxidative Damage. *Biochemistry* **2018**, *57*, 2958–2970. [CrossRef] [PubMed]
74. Jiang, Y.-C.; Feng, H.; Lin, Y.-C.; Guo, X.-R. New strategies against drug resistance to herpes simplex virus. *Int. J. Oral Sci.* **2016**, *8*, 1–6. [CrossRef] [PubMed]
75. Greenfield, N.J. Using circular dichroism collected as a function of temperature to determine the thermodynamics of protein unfolding and binding interactions. *Nat. Protoc.* **2006**, *1*, 2527–2535. [CrossRef] [PubMed]

Sample Availability: Not available.

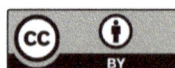

molecules

MDPI

Article

Intensive Distribution of G$_2$-Quaduplexes in the Pseudorabies Virus Genome and Their Sensitivity to Cations and G-Quadruplex Ligands

Hui Deng [1,†], Bowen Gong [1,†], Zhiquan Yang [2], Zhen Li [1], Huan Zhou [1], Yashu Zhang [3], Xiaohui Niu [2], Sisi Liu [1,*] and Dengguo Wei [1,*]

[1]   Laboratory of Medicinal Biophysical Chemistry, College of Science, Huazhong Agricultural University, Wuhan 430070, China; denghui0923@163.com (H.D.); night@webmail.hzau.edu.cn (B.G.); lizhen5a@163.com (Z.L.); zhouhuan@webmail.hzau.edu.cn (H.Z.)
[2]   Hubei Key Laboratory of Agricultural Bioinformatics, College of Informatics, Huazhong Agricultural University, Wuhan 430070, China; yang_zq@foxmail.com (Z.Y.); niuxiaoh@126.com (X.N.)
[3]   Laboratory of Medicinal Biophysical Chemistry, College of Plant Science and Technology, Huazhong Agricultural University, Wuhan 430070, China; yashu@webmail.hzau.edu.cn
*   Correspondence: liusisi@mail.hzau.edu.cn (S.L.); dgwei@mail.hzau.edu.cn (D.W.)
†   These authors contributed equally to this work.

Academic Editor: Sara N. Richter
Received: 17 January 2019; Accepted: 15 February 2019; Published: 21 February 2019

Abstract: Guanine-rich sequences in the genomes of herpesviruses can fold into G-quadruplexes. Compared with the widely-studied G$_3$-quadruplexes, the dynamic G$_2$-quadruplexes are more sensitive to the cell microenvironment, but they attract less attention. Pseudorabies virus (PRV) is the model species for the study of the latency and reactivation of herpesvirus in the nervous system. A total of 1722 G$_2$-PQSs and 205 G$_3$-PQSs without overlap were identified in the PRV genome. Twelve G$_2$-PQSs from the CDS region exhibited high conservation in the genomes of the *Varicellovirus* genus. Eleven G$_2$-PQSs were 100% conserved in the repeated region of the annotated PRV genomes. There were 212 non-redundant G$_2$-PQSs in the 3′ UTR and 19 non-redundant G$_2$-PQSs in the 5′ UTR, which would mediate gene expression in the post-transcription and translation processes. The majority of examined G$_2$-PQSs formed parallel structures and exhibited different sensitivities to cations and small molecules in vitro. Two G$_2$-PQSs, respectively, from 3′ UTR of *UL5* (encoding helicase motif) and *UL9* (encoding sequence-specific ori-binding protein) exhibited diverse regulatory activities with/without specific ligands in vivo. The G-quadruplex ligand, NMM, exhibited a potential for reducing the virulence of the PRV Ea strain. The systematic analysis of the distribution of G$_2$-PQSs in the PRV genomes could guide further studies of the G-quadruplexes' functions in the life cycle of herpesviruses.

Keywords: alphaherpesviruses; pseudorabies virus; genome; G-quadruplex; G-quadruplex ligand; nucleic acids conformation; regulatory element

---

1. Introduction

The life-long latency of herpesviruses poses potential threats to the host at any time, and the reason for the wide existence of the GC-rich sequences in herpesvirus genomes remains unknown [1]. Guanine-rich sequences have been discovered to form special DNA or RNA secondary structures called G-quadruplexes. They are composed of π-stacked G-quartets via hydrogen-bonded structure in DNA or RNA [2]. Each G-quartet contains four guanines held by eight hydrogen bonds, and coordinated with a central monovalent cation, such as K$^+$ and Na$^+$. The G$_3$-putative quadruplex sequences (G$_3$-PQSs) in the form of $(G_{3+}N_{1-7})_3G_{3+}$ form three or more G-quartets in the structures (Figure 1), and they exhibited good thermal stability under near-physiological conditions [3]. The function of these G_3-quadruplex sequences has been well-studied in the genomes of humans [3], maize [4] and human viruses [5,6]. Recently, some studies have reported on the regulatory function of G_2-quadruplexes (Figure 1), with two G-quartets in the viral mRNA translation of Epstein–Barr virus [7] and in the polyamine biosynthesis pathway of eukaryotic cells [8]. However, G_2-putative quadruplex sequences (G_2-PQSs) in the form of $(G_{2+}N_{1-7})_3G_{2+}$ have not attracted wide attention, due to their relatively low stability, even though they exhibit certain superiority in sensitivity. The systematic analysis of G_2-PQSs in the genomes of herpesviruses could explore more functions of G-rich sequences in herpesviruses, compared with that of G_3-PQSs.

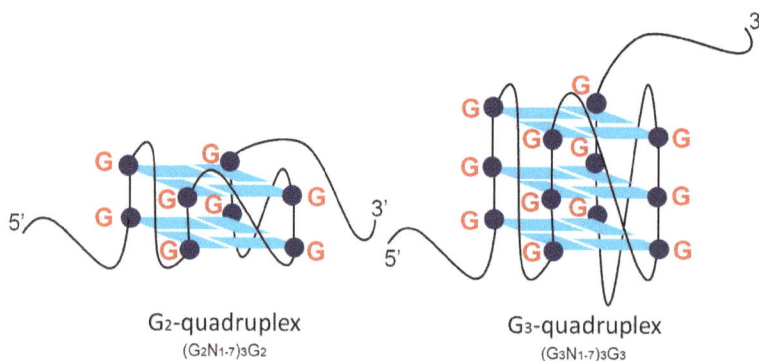

Figure 1. Schematic diagram of the G_2-quadruplex and the G_3-quadruplex.

Pseudorabies virus (PRV) represents a good model for the study of G_2-quadruplex functions in herpesvirus genomes. This virus is a herpesvirus of the *Varicellovirus* genus in the *Alphaherpesvirinae* subfamily that is included in the family *Herpesviridae*. The *Alphaherpesvirinae* chooses the nervous system for latency [9]. PRV causes neuronal and lethal infection in many animal species, yet posing little or no danger to humans [10–14]. PRV has been used as a model species for studying the cycle of infection, latency, and reactivation, which are critical processes for the survival of alphaherpesviruses [10]. Vaccination is the most effective approach to preventing virus infection. However, herpesviruses can establish latency in the host after the first infection, and they can reactivate to cause serious diseases in their host. Failure of vaccination will result in a big threat to humans and animals. For example, the Bartha-K61 vaccine has been used worldwide, and it played an important role in the eradication of pseudorabies virus in many countries. Nevertheless, it had failed to protect piglets from being infected by several virulent PRV strains in China, resulting in PRV re-outbreak in 2011 [15–23]. In order to prevent and cure herpesvirus infections successfully, it could be helpful to reveal the latency-reactivation mechanism, based on the characteristics of herpesvirus genomes and their feature in host cells. The Human gammaherpesvirus 4 (Epstein–Barr virus, EBV) was assumed to modulate immune evasion with a G_2-quadruplex forming in the coding sequence (CDS) of Epstein–Barr virus-encoded nuclear antigen 1 (EBNA1) [7]. The PRV may respond to the defense of the host cells, through the formation and resolution of G-quadruplexes to regulate latency and reactivation. This study is aimed to provide clues for vaccine and drug development at the nucleic acid level.

In this work, a systematic analysis will be carried out to locate the distribution of G_2/G_3-quadruplex sequences in the PRV genome. The conservation of the putative G-quadruplex-forming sequences will be evaluated in the PRV strains and in the *Varicellovirus* genus. The evolutionary differences in the G-quadruplexes between non-human infectious herpesvirus and human herpesviruses will be discussed further. G_2-PQSs structure types and their sensitivities to different cations and ligands will be examined, for their roles in regulating gene expression. The study of a classic G-quadruplex ligand, *N*-methyl mesoporphyrinIX (NMM), exhibited potential for inhibiting the virulence of the PRV Ea strain. This study will further investigate G_2-quadruplexes working as sensors in response to small molecules, proteins, and physiological cation conditions in the specific microenvironment, to reveal the latency-reactivation mechanism of herpesviruses.

2. Results

2.1. Bioinformatic Analysis

2.1.1. Genome-Wide Analysis of G_3-PQSs and G_2-PQSs Distributions in the PRV Genome

The putative G_3-quadruplex sequences (G_3-PQSs) in the PRV genome were predicted with the Quadparser program [3] in the form of the GnNm sequence (where $n \geq 3$ and $1 \leq m \leq 7$). The putative G_2-quadruplex sequences (G_2-PQSs) were predicted with the same program, but in the modified sequence form ($n \geq 2$). The genome size of PRV was 143,461 bp, and it encoded 69 proteins. The analysis of the PRV reference genome (NC_006151.1) indicated that 1722 G_2-PQSs and 205 G_3-PQSs were distributed in the PRV genome (Figure 2; File S1), with the density of the G_2-PQSs being 12 PQS/kb.

As the formation of the G-quadruplex could affect either transcription or translation, our analysis of PQSs was based on double strands with the well-annotated regions, and the predicted regulatory regions in the PRV reference genome (File S2). The 3′ end untranslated regions (3′ UTRs) from 63 genes, and the 5′ end untranslated regions (5′ UTRs) from 61 genes were annotated in the PRV reference genome in The National Center for Biotechnology Information (NCBI) Genome database [24]. The promoters of the annotated PRV genes were predicted to be 1 kb upstream of the annotated transcription start site of each gene. G_2-PQSs were higher in density in the CDS region and in the large latency transcript (LLT) than in the repeat region, while the G_3-PQSs were densely distributed in the repeat region (Table 1). The density of the G_2-PQSs in the 3′ UTR was higher than that in the 5′ UTR (Table 1). In the promoter regions, the G_2-PQSs density was 5.34 PQS/kb, and it was more than eight-fold that of the G_3-PQSs density (Table 1).

The PQS monomer was named the single G-quadruplex-forming sequence, and the sequences forming more than two possible simultaneous G-quadruplexes were defined as the PQS cluster. The G_3-quadruplex cluster, forming a highly stable structure, was identified in the repetitive region of the Herpes simplex virus type 1 (HSV-1) genome [25]. This study found that 86.8% of G_3-PQSs and 77% of G_2-PQSs were monomers in the genome of PRV (File S1). 27 non-redundant G_3-PQSs clusters were located in the regulatory regions, rather than in the coding region in the PRV genome. Sixty-nine G_2-PQS clusters were distributed in the repeat regions, and 122 G_2-PQS clusters were located in the coding region in the PRV genome (Table 1).

Molecules 2019, 24, 774

Table 1. Number of putative G-quadruplex sequences in three herpesvirus genomes.

Herpesviruses	Region †	Length (bp)	Putative G₂-quadruplex Sequences				Putative G₃-quadruplex Sequences			
			Number	Monomer	Cluster	Density (PQS/kb)	Number	Monomer	Cluster	Density (PQS/kb)
Pseudorabies virus (PRV, NC_006151.1)	coding sequence (CDS)	105,363	1126	1004	122	10.69	51	51	0	0.48
	3′ end untranslated region (3′ UTR)	35,688	166	149	17	4.65	6	6	0	0.17
	5′ end untranslated region (5′ UTR)	6760	19	18	1	2.81	5	3	2	0.74
	Promoter	56,324	301	276	25	5.34	36	32	4	0.64
	large latency transcript (LLT)	13,040	139	109	30	10.66	27	25	2	2.07
	Repeat region	36,234	338	269	69	9.33	131	109	22	3.62
Human alphaherpesvirus 1 (Herpes simplex virus type 1, HSV-1, NC_001806.2)	CDS	121,089	1351	1248	103	11.16	109	104	5	0.90
	3′ UTR	49,322	235	223	12	4.76	27	27	0	0.55
	5′ UTR	3434	18	18	0	5.24	3	1	2	0.87
	Promoter	64,966	346	317	29	5.33	64	56	8	0.99
	latency-associated transcript (LAT)	15,944	158	146	12	9.91	54	44	10	3.39
	Repeat region	31,875	338	307	31	10.60	120	87	33	3.76
Human alphaherpesvirus 3 (Varicella-zoster virus, VZV, NC_001348.1)	CDS	111,496	296	282	14	2.65	10	10	0	0.09
	3′ UTR	29,758	37	36	1	1.24	1	1	0	0.03
	5′ UTR *	496	0	0	0	0	0	0	0	0
	Promoter	60,900	71	69	2	1.17	5	3	2	0.08
	VZV latency-associated transcript (VLT)	2417	13	12	1	5.38	0	0	0	0
	Repeat region	15,514	119	111	8	7.67	11	9	2	0.71

†: The CDS, 3′ UTR, 5′ UTR and repeat regions were analyzed according to the annotation information in the reference genomes. The promoter regions were predicted as 1kb upstream of the transcription start site of each annotated gene. LLT: large latency transcript; LAT: latency-associated transcript; VLT: VZV latency-associated transcript; VLT: VZV latency-associated transcript [26]. *: The annotated 5′ UTR of the genes from the Human alphaherpesvirus 3 were analyzed for the PQSs.

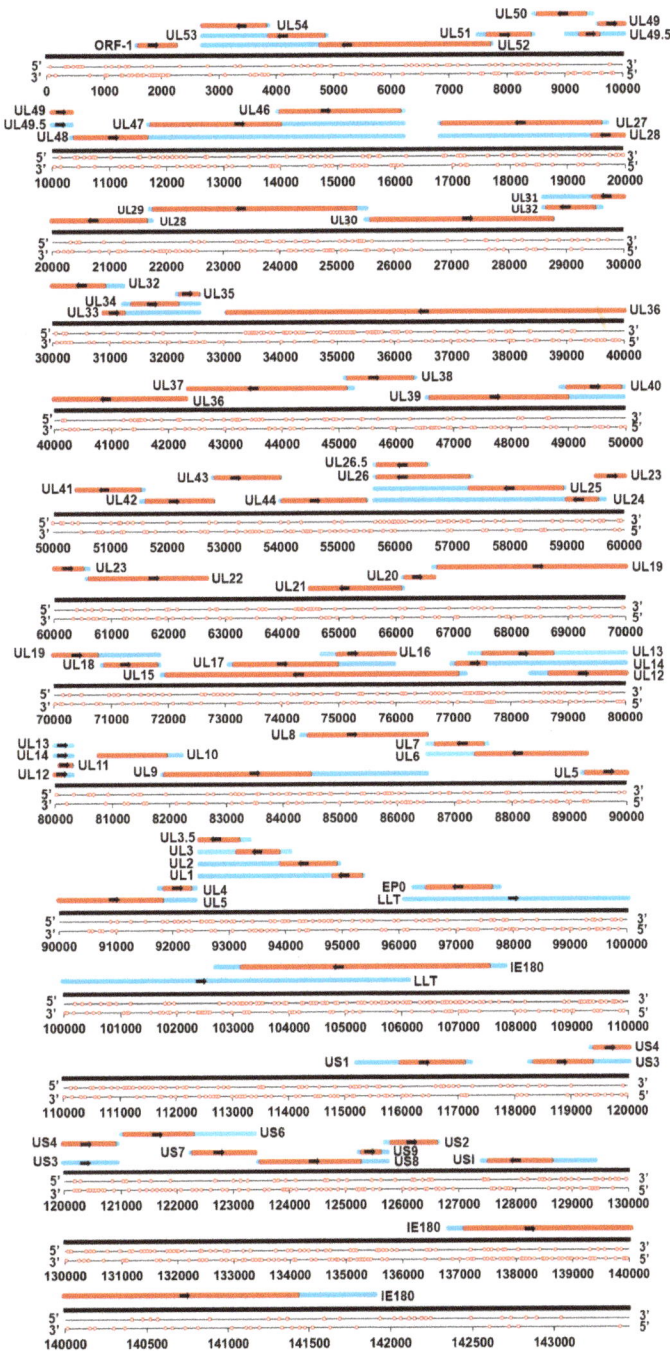

Figure 2. Distribution of G$_2$-putative quadruplex sequences (G$_2$-PQSs) in the double-strand genome of pseudorabies virus (PRV). One red circle indicates one G$_2$-PQS. The red bars indicate the coding sequence (CDS) region. The blue bars indicate the untranslated region.

2.1.2. Conserved G_2-PQSs in the Coding Sequences of PRV Genes

G_2-PQS Distribution in the Coding Regions of Genes Involved in the Replication Cycle of PRV

The G_2-quadruplex formation in the open reading frame (ORF) of Epstein–Barr virus-encoded nuclear antigen 1 (EBNA1) led to decreased mRNA translation in the Epstein–Barr virus (EBV), which suggested that the G-quadruplex in viral transcripts acts as a specific regulatory element to regulate translation level and immune evasion [7]. The PRV replication cycle contains five main processes, including entry, immediate early stage, early stage, late stage, and egress [10]. There were 481 G_2-PQSs in the ORFs of the genes in above five stages (Figure 3). 112 G_2-PQSs were found in the entry stage, and 30 of them were involved in important envelope glycoproteins recognizing host cells. After the entry stage, PRV is in the immediate early stage. It transcribes and expresses only one immediate early gene, *IE180*; this was different from human herpesviruses, which transcribe three to five immediate early genes. *IE180* is required for the effective transcription of early viral genes [10]. There were two copies of *IE180* in the PRV genome, and 22 G_2-PQSs were located in the coding sequence of each copy. The genes in the early stage contained 144 G_2-PQSs, which was twice as many as the total number of G_2-PQSs in the late stage ($n = 77$). The early-stage proteins had functions in transactivation and viral DNA synthesis, while the late-stage proteins were mainly responsible for DNA packaging and capsid maturation. A total of 104 G_2-PQSs were identified in the egress stage, and most of them were present in the tegument proteins, which are important for virion formation before cell-to-cell movement (Figure 3).

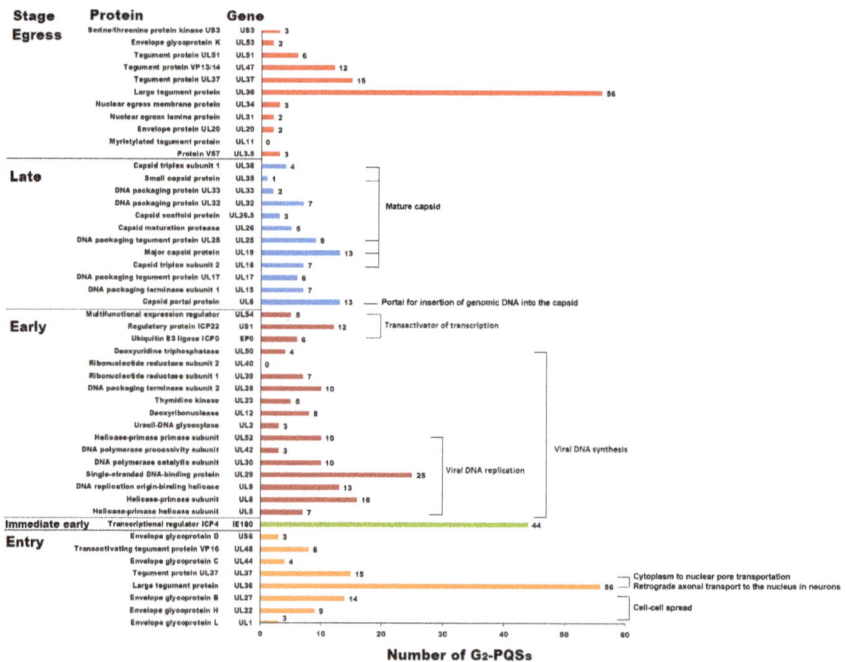

Figure 3. Number of G_2-PQSs in the coding sequences of the genes that are involved in the PRV replication cycle.

G_2-PQSs Involved in the Processes of DNA Replication and Encapsidation

Eighty-four G_2-PQSs were identified in the genes involved in the viral DNA replication process (Figure 3), including *UL5, UL8, UL9, UL29, UL30, UL42*, and *UL52*. In total, 39% of these G_2-PQSs were in the coding region of the helicase–primerase complex formed by *UL5*, *UL8*, and *UL52*. Twenty-five G_2-PQSs were found in the gene *UL29*, encoding the single-stranded DNA-binding protein ICP8. The DNA replication origin-binding helicase *UL9* contained 13 G_2-PQSs in its coding sequence, and the DNA polymerase complex *UL30/UL42* contained 13 G_2-PQSs in total.

In the late stage, *UL38*, *UL35*, *UL25*, *UL19*, *UL18*, and *UL6* encoded the proteins of the mature capsid constituents; these are required for the capsid assembly in the nucleus of the cell, and two scaffolding proteins (*UL26* and *UL26.5*) have been reported to have participated in capsid formation [10]. The above late proteins accounted for 61% of the G_2-PQSs in the late stage (Figure 3).

G_2-PQSs Involved in the Processes of Virus Entry and Egress

Both *UL36* and *UL37* were the tegument protein genes required in both the entry and egress stages [10]. The VP1/2 protein (*UL36*) is the important component of the inner layer of tegument proteins, and it was reported to be associated with the capsid during PRV transport across cytoplasm into the nuclear pore [27]. The production of VP1/2 protein is cut off by truncating the translation of *UL36* gene, resulting in the failed transportation of the virus particle. Fifty-six G_2-PQSs were observed in the CDS region of *UL36*, accounting for 50% of the total number of G_2-PQSs in the stages it involved (Figure 3). The viral glycoproteins gC (*UL44*), gD (*US6*), gB (*UL27*), gH (*UL22*), and gL (*UL1*) mediated a cascade required by PRV virions to enter specific cells, and totally there were 29 G_2-PQSs in the ORFs of glycoproteins (Figure 3).

Conservation and Potential Function of G_2-PQSs in CDS Region in the Varicellovirus Genus

Since coding sequences had higher conservation than regulatory regions among different viruses in the same genus, the inter-species analysis of the conservation of the G_2-PQSs in the coding region was performed within 11 *Varicellovirus* species including PRV. The conservation of the 494 G_2-PQSs in the CDS region was analyzed. The analysis indicated that 55.3% of G_2-PQSs exhibited the conservation score higher than 0.2 (Figure S1). Twelve of these 494 G_2-PQSs were found with the conservation score higher than 0.7 (Table 2). Five G_2-PQSs of them were derived from the immediate early gene *IE180*, and two G_2-PQSs were derived from the gene *UL30* encoding the DNA polymerase catalytic subunit. One G_2-PQS derived from the gene *UL13* encoding protein-serine/threonine kinase was 100% conserved in the *Varicellovirus* genus (Table 2). The other G_2-PQSs with their conservation scored as 1.0 were from the gene *UL33* associated with *UL28* and *UL15* to contribute to DNA cleavage and PRV package. The DNA cleavage and encapsidation related gene *UL17* and major capsid protein gene *UL19* contained one conserved G_2-PQS in their coding sequences. Two tegument protein genes *UL16* and *UL47* also contained one conserved G_2-PQS, respectively (Table 2).

Table 2. G_2-PQS with high conservation score in the coding sequence of *Varicellovirus* genes.

Gene Common Name	Function	Putative G_2-quadruplex Sequence (5'-3')	Score	Nucleotide Identity
IE180	Transactivator, homolog of ICP4	GGGCCGGGAACTGGACCGGG	1.000	0.579
		GGACTGGCCCGCGGACGGCCCGGCCGTGGGGG	0.900	0.579
		GGCTCGGCGCGGCGCGGCGCCGG	0.800	0.579
		GGCCAACGTGGCCGCGGCCCGG	0.700	0.579
		GGGCCCCGGTCCCGGGCCGGCTCCGGGCCCCGG	0.700	0.579
UL30	DNA replication	GGACGACGGCGGCGGCTACCAGGGCGCCAAGG	0.727	0.678
		GGTGTACGGGTTCACGGGCGTGGCCAACGGG	0.727	0.678
UL33	DNA cleavage and packaging	GGGGAGGCGCTGCGGGCGCGG	1.000	0.664
UL17	DNA cleavage and encapsidation	GGGGCGGCCGGCGCGGGCCCCGG	0.778	0.589
UL16	Tegument protein	GGTCCTGGCCCCCGGCGCGTGGTGGGCGCGCGG	0.800	0.580
UL47	Tegument protein	GGGGACGAGGAGGAGGAGGAGGAGGAGGAG AGAGCGAGGGGGGCGCGTGGTCCGACGGGG	0.700	0.486
UL13	Protein-serine/threonine kinase	GGCCGTCGGGGCCGGATCGTACGG	1.000	0.525

2.1.3. Distribution Analysis of G_2-PQSs in Regulatory Regions in PRV Genomes

Promoter, untranslated region, and intergenic region, which were important regulatory regions, had multiple functions in gene regulation. G_3-PQSs were reported to be mainly located in the regulatory regions in the genomes of human herpesviruses [5], while less report on G_2-PQSs was available. Systematic analysis of G_2-PQS could be conducive to the exploration of their regulatory function. In this study, PRV was found to have higher density of G_2-PQS than G_3-PQS in the repeat regions (Table 1).

Dozens of Conserved G_2-PQSs in the Repeat Regions Related to Genome Recombination

Terminal repeat (TR) region is important for genome replication in some herpesviruses. The G-quadruplex in the TR region of gammaherpesvirus Kaposi sarcoma-associated herpesvirus (KSHV) altered the latent DNA replication and episomal persistence [28]. Furthermore, the stabilization of HSV-1 G-quadruplexes in the repeat region inhibited DNA polymerase processing and viral DNA replication [25]. The PRV genome was similar to the HSV-1 genome which was characterized by two unique regions (UL and US), and the US region was flanked by the internal and terminal repeat sequences (IRS and TRS, respectively). During PRV infection, the recombination between the inverted repeats produced two possible isomers of the genome with the U_S region in opposite orientation. Both isomers were infectious and were in equimolar amount after infection, and the PRV genome was circularized upon entry into the host nucleus through blunt end ligation independent of any viral protein synthesis (reviewed in [10]).

4 G_2-PQSs were located in 0–656 bp region, and 208 G_2-PQSs were located in the two regions between genes *IE180* and *US1* (Figure 4). The conservation percentage of 117 G_2-PQSs on the sense strand of PRV genome ranged from 4% to 100% (Figure 5). There were 38 G_2-PQSs in the repeated region between *IE180* and *US1* with conservation percentage more than 90% (Figure 5), including 11 G_2-PQSs with 100% conservation rate (Table S1). These conserved GC-rich sequences might form G-quadruplexes in the inverted repeat region, mediating the genome recombination after infection. 14 G_2-PQSs existing between *IE180* and *ORF1* may be switches of PRV replication in circular genome.

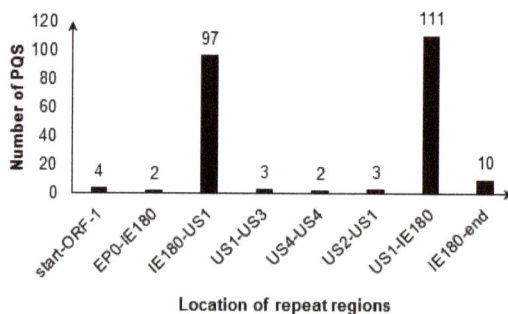

Figure 4. Distribution of G_2-PQS in repeat regions in PRV genome.

G_2-PQSs in the Untranslated Regions of PRV Genes

The untranslated regions (UTR) are important regulatory region for gene expression. G-quadruplex-forming sequences in the 5′ UTR acting as translational repressor have been reported in several human genes [29,30]. The 3′ UTR is related to mRNA stability, alternative splicing, polyadenylation, and localization. G-quadruplexes in the 3′ UTR of CaMKIIa (Ca²⁺/calmodulin-dependent protein kinase II) and PDS-95 (post-synaptic density protein 95) mRNAs are responsible for the transport of those mRNA in neurites in vivo [31].

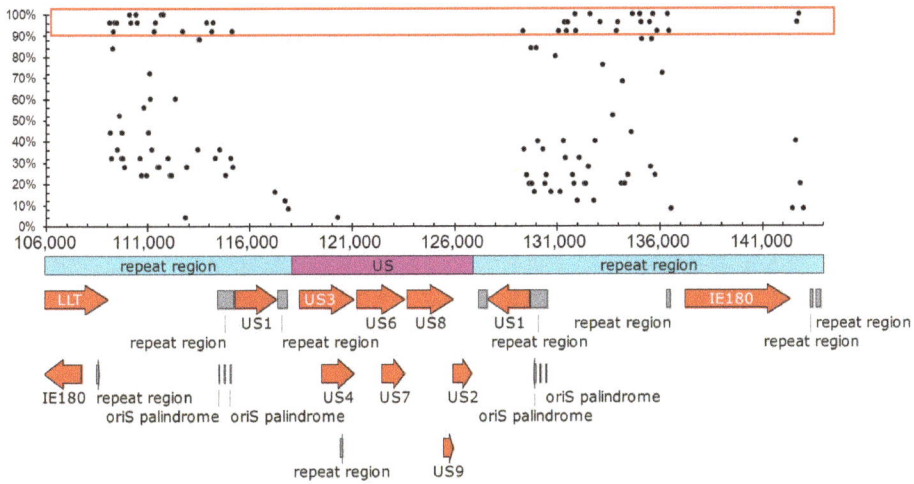

Figure 5. Conservation percentage of putative G-quadruplex sequences in the repeat region. Red block indicated the G_2-PQSs with conservation percentage more than 90%.

Nineteen non-redundant G_2-PQSs and five G_3-PQSs were found in the 5′ UTR of the annotated PRV genes (Figure S2). Among all the genes in PRV genome, the gene *UL13* contained four G_2-PQSs in its 212-bp 5′ UTR with the highest density of G_2-PQS in the 5′ UTR regions, and the gene *UL28* contained one G_3-PQS in its 72-bp 5′ UTR with the highest density of G_3-PQS in the 5′ UTR (Figure 6). The transactivator gene *US1* contained four G_2-PQSs in its 5′ UTR, accounting for 17% of G_2-PQS monomers found in 5′ UTR region in the whole genome (Figure 7A). *UL13* had three G_2-PQS monomers in its 5′ UTR, accounting for 13% of G_2-PQS monomers in 5′ UTR in the PRV genome (Figure 7A). In the early protein genes, the deoxyribonuclease gene *UL12* and dUTPase gene *UL50* had two G_2-PQS monomers in their 5′ UTR, respectively (Figure 7A). One G_2-PQS cluster was found in the gene *UL13*, which was the unique G_2-PQS cluster in the all annotated 5′ UTR of PRV genes (File S2).

The G_2-PQSs in the 3′ UTR of annotated PRV genes were more than ten folds of those found in the 5′ UTR of the annotated PRV genes. There existed 212 non-redundant G_2-PQSs and 8 G_3-PQSs in the 3′ UTR of PRV genes (Figure S2). These results suggested that G_2-quadruplexes might regulate gene expression frequently by effecting 3′ UTR secondary structure. The genes *UL51* and *UL29* had the highest density of G_3-PQSs in their 3′ UTR regions (Figure 6).

More than 70 G_2-PQS monomers were found in the 3′ UTR of the genes related to viral genome replication, envelopment, and packaging processes (Figure S2). *UL48* encoded the VP16 protein exerting multiple functions in the PRV, including transactivation in gene regulation and secondary envelopment in viral egress [10]. 21 G_2-PQS monomers were found in the 3′ UTR of gene *UL48*, accounting for 11% of all the G_2-PQS monomers in the 3′ UTR in the PRV genome (Figure 7B). The late stage gene *UL15* encoding DNA packaging terminase subunit 1 had 15 G_2-PQS monomers in its 3′ UTR. The *UL9* encoded the sequence-specific ori-binding protein OBP which formed the ATP-dependent helicase motif. OBP was essential for the replication of the viral DNA [10]. *UL9* had 13 G_2-PQS monomers in its 3′ UTR. The tegument protein coding gene *UL14* and type III membrane protein coding gene *UL24* had the same number of G_2-PQSs in their 3′ UTR (Figure S2). The G_2-PQS monomers from *UL9*, *UL14* and *UL24* accounted for 21% of the entire number of G_2-PQS monomers in the 3′ UTR (Figure 7B).

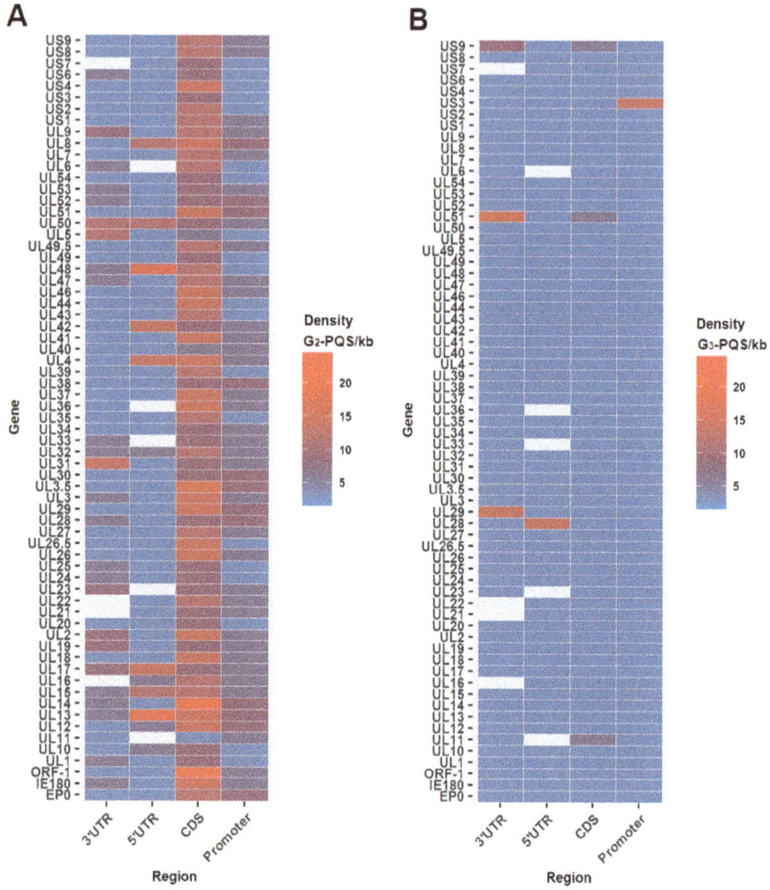

Figure 6. Heat maps of PQS density in coding sequence and regulatory regions of each PRV gene. (**A**) Heat map of G_2-PQSs; (**B**) Heat map of G_3-PQSs.

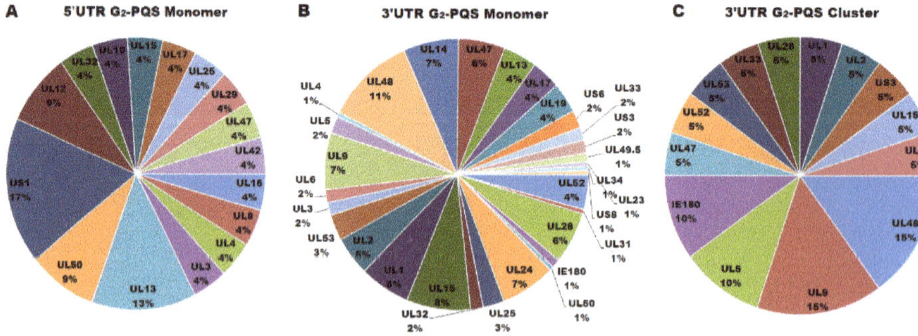

Figure 7. Quantitative distribution of G_2-PQSs in the untranslated regions of annotated genes in PRV genome. (**A**) G_2-PQS monomers in the 5′ UTR of the PRV genes. (**B**) G_2-PQS monomers in the 3′ UTR of the PRV genes. (**C**) G_2-PQS clusters in the 3′ UTR of the PRV genes.

Another important characteristic was that G_2-PQS clusters existed in the 3′ UTR of PRV gene densely. The gene *UL48* had 3 G_2-PQS clusters in its 3′ UTR. The DNA replication related gene group had far more G_2-PQS clusters than other functional gene groups. The *UL9/UL5/UL52* group had 6 G_2-PQS clusters in the 3′ UTR region (Figure 7C). The proteins coded by above three genes included the sequence-specific ori-binding protein, helicase motif, and primase subunit. The G_2-PQSs from 3′ UTR of *UL5* and *UL9* were validated in further experiments. The identification of the functional G_2-PQSs in the untranslated regions of genes in transactivation, and viral DNA synthesis processes will provide the elements for post-transcriptional regulation of virus genes.

A Wide Distribution of G_2-PQSs in the Large Latency Transcript

The large latency transcript was the only gene reported to be transcribed during PRV latency [10]. It overlapped with the oppositely transcribed *IE180* gene and *EP0* gene, and it was one of the spliced transcripts in the PRV genome [9]. Sixty-seven G_2-PQSs and 72 G_2-PQSs were predicted, respectively, in the positive strand and in the negative strand of the LLT (Figure 8). Forty G_2-PQSs were found to be 100% conserved among the annotated PRV genomes (Table S2). Thirty G_2-PQSs in the negative strand were overlapped with the G_2-PQSs in the *EP0* and *IE180* transcripts, suggesting that these overlapped G_2-PQSs could be potential dual-functional regulatory elements. Twenty-seven G_3-PQSs were found in the LLT transcription region (Figure S3), and only one G_3-PQS was overlapped with *EP0* transcript, while the *IE180* transcript did not have any overlapped G_3-PQS. The LLT intron had a microRNA cluster that was involved in PRV replication and affecting virulence [32,33]. Fifteen G_3-PQSs and 35 G_2-PQSs were found to be located in the intron of LLT. Thus, it could be speculated that these PQSs in the intron might be involved in the transcription regulation of microRNAs during PRV latency.

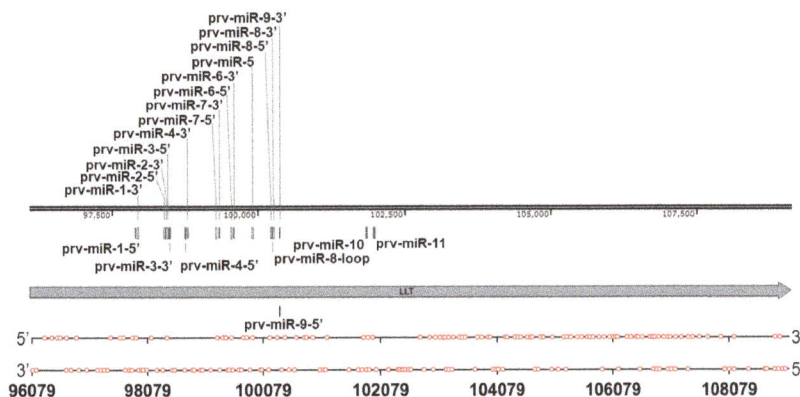

Figure 8. Distribution of G_2-PQSs in the double-strands of the PRV large latency transcript region. One red circle indicates one G_2-PQS.

Density of the G_2-PQSs in the Promoter Regions

The G_3-quadruplexes in the promoter regions of Human immunodeficiency virus 1 (HIV-1) and human herpesviruses were reported to negatively regulate gene expression [5,34–36]. Since the promoters of PRV genes were not annotated in the reference genome, we predicted the promoters to be 1 kb upstream of the transcription start site of each gene. The gene *UL14* coding tegument protein and the gene *UL28*, coding DNA packaging terminase subunit 2, were found to contain nine G_2-PQSs in their promoters, respectively, which was the largest number among all of the PRV genes. Viral DNA replication-related genes *UL29/UL30/UL8* had eight G_2-PQSs in each promoter (Figure 6).

2.1.4. Comparison of PQS Distribution among Three Herpesvirus Genomes

Inter-species comparison was performed among PRV, HHV-1 (Herpes simplex virus type 1, HSV-1) and HHV-3 (Varicella-zoster virus, VZV). These three viruses were neurotropic alphaherpesviruses. PRV and HHV-3 belonged to the same genus called *Varicellovirus*. These herpesviruses always caused serious diseases after reactivation from latency. Trigeminal ganglia (TG) was the common latency site for these three herpesviruses, and the dorsal root ganglia (DRG) was another latency site for HHV-3 [10,25,37]. It was difficult to control the switch between latency and reactivation of these herpesviruses. An analysis of the common features and differences in the PQS distribution among these herpesviruses will provide an insight into latency modulation.

G_3-PQSs with the highest density among three herpesviruses were located in the repeat regions (Table 1) related to genome recombination during infection. Though they were in different genuses, PRV and HHV-1 shared similar features in the distribution and high density of G_2-PQSs, which were different from HHV-3. G_2-PQSs with the highest density in PRV and HHV-1 were located in the coding regions. The density of G_2-PQSs in the coding regions of PRV and HHV-1 genes was found to be five-fold as much as that of HHV-3 (Table 1). In the PRV and HHV-1 genomes, the number of the G_2-PQS monomers in the 3' UTR regions was 8–12 fold of that of the 5' UTR region. The latency-associated transcripts in HHV-1 and PRV were much longer than that in HHV-3. In PRV, the densities of G_2-PQSs and G_3-PQSs were 10.66 G_2-PQS/kb and 2.07 G_3-PQS/kb in its LLT, respectively. In HHV-1, it was 9.91 G_2-PQS/kb and 3.39 G_3-PQS/kb in its LAT, while in HHV-3, no G_3-PQS was observed in its VLT, and the density of G_2-PQS was half that of PRV (Table 1). Compared with HHV-1, the PRV had more G_3-PQS monomers distributed in the repeat region, but less G_3-PQS monomers in the CDS, UTR, promoter, and LLT regions (Table 1).

2.1.5. Summary of Bioinformatics Analysis

In herpesvirus genomes, G_3-PQSs were especially abundant in the repeat regions, while G_2-PQSs were distributed genome-wide. The non-coding region had many more G_2-PQSs than G_3-PQSs, and G_2-PQSs showed a higher density in the CDS region and LLT than in the repeat region. The genes involved in transactivation, genomic DNA replication, and the virus maturation processes had rich and conserved G_2-PQSs in their mRNA sequences. In the *Varicellovirus* genus, some G_2-PQSs in the coding sequences of the immediate early protein ICP4, DNA cleavage and packaging protein (*UL33*), and serine/threonine kinase (*UL13*) exhibited conservations of 100%. The highly conserved G_2-PQSs provide universal target sites to control *Varicellovirus* by disturbing the translation of the above proteins. The density of G_2-PQS in 3' UTR was higher than that in the 5' UTR, and more G_2-PQS clusters were found in the 3' UTR of PRV genes than those in the 5' UTR. The 38 G_2-PQSs in the repeated region between *IE180* and *US1* exhibited conservations of higher than 90% among all the annotated PRV genomes, indicating that the conserved elements might be involved in PRV genome recombination. The LLT overlapped with the oppositely transcribed *IE180* gene and the *EP0* gene. The PQSs in the overlapped regions might be potential dual-functional regulatory elements.

2.2. Experimental Validation

The genome-wide analysis of the G_2-PQS distribution indicated that one-third of the PRV G_2-PQSs were distributed in the non-coding regions of PRV genome, such as the regions of UTR, IRS, TRS, and LLT (File S1). Further study is needed to determine whether these PQSs could serve as *cis*-regulatory elements in gene expression.

2.2.1. Parallel G-Quadruplexes formed by G_2-PQSs In Vitro

Circular dichroism (CD) spectroscopy is widely used to distinguish parallel, anti-parallel or hybrid G-quadruplex structures [38]. A parallel G-quadruplex showed a negative peak near 240 nm, and a positive peak near 260 nm. An anti-parallel G-quadruplex exhibited a negative peak near 260 nm and a positive peak around 290 nm. The hybrid G-quadruplex always displayed one negative peak at 240 nm and two positive peaks at 260 nm and 290 nm. Of the 15 G_2-PQS oligonucleotides (details in Table S3) selected from the regulatory regions of the PRV genome, 13 G_2-PQS folded into parallel G-quadruplexes in a buffer containing 100 mM potassium. LLT-PQS1 and LLT-PQS2, between the start of LLT and the Prv-miR-1-5′, formed hybrid G-quadruplexes, while other LLT-PQSs between Prv-miR-11-1 and the end of LLT formed parallel G-quadruplexes (Figure 9A). The three G_2-PQSs were located in the repeat region between *IE180* and *US1*, and the five G_2-PQSs were located in the repeat region complementary to *US1* CDS, and all of these eight G_2-PQSs mentioned above formed parallel G-quadruplexes (Figure 9B,C). One G_2-PQS from the 3′ UTR of *UL5*, and another from the 5′ UTR of *US1* exhibited typical parallel G-quadruplex peaks (Figure 9D).

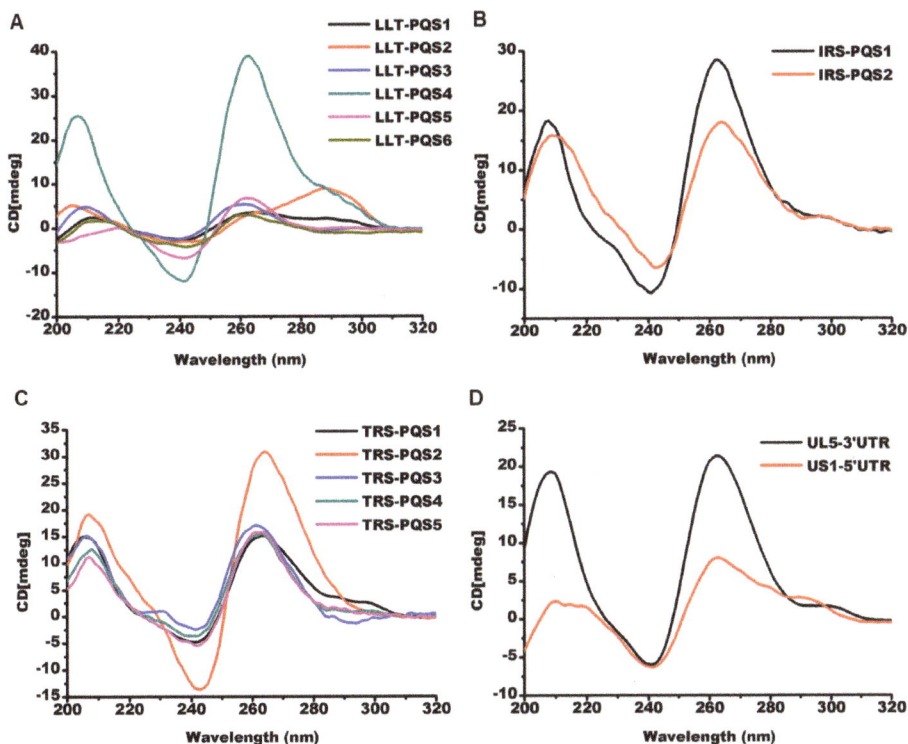

Figure 9. Circular dichroism (CD) spectra of G-quadruplex structures formed by selected oligonucleotides. (**A**) G_2-PQS from the large latency-associated transcript (LLT) region. The LLT-PQS1 and LLT-PQS2 are located between the start site of LLT and the Prv-miR-1-5′; the LLT-PQS3, LLT-PQS4, LLT-PQS5, and LLT-PQS6 are located between Prv-miR-11-1 and the end of the LLT. (**B**) G_2-PQS from the internal repeat sequence (IRS) region. The IRS-PQS1 and IRS-PQS2 are located between *IE180* and *US1*. (**C**) G_2-PQS from the terminal repeat sequence (TRS) region. TRS-PQS1, TRS-PQS2, TRS-PQS3, and TRS-PQS4 are located in the sequence complementary to *US1* CDS; TRS-PQS5 is located between *IE180* and *US1*. (**D**) G_2-PQS from the untranslated region (UTR). The UL5-3UTR is from the 3′ UTR of the gene *UL5*; US1-5UTR is from the 5′ UTR of the gene *US1*.

2.2.2. G_2-quadruplexes in the 3′ UTR Affects Gene Expression In Vivo with Varying Sensitivities

The formation of a G-quadruplex in the 3′ UTR was reported to result in gene expression decrease, alternative polyadenylation [39], and retrotransposition [40].This study found that there were more

G_2-PQSs in the 3′ UTR than in the 5′ UTR, in PRV (Table 1). In this study, G_2-PQSs from the 3′ UTR were inserted into the dual luciferase vector, to check their functions.

In the Circular dichroism (CD) experiment, the PQS UL9-3′UTR-2G exhibited no G-quadruplex signal in 100 mM sodium solution, while it folded into a parallel G-quadruplex in the buffer containing 100 mM potassium (Figure 10A). The stability of the G-quadruplex increased with the addition of the potassium cation. (Figure 10B). UL9-3′UTR-2G showed a higher sensitivity to the increase of the potassium than the 3G mutant oligonucleotide obtained by replacing "GG" with "GGG" (Figure 10C). The insertion of PQS UL9-3′UTR-2G into the 3′ UTR region of the renilla luciferase gene in the psiCHECK-2 vector resulted in a 38% decrease in relative luciferase activity (Figure 11A). The PQS UL5-3′UTR-2G folded into a parallel G-quadruplex in a buffer with 100 mM K$^+$ (Figure 10D), and the addition of the G-quadruplex ligand NMM stabilized the structure. The insertion of PQS UL5-3′UTR into the 3′ UTR region of renilla luciferase gene in the psiCHECK-2 vector made no difference in the protein expression (Figure 11A). The addition of NMM at 20 μM increased the relative luciferase activity ($p < 0.01$) (Figure 11B, Figures S5). The addition of other typical G-quadruplex ligands such as PDS and BRACO-19 made no significant difference in structural stability (Figures S5, S6A, S6B) and relative luciferase activity (Figures S5, S7A, S7B). The above results suggested that the G-quadruplex formed from G_2-PQSs in 3′ UTR affected the protein expression, and that G_2-PQSs were more sensitive to different cations and ligands than G_3-PQSs. These features made the G_2-quadruplex suitable as sensitive switches for gene expression regulation in response to different environmental factors, such as various proteins, small molecules, and signal cations.

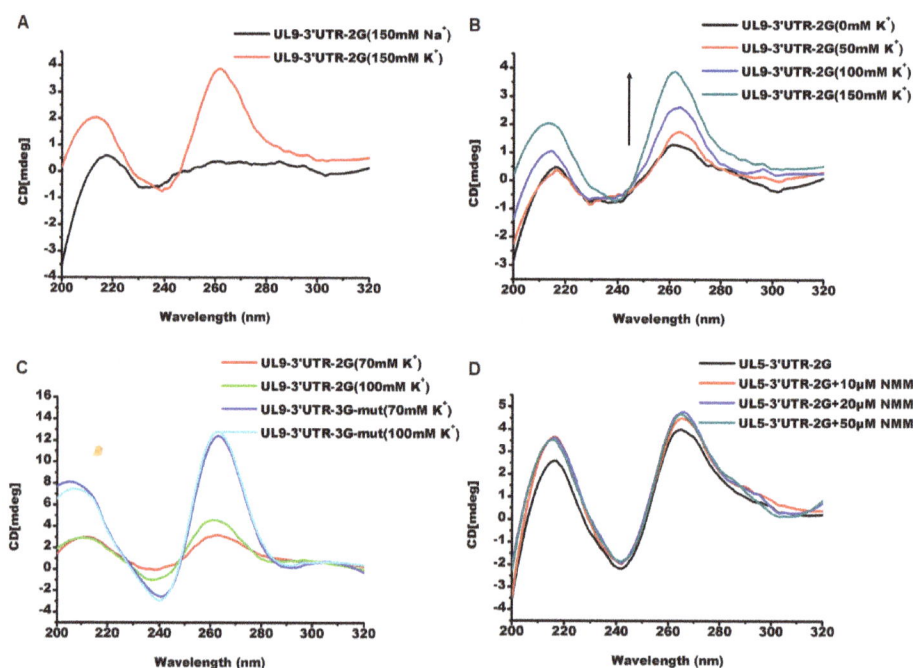

Figure 10. G_2-PQSs from UL5-3′UTR and UL9-3′UTR are sensitive to cations and ligands. (**A**) CD spectroscopy of the G_2-PQS (UL9-3′UTR-2G) in the presence of 150 mM NaCl or KCl. (**B**) CD spectroscopy of the G_2-PQS (UL9-3′UTR-2G) with increasing KCl concentration (0–150 mM). (**C**) CD spectroscopy of G_2-PQS (UL9-3′UTR-2G) and the G_3-PQS mutant (UL9-3′UTR-3G-mut) with increasing KCl concentration (70–100 mM). (**D**) CD spectroscopy of the G_2-PQS (UL5-3′UTR-2G) with increasing NMM concentration (10–50 μM).

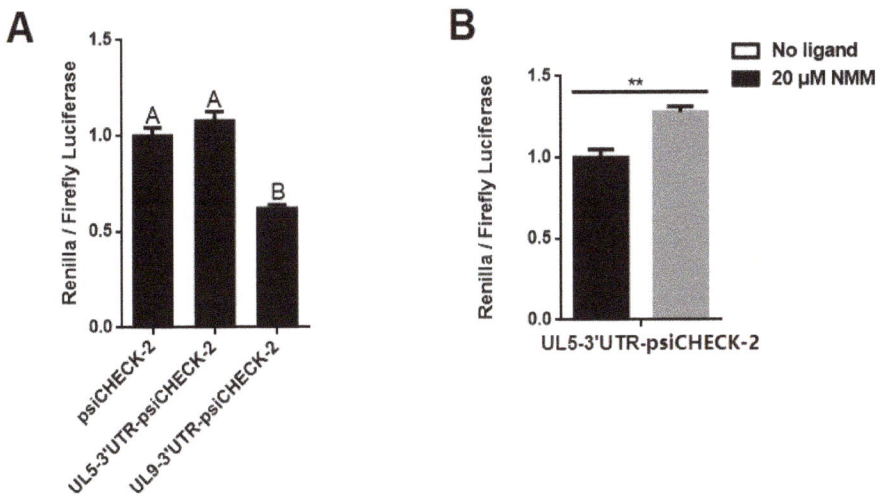

Figure 11. G_2-PQSs from UL5-3'UTR- and UL9-3'UTR-regulated gene expression. (**A**) Dual-luciferase assay of G_2-PQS from *UL5* and *UL9* in gene expression regulation. Different uppercase letters indicate the significant differences among the different constructs ($p < 0.05$, Tukey's honestly significant difference (HSD) test) (**B**) Dual-luciferase assay of G_2-PQS from *UL5* in gene expression regulation with the ligand NMM. ** $p < 0.01$, Student *t*-test.

2.2.3. The G-Quadruplex Ligand Decreases the Virulence of PRV

G-quadruplex ligands were reported to interfere with biological processes related to tumor growth, by binding, stabilizing, converting, or unwinding G-quadruplex structures [41–43]. NMM at a series of concentrations (150 nM, 100 nM, 50 nM) was employed to treat the PRV-infected PK15 cells for 24 h. The plaque assay indicated that the NMM had the potential for reducing the virus titer at 24 h post-treatment (Figure S8).

3. Discussion

A high density of G_2-PQSs was distributed widely in the genomes of PRV, HHV-1, and HHV-3, and they could provide sensitive regulatory switches in response to environmental factors in gene expression regulation. Compared to the G_3-quadruplexes, the G_2-quadruplexes exhibited less thermal stability and higher sensitivity to loop size and compositions, and they presented multiple conformations in different solutions [44]. As they were sensitive to the microenvironment in the cells, the G_2-quadruplexes could act as the receptors of specific proteins or metabolites in the cells, to identify the cells that are suitable for PRV latency. In this study, PQS UL9-3'UTR-2G exhibited a parallel structure in potassium solution, while it could not fold into a G-quadruplex in a sodium cation solution (Figure 9A). The insertion of PQS UL9-3'UTR-2G into the psiCHECK-2 vector led to the decrease in reporter gene expression, while the insertion of PQS UL5-3'UTR-2G resulted in an increase in gene expression only with the addition of the ligand NMM (Figure 11, Figure S4). The G-quadruplex structural sensitivity enabled the virus to be easily mediated by physiological cations, different small molecules, or proteins. These findings are conducive to revealing the latency–reactivation mechanism of PRV in specific tissues under certain conditions.

Highly conserved G_2-PQSs were discovered in the coding regions of genes related to virus replication and maturation, in the *Varicellovirus* genus. The formation of the RNA G_2-quadruplex in the open reading frame of EBNA1 of EBV resulted in a downregulation of the expression level of the maintenance protein, facilitating virus escape from immune recognition [7]. The conserved G_2-PQSs in the *Varicellovirus* genus were located in the unique immediate early protein (*IE180*), viral DNA replication protein (*UL30*), DNA cleavage and package proteins (*UL33/UL17*), and tegument proteins (*UL16/UL47*). *IE180* had five conserved G_2-PQSs among all the *Varicellovirus* (Table 2). *IE180* was found to be a unique immediate early gene of PRV and the first viral gene transcribed during PRV infection. *IE180* is reported to mediate latency and reactivation by regulating early genes, and it activates *US4*, *UL12* (alkaline exonuclease), *UL22* (type I membrane protein), *UL23* (thymidine kinase), and *UL41* (RNAse) [10]. Based on previous reports, we speculated that the formation of the G-quadruplex in the CDS region of *IE180* would result in a reduction of immediate early protein levels, disturbing downstream gene expression in the life-cycle of PRV. Therefore, it could be further inferred that the G_2-quadruplex might have a significant regulatory effect on the *Varicellovirus* genus, especially for the immediate early protein ICP4, the homolog of immediate early protein from PRV.

A high density of G_2-PQSs in the untranslated regions of the PRV genes could provide cis-elements to regulate the post-transcription and translation processes. Though the G_3-quadruplexes in 3′ UTR and 5′ UTR were widely reported to have regulated human gene translation [5,29–31,45], few reports on the G-quadruplexes in the untranslated regions of human herpesvirus genes are available. In this study, many G_2-PQSs were found in the untranslated regions of herpesvirus genes (Figure 7). Various G-quadruplexes formed by those G_2-PQSs regulated gene expression diversely, either under physiological conditions or with a stabilizing ligand (Figure 11). The data suggested that the formation of these G_2-quadruplexes might result in the truncated 3′ UTR, and in turn, disturb 3′-end polyadenylation, finally leading to unstable virus mRNA. The G-quadruplex in the 3′ UTR was also reported to have played a role in regulating microRNA binding in humans [46,47], suggesting that the G-quadruplex might be involved in the interaction between virus/host microRNAs and virus genes.

A large number of G_2-PQSs and G_3-PQSs in the repeat regions of the herpesvirus genomes might play an important role in genomic integration or recombination during herpesvirus latency. Some conserved G_3-PQSs in herpesviruses were reported to have played important role in virus integration, latent DNA replication, and episomal persistence. Several herpesviruses, like Marek's Disease virus (MDV) [48], gallid herpesvirus 2 (GaHV-2) [49], and human herpesvirus 6 (HHV6) [50], were found to establish latent infections, with viral genomes integrated into telomere repeat tracts in host chromosomes through homologous recombination. In this study, the pseudorabies virus had 205 G_3-PQSs in the genome, with 43.9% located in the repeat region (File S1). A high density of conserved G_2-PQSs existed in the repeat regions between the two diverging transcripts *IE180* and *US1*, which were close to the origin of replication (OriS) (Figure 5). Telomeres were reported to form G-quadruplex clusters with a repeated sequence of (GGGTTA)n [51]. This study found that the PRV genome had imperfect telomeric repeats, with the unit sequence 5′-GGGGTGGAGACGGTGGAGGGAGAGGGGAGTGGG-3′ repeated 12 times. Thus, these G_2-PQSs were speculated to be related to genomic recombination and integration during latency.

4. Methods and Materials

4.1. Virus Sequences

The complete genome sequence of the Suid herpesvirus 1 (Pseudorabies virus, PRV) (NC_006151.1) was retrieved from NCBI Genome database [24]. It was annotated into 12 features, including 69 CDS regions, 70 genes, four introns, 119 misc. feature regions, one misc. RNA, 20 polyA sites, 14 protein binding sites, 117 regulatory region, 28 repeat regions, seven stem loop regions, one sequence tagged sites (STS), and one variation. The UTR was determined through alignment between the CDS sequence and the gene sequence. The sequences included in the gene sequences and located upstream of the CDS sequence were designated as 5′ UTRs, and the sequences downstream of the CDS were defined as 3′ UTRs. The putative G-quadruplex sequences (PQS) were searched in the standard genome sequence of PRV. The number of PQSs in the CDS, 3′ UTR, 5′ UTR and repeat regions was counted, respectively.

The standard genome sequences of the *Varicellovirus* genus retrieved from the NCBI Genome database [24] for conservation analysis were Human herpesvirus 3 (NC_001348.1), Equid herpesvirus 1 (NC_001491.2), Equid herpesvirus 3 strain AR/2007/C3A (NC_024771.1), Equid herpesvirus 4 (NC_001844.1), Equid herpesvirus 8 (NC_017826.1), Equid herpesvirus 9 (NC_011644.1), Bovine herpesvirus 1 (NC_001847.1), Bovine herpesvirus 5 (NC_005261.2), Suid herpesvirus 1 (NC_006151.1), Cercopithecine herpesvirus 9 (NC_002686.2), and Felid herpesvirus 1 (NC_013590.2).

4.2. Identification of Putative G-Quadruplex Sequences in the PRV Genome

The putative G_3-quadruplex sequences were searched by Quadparser software [3]. The formula of the putative G_2-quadruplex sequence was defined as $G_{2+}N_{1-7}G_{2+}N_{1-7}G_{2+}N_{1-7}G_{2+}$, where G is guanine, and N is any nucleotide including G. With the same software, the putative I-motif sequences were searched with the formula $C_{2+}N_{1-7}C_{2+}N_{1-7}C_{2+}N_{1-7}C_{2+}$, where C is cytosine, and N is any nucleotide including C. The Quadparser coded the sequence in the format $x{:}y{:}z$, where x stands for the number of guanine tracts or C-runs, y stands for the number of locations of putative G4 or I-motif formations, and z stands for the number of possible simultaneous G4- or I-motif structures.

The number of I-motif sequences in the sense strand was the same as the number of G_2-PQSs in its complementary strand. The sum of the G_2-PQSs and I-motif sequences in the sense strand was the total number of G_2-PQSs in the double-stranded genome of PRV. The density of G_2-PQS in the PRV standard genome was calculated by dividing the total number of G_2-PQSs in the double-stranded genome of PRV by the genome size. If $z = 1$, the G_2-PQS was counted as a PQS monomer. If $z \geq 2$, the G_2-PQS was counted as a PQS cluster.

4.3. Comparison of the Distribution of G_2-PQS and G_3-PQS between PRV and Two Herpesviruses

The G_3-PQS preferred to be located in the repeat regions in human herpesvirus genomes and some repeated G_3-PQS clusters among the analyzed genomes were reported to be conserved [5]. In order to determine the distribution features of PQSs in PRV genome, we compared PRV, Human herpesvirus 1 (HHV-1), also known as Herpes simplex virus type 1 (HSV-1), and Human herpesvirus 3 (HHV-3), also known as Varicella-zoster virus (VZV). The reference genome sequences of PRV (NC_006151.1), HHV-1 (NC_001806.2) and HHV-3 (NC_001348.1) were downloaded from NCBI [24] and saved as FASTA files. The genome features of viruses above were analyzed with the software BEDTools (https://github.com/arq5x/bedtools2) [52] and the length of CDS region, 3′ UTR region, 5′ UTR region, repeat region, and latency associate transcript was recorded. The promoter region of each gene was predicted as 1kb upstream of the transcription start site of each gene. The PQSs in CDS, latency associate transcript, and repeat regions were counted in both positive strand and negative strand, and the PQSs in the untranslated regions and promoters were counted in terms of the transcription direction of each PRV gene. The number of G_3-PQS monomer, G_3-PQS cluster, G_2-PQS monomer and G_2-PQS cluster was counted with the Quadparser software. Quadparser was modified as described in last section. The density of PQSs was calculated by dividing the total number of PQSs located in each region or gene by the length of the corresponding region or gene.

4.4. Conservation of Putative G-Quadruplex Sequences and I-Motif Sequences in the PRV CDS Region in the Varicellovirus Genus

The reference genome sequences of 11 virus species from the *Varicellovirus* genus were downloaded from NCBI. All the PQS and I-motif sequences in the genome of viruses from *Varicellovirus* genus were searched with Quadparser software and output into file g4_cds.txt (File S3). The protein sequences in each genome were listed in file common_protein.txt (File S4). Following data preparation, CDS and amino acid sequences of all proteins in the eleven virus species were used for multiple sequence alignment with MAFFT software (https://www.ebi.ac.uk/Tools/msa/mafft/). The identity of the above nucleotide sequences and amino acid sequences of each protein was calculated with infoalign program of the EMBOSS package (http://emboss.sourceforge.net/apps/release/6.

6/emboss/apps/infoalign.html). The PQS sequences (GG**GG**GG**GG) and I-motif sequences (CC**CC**CC**CC) from the multiple alignment result of nucleotide sequences were identified and counted, and then the ratio of the common PQSs and I-motif sequences to the nucleotide sequences of all the proteins was calculated and output as conservation score of each PQS and I-motif sequence. The conservation of PQS in PRV CDS in the *Varicellovirus* genus was analyzed.

4.5. Percentage Conservation of Putative G-Quadruplex Sequences in the Repeat Regions and LLTs of the PRV Genomes

Twenty-five PRV complete genome sequences from different strains were downloaded from the NCBI Genome database [24]. These sequences were Suid herpesvirus 1 (NC_006151.1, KU056477.1, BK001744.1), Suid alphaherpesvirus 1 isolate Ea (Hubei) (KX423960.1), Suid alphaherpesvirus 1 isolate LA (KU552118.1), Suid herpesvirus 1 strain NIA3 (KU900059.1), Suid herpesvirus 1 isolate DL14/08 (KU360259.1), Suid herpesvirus 1 strain Ea (KU315430.1), Suid herpesvirus 1 strain ADV32751/Italy2014 (KU198433.1), Suid herpesvirus 1 strain Kolchis (KT983811.1), Suid herpesvirus 1 isolate HLJ8 (KT824771.1), Suid herpesvirus 1 strain HN1201 (KP722022.1), Suid herpesvirus 1 strain HNB (KM189914.3), Suid herpesvirus 1 strain Fa (KM189913.1), Suid herpesvirus 1 strain Kaplan (KJ717942.1, JF797218.1, JQ809328.1), Suid herpesvirus 1 strain HNX (KM189912.1), Suid herpesvirus 1 isolate SC (KT809429.1), Suid herpesvirus 1 strain JS-2012 (KP257591.1), Suid herpesvirus 1 strain HeN1 (KP098534.1), Suid herpesvirus 1 isolate ZJ01 (KM061380.1), Suid herpesvirus 1 strain TJ (KJ789182.1), Suid herpesvirus 1 strain Becker (JF797219.1), and Suid herpesvirus 1 strain Bartha (JF797217.1). All of the putative G-quadruplex sequences located in the repeat regions or LLT of the reference genome sequence (Accession Number: NC_006151.1) were searched from the other 24 genome sequences, and the percentage conservation was calculated through dividing the number of genome sequences containing the same putative G-quadruplex sequences by the total number of genome sequences.

4.6. Oligonucleotide Folding Conditions

All oligonucleotides purchased from Sangon Biotech, Shanghai, China were salt-free, purified, and dissolved in ddH$_2$O to a concentration of 100 μM. Oligonucleotide sequences of PQS in regulatory region were selected from the PQSs predicted by Quadparser (Table S3). G$_2$-PQSs from the *UL5* 3' UTR, *UL9* 3' UTR, and mutant sequences (Table S4) were folded under the same conditions, as follows. Oligonucleotides were diluted to 10 μM in 10 mM phosphate buffer at pH 7.0 supplemented with 100 mM KCl, then they were heated to 95 °C for 5 min in a 1.5 mL Eppendorf tube in water bath, and subsequently slowly cooled for ~8 h to room temperature, then used for spectra or stored at 4 °C.

Under the induced folding conditions for G$_2$-PQS from *UL9* 3' UTR, the G$_2$-PQS was diluted to 10 μM in 10mM Tris-HCl buffer at pH 7.0, supplemented with an increasing concentration of KCl (50 mM, 100 mM, and 150 mM). The G$_2$-PQS in 10mM sodium phosphate buffer at pH 7.0 supplemented with 100 mM NaCl was tested. These samples were placed at room temperature for 30 min, and then applied to CD spectra.

Under the induced folding condition for G$_2$-PQS from *UL5* 3' UTR, the G$_2$-PQS was diluted to 10 μM in 10 mM phosphate buffer at pH 7.0, supplemented with 100 mM KCl, and then incubated with different ligands at room temperature for 30 min before CD spectroscopy.

4.7. Circular Dichroism Spectroscopy

CD spectra of the 10 μM folded oligonucleotide samples were collected at 25 °C on a JASCO 1500 CD spectrometer by using a quartz cuvette with 1 mm optical path. Data within a 200–320 nm range were collected using two scans at 100 nm/min with 1 s settling time and 1 nm bandwidth. The buffer baseline was recorded with the same parameters, and it was subtracted from the sample spectra before plotting.

4.8. Plasmid Construction

The plasmids UL5-3′UTR-psiCHECK-2 and UL9-3′UTR-psiCHECK-2 were constructed by using specific oligonucleotides (Table S5), with the ClonExpress II One Step Cloning Kit (Vazyme, Nanjing, China) according to the manufacturer's instructions.

4.9. Cell Culture

Cell lines, human embryonic kidney (HEK) 293T, porcine kidney cell (PK-15), and bovine kidney cells (MDBK) were provided by the State Key Laboratory of Agricultural Microbiology, College of Veterinary Medicine, Huazhong Agricultural University in China. The above cell lines were cultured in Dulbecco's modified Eagle medium (DMEM) containing 10% fetal bovine serum (FBS), 0.044 M NaHCO$_3$, and 0.025 M HEPES. Cells were grown at 37 °C in a humidified atmosphere with 5% CO$_2$.

4.10. Cytotoxicity Assay

The cytotoxicity of the G-quadruplex ligands, N-methyl mesoporphyrin IX (NMM) [53] (J&K Scientific, Beijing, China), BRACO-19 [54] (Sigma-Aldrich, Saint Louis, MO, USA), and pyridostatin (PDS) [55] (J&K Scientific, Beijing, China) to HEK293T was determined by the MTT assay, which is dependent on the measurement of mitochondrial dehydrogenase enzyme activity of viable cells. MTT, 3-(4,5-dimethylthiazol-2-yl)-2,5-diphenyltetrazolium bromide, is a yellow tetrazole, and it can be reduced to a purple formazan in living cells. The HEK293T cells, at a density of 1×10^4 cells per well were seeded into a 96-well microplate. When the cell confluence reached 90%, the growth medium was replaced with 100 μL of DMEM containing 2% FBS and G-quadruplex ligands at a series of final concentrations (Figure S5), and the cells were incubated at 37 °C for 24 h. Then, 50 μL of MTT solution was added into each well, and the cells were incubated at 37 °C for another 4 h. After incubation, the supernatant was removed and 150 μL of dimethyl sulfoxide (DMSO) was added into each well to dissolve the formazan. The relative cell viability was analyzed by measuring the absorbance of formazan at 570 nm on the Synergy™ HTX microplate reader (BioTek, Winooski, VT, USA). The cytostatic concentration, which will be applied in the subsequent dual luciferase assays, was required to maintain a cell viability of more than 90%.

4.11. Transfection and Dual Luciferase Assays

The HEK293T cells were seeded in the 24-well plates at the concentration of 1×10^5 cells/well. The cells were transfected with 0.8 μg of psiCHECK-2 reporter plasmids and Lipofectamine 2000 (Thermo Fisher Scientific, Carlsbad, CA, USA) according to the manufacturer's instructions. NMM at 20 μM, BRACO-19 at 10 μM, or PDS at 10 μM was respectively added to the cells, with the medium being replaced at 6 h after transfection. The activities of firefly and renilla luciferase were measured 24 h after addition of the above G-quadruplex ligands, using the Dual-Luciferase Reporter Assay Kit (Promega, Madison, WI, USA) on a GloMax 20/20 luminometer (Promega, Madison, WI, USA).

4.12. Plaque Assay

The antiviral activity of NMM to PRV Ea strain was examined through plaque assay. The PK15 cells at the density of 1.2×10^6 cells per well were seeded in the 6-well plate. When cell confluence reached 80–90%, the cells were placed in 4 °C for 1 h, and then the PRV Ea strain virus solution (MOI = 5) was added into each well. Then, the cells were placed back to 4 °C for 2 h, and the plate with cells was shacked once every 15 min during the incubation. After the incubation at 4 °C, the virus solution was removed and replaced with 2 mL of DMEM supplemented with NMM at different final concentrations (150 nM, 100 nM, 50 nM). Afterwards, the cells were incubated at 37 °C for 24 h. After incubation, the infectious viral particles were isolated from each well and prepared for plaque assay.

MDBK cells at the density of 2×10^5 cells per well were seeded in the 12-well plate. When the cell confluence reached 90%, the cells were used for the plaque assay. Exactly 200 μL of virus solution was added into each well. Afterwards, the cells were incubated at 37 °C for 2 h. Then, the infected cells were covered by 4% sodium carboxymethylcellulose (CMC-Na) supplemented with 3% FBS and 1% penicillin–streptomycin solution. After incubation at 37 °C for another 48 h, the infected cells were fixed and stained with the crystal violet solution (0.35%, *w/v* in ethanol) at room temperature. After 15 min, the crystal violet solution was removed, and the plate was washed with tap water. Then, the plate was put in the dry oven for a few minutes. Finally, the viral titer was determined by the plaque assay.

4.13. Statistical Analysis

A Student's *t*-test was used to determine the significant differences in luciferase activity between the ligand treatment and control of each construct. One-way analysis of variance (ANOVA) with Tukey's multiple comparison was applied to determining the significant difference among various treatments dual luciferase assay.

5. Conclusions

In summary, the systematic analysis of the distribution of G_2-PQS in the PRV genomes provides a clear guide for elaborated studies of their functions, related to the establishment of latency and its reactivation in herpesviruses. We analyzed the putative G_2-quadruplex and G_3-quadruplex sequences in the PRV genome systematically, and then compared it with typical human herpesviruses in the same subfamily, then evaluated the structures and functions of G_2-quadruplexes. G_2-quadruplex sequences in the form of both monomers and clusters were found to be distributed in the entire PRV genome, especially in the CDS, LLT, and repeat regions. Extremely conserved G_2-quadruplex sequences existed in the CDS of the genes related to viral genome replication and maturation processes. G_2-quadruplex sequences tended to be located in the repeat regions close to the origin of replication site, which may contribute to genome replication and recombination. Most G_2-quadruplexes from the regulatory regions formed parallel-type G-quadruplex. There were more G_2-quadruplex sequences in the $3'$ UTR regions than in the $5'$ UTR regions. These G_2-quadruplexes showed different sensitivities to physiological cations and small molecules. Thus, it could be inferred that the G_2-quadruplex could act as a switch to control the expression of genes involved in virus latency establishment, viral genome replication cascade, and virus cell-to-cell movement. The G-quadruplex ligand, NMM, exhibited the potential for inhibition of the proliferation of PRV in its host cells. These massive and sensitive G_2-quadruplexes could serve as a class of receptors in response to intracellular environments, guiding herpesviruses to choose specific cells or conditions for latency or reactivation.

Supplementary Materials: The following are available online.

Author Contributions: Conceptualization, S.L., X.N. and D.W.; methodology, S.L., X.N. and D.W.; software, B.G., Z.L., Z.Y. and X.N.; validation, H.Z. and Y.Z.; formal analysis, S.L., H.D. and B.G.; investigation, H.D., B.G., Z.L., and Z.Y.; resources, D.W.; data curation, Z.L.; writing—original draft preparation, H.D. and B.G.; writing—review and editing, S.L. and D.W.; visualization, S.L., H.D., B.G. and Z.L.; supervision, D.W.; project administration, S.L. and D.W.; funding acquisition, S.L. and D.W.

Funding: This research was funded by the National Natural Science Foundation of China awarded to D.W. (grant number 31672558, 21502060 and 21732002) and S.L. (grant number 31701791); Huazhong Agricultural University Scientific & Technological Self-innovation Foundation (grant number 2015RC013, 2662017PY113 and 2662015PY208), and the Open fund of The State Key Laboratory of Bio-organic and Natural Products Chemistry, Chinese Academy of Sciences (grant number SKLBNPC16343) to D.W.; Hubei Provincial Natural Science Foundation of China (grant number 2017CFB233) and Fundamental Research Funds for the Central Universities (grant number 2662015QD046) to S.L.

Acknowledgments: The authors thank Shaobo Xiao and Zhengfei Liu in Huazhong Agricultural University for providing equipment for the cell culture and luciferase assay. The authors thank Huazhong Agricultural University and the State Key Laboratory of Agricultural Microbiology for providing access to the JASCO 1500 CD spectrometer.

Conflicts of Interest: The authors declare no conflict of interest.

References

1. Lee, K.; Kolb, A.W.; Sverchkov, Y.; Cuellar, J.A.; Craven, M.; Brandt, C.R. Recombination Analysis of Herpes Simplex Virus 1 Reveals a Bias toward GC Content and the Inverted Repeat Regions. *J. Virol.* **2015**, *89*, 7214–7223. [CrossRef]
2. Balasubramanian, S.; Neidle, S. G-quadruplex nucleic acids as therapeutic targets. *Curr. Opin. Chem. Biol.* **2009**, *13*, 345–353. [CrossRef]
3. Huppert, J.L.; Balasubramanian, S. Prevalence of quadruplexes in the human genome. *Nucleic Acids Res.* **2005**, *33*, 2908–2916. [CrossRef]
4. Andorf, C.M.; Kopylov, M.; Dobbs, D.; Koch, K.E.; Stroupe, M.E.; Lawrence, C.J.; Bass, H.W. G-Quadruplex (G4) Motifs in the Maize (*Zea mays* L.) Genome Are Enriched at Specific Locations in Thousands of Genes Coupled to Energy Status, Hypoxia, Low Sugar, and Nutrient Deprivation. *J. Genet. Genomics* **2014**, *41*, 627–647. [CrossRef]
5. Biswas, B.; Kandpal, M.; Jauhari, U.K.; Vivekanandan, P. Genome-wide analysis of G-quadruplexes in herpesvirus genomes. *BMC Genomics* **2016**, *17*. [CrossRef]
6. Lavezzo, E.; Berselli, M.; Frasson, I.; Perrone, R.; Palu, G.; Brazzale, A.R.; Richter, S.N.; Toppo, S. G-quadruplex forming sequences in the genome of all known human viruses: A comprehensive guide. *PLoS Comput. Biol.* **2018**, *14*, e1006675. [CrossRef]
7. Murat, P.; Zhong, J.; Lekieffre, L.; Cowieson, N.P.; Clancy, J.L.; Preiss, T.; Balasubramanian, S.; Khanna, R.; Tellam, J. G-quadruplexes regulate Epstein-Barr virus-encoded nuclear antigen 1 mRNA translation. *Nat. Chem. Biol.* **2014**, *10*, 358–364. [CrossRef]
8. Lightfoot, H.L.; Hagen, T.; Clery, A.; Allain, F.H.; Hall, J. Control of the polyamine biosynthesis pathway by G2-quadruplexes. *eLife* **2018**, *7*. [CrossRef]
9. Adler, B.; Sattler, C.; Adler, H. Herpesviruses and Their Host Cells: A Successful Liaison. *Trends Microbiol* **2017**, *25*, 229–241. [CrossRef]
10. Pomeranz, L.E.; Reynolds, A.E.; Hengartner, C.J. Molecular biology of pseudorabies virus: Impact on neurovirology and veterinary medicine. *Microbiol Mol. Biol. Rev.* **2005**, *69*, 462–500. [CrossRef]
11. Muller, T.; Hahn, E.C.; Tottewitz, F.; Kramer, M.; Klupp, B.G.; Mettenleiter, T.C.; Freuling, C. Pseudorabies virus in wild swine: A global perspective. *Arch. Virol* **2011**, *156*, 1691–1705. [CrossRef]
12. Masot, A.J.; Gil, M.; Risco, D.; Jimenez, O.M.; Nunez, J.I.; Redondo, E. Pseudorabies virus infection (Aujeszky's disease) in an Iberian lynx (Lynx pardinus) in Spain: A case report. *BMC Vet. Res.* **2017**, *13*, 6. [CrossRef]
13. Musante, A.R.; Pedersen, K.; Hall, P. First reports of pseudorabies and winter ticks (Dermacentor albipictus) associated with an emerging feral swine (Sus scrofa) population in New Hampshire. *J. Wildlife Dis.* **2014**, *50*, 121–124. [CrossRef]
14. Pedersen, K.; Bevins, S.N.; Baroch, J.A.; Cumbee, J.C., Jr.; Chandler, S.C.; Woodruff, B.S.; Bigelow, T.T.; DeLiberto, T.J. Pseudorabies in feral swine in the United States, 2009–2012. *J. Wildlife Dis.* **2013**, *49*, 709–713. [CrossRef]
15. An, T.Q.; Peng, J.M.; Tian, Z.J.; Zhao, H.Y.; Li, N.; Liu, Y.M.; Chen, J.Z.; Leng, C.L.; Sun, Y.; Chang, D.; et al. Pseudorabies virus variant in Bartha-K61-vaccinated pigs, China, 2012. *Emerg. Infect. Dis.* **2013**, *19*, 1749–1755. [CrossRef]
16. Hu, H.; Yu, T.; Fan, J.; Cheng, S.; Liu, C.; Deng, F.; Guo, N.; Wu, B.; He, Q.G. Genetic Properties of the New Pseudorabies Virus Isolates in China in 2012. *Pak. Vet. J.* **2016**, *36*, 264–269.
17. Liu, H.; Li, X.T.; Hu, B.; Deng, X.Y.; Zhang, L.; Lian, S.Z.; Zhang, H.L.; Lv, S.; Xue, X.H.; Lu, R.G.; et al. Outbreak of severe pseudorabies virus infection in pig-offal-fed farmed mink in Liaoning Province, China. *Arch. Virol* **2017**, *162*, 863–866. [CrossRef]
18. Wang, X.; Wu, C.X.; Song, X.R.; Chen, H.C.; Liu, Z.F. Comparison of pseudorabies virus China reference strain with emerging variants reveals independent virus evolution within specific geographic regions. *Virology* **2017**, *506*, 92–98. [CrossRef]
19. Wu, R.; Bai, C.; Sun, J.; Chang, S.; Zhang, X. Emergence of virulent pseudorabies virus infection in northern China. *J. Vet. Sci.* **2013**, *14*, 363–365. [CrossRef]

20. Yu, T.; Chen, F.; Ku, X.; Fan, J.; Zhu, Y.; Ma, H.; Li, S.; Wu, B.; He, Q. Growth characteristics and complete genomic sequence analysis of a novel pseudorabies virus in China. *Virus Genes* **2016**, *52*, 474–483. [CrossRef]
21. Yu, T.; Chen, F.; Ku, X.; Zhu, Y.; Ma, H.; Li, S.; He, Q. Complete Genome Sequence of Novel Pseudorabies Virus Strain HNB Isolated in China. *Genome. Announc.* **2016**, *4*. [CrossRef]
22. Yu, X.; Zhou, Z.; Hu, D.; Zhang, Q.; Han, T.; Li, X.; Gu, X.; Yuan, L.; Zhang, S.; Wang, B.; et al. Pathogenic pseudorabies virus, China, 2012. *Emerg. Infect. Dis.* **2014**, *20*, 102–104. [CrossRef]
23. Dong, B.; Zarlenga, D.S.; Ren, X. An overview of live attenuated recombinant pseudorabies viruses for use as novel vaccines. *J. Immunol. Res.* **2014**, *2014*, 824630. [CrossRef]
24. The National Center for Biotechnology Information Genome Home Page. Available online: https://www.ncbi.nlm.nih.gov/genome (accessed on 13 August 2018).
25. Artusi, S.; Nadai, M.; Perrone, R.; Biasolo, M.A.; Palu, G.; Flamand, L.; Calistri, A.; Richter, S.N. The Herpes Simplex Virus-1 genome contains multiple clusters of repeated G-quadruplex: Implications for the antiviral activity of a G-quadruplex ligand. *Antiviral. Res.* **2015**, *118*, 123–131. [CrossRef]
26. Depledge, D.P.; Ouwendijk, W.J.D.; Sadaoka, T.; Braspenning, S.E.; Mori, Y.; Cohrs, R.J.; Verjans, G.; Breuer, J. A spliced latency-associated VZV transcript maps antisense to the viral transactivator gene 61. *Nat. Commun* **2018**, *9*, 1167. [CrossRef]
27. Granzow, H.; Klupp, B.G.; Mettenleiter, T.C. Entry of pseudorabies virus: An immunogold-labeling study. *J. Virol.* **2005**, *79*, 3200–3205. [CrossRef]
28. Madireddy, A.; Purushothaman, P.; Loosbroock, C.P.; Robertson, E.S.; Schildkraut, C.L.; Verma, S.C. G-quadruplex-interacting compounds alter latent DNA replication and episomal persistence of KSHV. *Nucleic Acids Res.* **2016**, *44*, 3675–3694. [CrossRef]
29. Bugaut, A.; Balasubramanian, S. 5′-UTR RNA G-quadruplexes: Translation regulation and targeting. *Nucleic Acids Res.* **2012**, *40*, 4727–4741. [CrossRef]
30. Kumari, S.; Bugaut, A.; Huppert, J.L.; Balasubramanian, S. An RNA G-quadruplex in the 5′ UTR of the NRAS proto-oncogene modulates translation. *Nat. Chem. Biol.* **2007**, *3*, 218–221. [CrossRef]
31. Subramanian, M.; Rage, F.; Tabet, R.; Flatter, E.; Mandel, J.L.; Moine, H. G-quadruplex RNA structure as a signal for neurite mRNA targeting. *EMBO Rep.* **2011**, *12*, 697–704. [CrossRef]
32. Wang, X.; Zhang, M.M.; Yan, K.; Tang, Q.; Wu, Y.Q.; He, W.B.; Chen, H.C.; Liu, Z.F. The full-length microRNA cluster in the intron of large latency transcript is associated with the virulence of pseudorabies virus. *Virology* **2018**, *520*, 59–66. [CrossRef]
33. Mahjoub, N.; Dhorne-Pollet, S.; Fuchs, W.; Endale Ahanda, M.L.; Lange, E.; Klupp, B.; Arya, A.; Loveland, J.E.; Lefevre, F.; Mettenleiter, T.C.; et al. A 2.5-kilobase deletion containing a cluster of nine microRNAs in the latency-associated-transcript locus of the pseudorabies virus affects the host response of porcine trigeminal ganglia during established latency. *J. Virol.* **2015**, *89*, 428–442. [CrossRef]
34. Amrane, S.; Kerkour, A.; Bedrat, A.; Vialet, B.; Andreola, M.L.; Mergny, J.L. Topology of a DNA G-quadruplex structure formed in the HIV-1 promoter: A potential target for anti-HIV drug development. *J. Am. Chem. Soc.* **2014**, *136*, 5249–5252. [CrossRef]
35. Perrone, R.; Nadai, M.; Frasson, I.; Poe, J.A.; Butovskaya, E.; Smithgall, T.E.; Palumbo, M.; Palu, G.; Richter, S.N. A dynamic G-quadruplex region regulates the HIV-1 long terminal repeat promoter. *J. Med. Chem.* **2013**, *56*, 6521–6530. [CrossRef]
36. Kong, J.N.; Zhang, C.; Zhu, Y.C.; Zhong, K.; Wang, J.; Chu, B.B.; Yang, G.Y. Identification and characterization of G-quadruplex formation within the EP0 promoter of pseudorabies virus. *Sci. Rep.* **2018**, *8*, 14029. [CrossRef]
37. Depledge, D.P.; Sadaoka, T.; Ouwendijk, W.J.D. Molecular aspects of Varicella-Zoster Virus latency. *Viruses* **2018**, *10*. [CrossRef]
38. Kypr, J.; Kejnovska, I.; Renciuk, D.; Vorlickova, M. Circular dichroism and conformational polymorphism of DNA. *Nucleic Acids Res.* **2009**, *37*, 1713–1725. [CrossRef]
39. Beaudoin, J.D.; Perreault, J.P. Exploring mRNA 3′-UTR G-quadruplexes: Evidence of roles in both alternative polyadenylation and mRNA shortening. *Nucleic Acids Res.* **2013**, *41*, 5898–5911. [CrossRef]
40. Sahakyan, A.B.; Murat, P.; Mayer, C.; Balasubramanian, S. G-quadruplex structures within the 3′ UTR of LINE-1 elements stimulate retrotransposition. *Nat. Struct. Mol. Biol.* **2017**, *24*, 243–247. [CrossRef]

41. Kim, M.Y.; Gleason-Guzman, M.; Izbicka, E.; Nishioka, D.; Hurley, L.H. The different biological effects of telomestatin and TMPyP4 can be attributed to their selectivity for interaction with intramolecular or intermolecular G-quadruplex structures. *Cancer Res.* **2003**, *63*, 3247–3256.

42. Grand, C.L.; Han, H.; Munoz, R.M.; Weitman, S.; Von Hoff, D.D.; Hurley, L.H.; Bearss, D.J. The cationic porphyrin TMPyP4 down-regulates c-MYC and human telomerase reverse transcriptase expression and inhibits tumor growth in vivo. *Mol. Cancer Ther.* **2002**, *1*, 565–573.

43. Mikami-Terao, Y.; Akiyama, M.; Yuza, Y.; Yanagisawa, T.; Yamada, O.; Yamada, H. Antitumor activity of G-quadruplex-interactive agent TMPyP4 in K562 leukemic cells. *Cancer Lett.* **2008**, *261*, 226–234. [CrossRef]

44. Varizhuk, A.M.; Protopopova, A.D.; Tsvetkov, V.B.; Barinov, N.A.; Podgorsky, V.V.; Tankevich, M.V.; Vlasenok, M.A.; Severov, V.V.; Smirnov, I.P.; Dubrovin, E.V.; et al. Polymorphism of G4 associates: From stacks to wires via interlocks. *Nucleic Acids Res.* **2018**, *46*, 8978–8992. [CrossRef]

45. Beaudoin, J.D.; Perreault, J.P. 5′-UTR G-quadruplex structures acting as translational repressors. *Nucleic Acids Res.* **2010**, *38*, 7022–7036. [CrossRef]

46. Rouleau, S.; Glouzon, J.S.; Brumwell, A.; Bisaillon, M.; Perreault, J.P. 3′ UTR G-quadruplexes regulate miRNA binding. *RNA* **2017**, *23*, 1172–1179. [CrossRef]

47. Bolduc, F.; Garant, J.M.; Allard, F.; Perreault, J.P. Irregular G-quadruplexes Found in the Untranslated Regions of Human mRNAs Influence Translation. *J. Biol. Chem.* **2016**, *291*, 21751–21760. [CrossRef]

48. Greco, A.; Fester, N.; Engel, A.T.; Kaufer, B.B. Role of the short telomeric repeat region in Marek's disease virus replication, genomic integration, and lymphomagenesis. *J. Virol.* **2014**, *88*, 14138–14147. [CrossRef]

49. Lieberman, P.M. Epigenetics and Genetics of Viral Latency. *Cell Host Microbe* **2016**, *19*, 619–628. [CrossRef]

50. Gilbert-Girard, S.; Gravel, A.; Artusi, S.; Richter, S.N.; Wallaschek, N.; Kaufer, B.B.; Flamand, L. Stabilization of Telomere G-Quadruplexes Interferes with Human Herpesvirus 6A Chromosomal Integration. *J. Virol.* **2017**, *91*. [CrossRef]

51. Sun, D.; Thompson, B.; Cathers, B.E.; Salazar, M.; Kerwin, S.M.; Trent, J.O.; Jenkins, T.C.; Neidle, S.; Hurley, L.H. Inhibition of human telomerase by a G-quadruplex-interactive compound. *J. Med. Chem.* **1997**, *40*, 2113–2116. [CrossRef]

52. Quinlan, A.R.; Hall, I.M. BEDTools: A flexible suite of utilities for comparing genomic features. *Bioinformatics* **2010**, *26*, 841–842. [CrossRef]

53. Nicoludis, J.M.; Miller, S.T.; Jeffrey, P.D.; Barrett, S.P.; Rablen, P.R.; Lawton, T.J.; Yatsunyk, L.A. Optimized end-stacking provides specificity of N-methyl mesoporphyrin IX for human telomeric G-quadruplex DNA. *J. Am. Chem. Soc.* **2012**, *134*, 20446–20456. [CrossRef]

54. Campbell, N.H.; Parkinson, G.N.; Reszka, A.P.; Neidle, S. Structural basis of DNA quadruplex recognition by an acridine drug. *J. Am. Chem. Soc.* **2008**, *130*, 6722–6724. [CrossRef]

55. Koirala, D.; Dhakal, S.; Ashbridge, B.; Sannohe, Y.; Rodriguez, R.; Sugiyama, H.; Balasubramanian, S.; Mao, H. A single-molecule platform for investigation of interactions between G-quadruplexes and small-molecule ligands. *Nat. Chem.* **2011**, *3*, 782–787. [CrossRef]

Sample Availability: Samples of the compounds are not available from the authors.

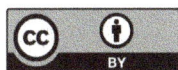

![molecules logo] *molecules*

MDPI

Article

Towards Understanding of Polymorphism of the G-rich Region of Human Papillomavirus Type 52

Maja Marušič [1] and Janez Plavec [1,2,3,*]

1   Slovenian NMR Center, National Institute of Chemistry, Hajdrihova 19, SI-1000 Ljubljana, Slovenia; marusic.maja@ki.si
2   EN-FIST Center of Excellence, SI-1000 Ljubljana, Slovenia
3   Faculty of Chemistry and Chemical Technology, University of Ljubljana, SI-1000 Ljubljana, Slovenia
*   Correspondence: janez.plavec@ki.si; Tel.: +3861-4760-353; Fax: +3861-4760-300

Academic Editor: Sara N. Richter
Received: 16 March 2019; Accepted: 31 March 2019; Published: 2 April 2019

Abstract: The potential to affect gene expression via G-quadruplex stabilization has been extended to all domains of life, including viruses. Here, we investigate the polymorphism and structures of G-quadruplexes of the human papillomavirus type 52 with UV, CD and NMR spectroscopy and gel electrophoresis. We show that oligonucleotide with five G-tracts folds into several structures and that naturally occurring single nucleotide polymorphisms (SNPs) have profound effects on the structural polymorphism in the context of G-quadruplex forming propensity, conformational heterogeneity and folding stability. With help of SNP analysis, we were able to select one of the predominant forms, formed by G-rich sequence d(G$_3$TAG$_3$CAG$_4$ACACAG$_3$T). This oligonucleotide termed HPV52$_{(1-4)}$ adopts a three G-quartet snap back (3 + 1) type scaffold with four *syn* guanine residues, two edgewise loops spanning the same groove, a no-residue V loop and a propeller type loop. The first guanine residue is incorporated in the central G-quartet and all four-guanine residues from G4 stretch are included in the three quartet G-quadruplex core. Modification studies identified several structural elements that are important for stabilization of the described G-quadruplex fold. Our results expand set of G-rich targets in viral genomes and address the fundamental questions regarding folding of G-rich sequences.

Keywords: G-quadruplex; NMR; folding; DNA; structure; human papillomaviruses

1. Introduction

Human papillomaviruses (HPV) are pathogens infecting skin and mucosa that have co-evolved with human species and are therefore well adapted to cause infection with minimal damage to their host. Even though there are currently more than 200 different types of HPVs described [1], only a fraction of those are responsible for the development of diseases in humans. Their life-cycle unravels in synchrony with differentiation of keratinocytes, starting from increased copy number of viral episome in the basal layer, through production of viral protein and finally assembly of viral particles that are shed from mature keratinocytes when they die [2]. In most cases the infection passes unnoticed and is quickly resolved by immune system [3]. A subgroup of HPVs designated as 'high-risk' are more potent in driving differentiating keratinocytes into the unscheduled and therefore potentially erroneous cell cycle due to a wider range of binding partners of main viral oncoproteins E6 and E7 [4–6]. Consequently, persistent infection with high-risk HPVs can eventually lead to development of neoplasms and even cancer, most commonly cancer of skin, head and neck and anogenital regions [7,8]. Among most potent high-risk HPVs are HPV16, HPV18, HPV52 and HPV58 with different regional distribution around the world and ability to cause disease [9].

We have recently examined ability of G-rich sequences in several high-risk HPV types to fold into G-quadruplexes [10], four stranded DNA structures with square planar arrangements of guanine residues [11] stacked on each other and stabilized with cations. Stabilization of G-quadruplexes in cells was shown to induce breaks in double-stranded DNA and lead to genome instability [12–14], while reporter assays in different expression systems confirmed effect on protein expression for a wide range of G-rich sequences [15]. Analogously, several G-rich sequences with G-quadruplex forming potential were identified in viruses [16–18] and stabilization of G-quadruplexes with ligands could have potential effect on expression and/or stability of viral DNA [19–24], especially in viruses with double stranded DNA genomes, such as HPV. However, designing ligands that would specifically bind to G-quadruplexes and lock their structure is hampered due to a large number of potential G-quadruplex-forming sequences in the human genome [25–28], highlighting the importance of structural characterization of G-rich oligonucleotides to guide ligand design. Most promising G-quadruplex targets possess specific structural features found in loops that could promote specific binding in tandem with large planar surface of G-quartets [29]. Additionally, as G-rich oligonucleotides are notoriously polymorphic, their structure can change with variations in solution conditions (pH, T, oligonucleotide and cation concentrations) and intrinsic attributes of G-rich sequence (length of G-tracts, type of connecting loop residues and 5′- and/or 3′-end flanking residues) [30–32]. Selective stabilization of predominant fold and its characterization therefore still represent the main obstacle on the way to design structurally discriminating ligands. Moreover, point mutations or single nucleotide polymorphisms (SNPs) inevitably present in G-rich sequences from natural sources might drastically affect structure and therefore cannot be neglected when assessing structural polymorphism of a given G-rich oligonucleotide.

In the current study, we have concentrated our efforts on structure determination of the predominant form of G-rich oligonucleotide from HPV type 52, as well as the characterization of other folds that might exist in dynamic equilibrium and may also be important in the cellular environment. HPV 52 is one of the most relevant HPV types especially in (Southeast) Asia, where it causes up to 20% of all cervical cancer [33]. G-rich oligonucleotide found in the genome of HPV52 forms several different structures due to its five G-rich tracts of different lengths (3, 3, 4, 3, and 3 nt, Figure 1A) [10]. Shortening of the G-rich sequence to four G-tracts was considered as the first approach to reduce polymorphism and be able to identify predominant form(s). By this approach we obtained two shorter oligonucleotides that comprise first to the fourth and the second to the fifth G-tract. The second approach utilizes introduction of point mutations, which can drastically affect number and type of G-quadruplex structure(s). Specifically, three SNPs were found in the genomes of different HPV type 52 isolates in GenBank [34] (Figure 1A) that can be exploited to study effect of nucleotide changes without introduction of artificial sequence changes. SNPs in the G-rich tracts (8G > A and 22G > A) were expected to substantially reduce number of structures in solution, while SNP in loop region (18C > T) was expected to have minimal effect. Selection of the predominant species and its characterization followed by determination of 3D structure to the level of atomic resolution offers a rich collection of NMR parameters uncovering structural elements that are important for stabilization of described G-quadruplex fold and for their recognition by cellular partners or ligands. With introduction of modifications we were able to assess the importance of several structural elements, particularly a four-guanine tract adopting a V loop and a GNA type loop that have been well studied in the context of nucleic acid's structure and can potentially drive formation of G-quadruplex structure.

2. Results

2.1. SNPs Reduce Polymorphism of HPV52$_{(1-5)}$ and Assist Identification of Predominant Species

Twenty seven (27) nt long oligonucleotide originating from the genome of HPV type 52 with its five G-rich tracts was expected to adopt a large number of structures, thus posing a challenge for structural studies. Indeed, after titration with aqueous solution of KCl a high number of signals of different intensities was observed in the region between δ 10.0 and 12.2 ppm in the ^{1}H-NMR spectrum of HPV52(1–5) (Figure 1B), which indicated its folding into several G-quadruplex structures. Comparison of NMR and CD spectra of HPV52$_{(1-5)}$ without and with SNPs enabled several interesting observations (Figure 1B–D). Spectra of HPV52$_{(1-5)}$ and HPV52$_{(1-5)}$ 18C > T are very similar, which suggests that SNP 18C > T in the third loop does not affect structures formed by the HPV52$_{(1-5)}$ or reduce their number. In contrast, for HPV52$_{(1-5)}$ 8G > A and HPV52$_{(1-5)}$ 22G > A the number of ^{1}H-NMR signals in imino region decreases to 24, suggesting reduction of a number of G-quadruplex structures to two in each case. PAGE gel for all four oligonucleotides shows fast moving bands, which are suggestive of formation of monomeric species (Figure S1 and [30]).

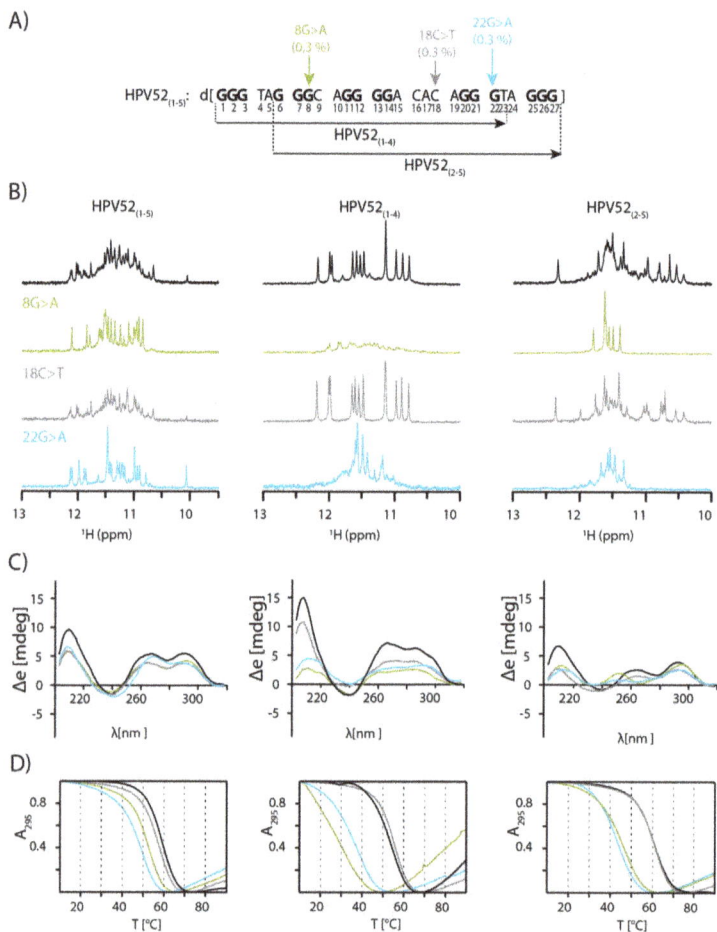

Figure 1. Characterization of G-rich oligonucleotides HPV52$_{(1-5)}$, HPV52$_{(1-4)}$ and HPV52$_{(2-5)}$. (**A**) G-rich sequence of HPV type 52 with indicated position and frequency (in %) of occurrence of observed SNPs in the sequence. (**B**) NMR, (**C**) CD spectra and (**D**) UV melting curves of twelve different oligonucleotides derived from G-rich sequence of HPV type 52. Spectra were recorded at 25 °C, pH 7, 50 mM [K$^+$] and c_{oligo} between 0.26 and 0.41 mM (NMR) and 10 μM (CD, UV).

From the analysis of the fingerprint imino region it can be inferred that most likely four different structures present for HPV52$_{(1-5)}$ 8G > A and HPV52$_{(1-5)}$ 22G > A are also observed for HPV52$_{(1-5)}$. Especially one of the structures adopted by HPV52$_{(1-5)}$ 22G > A can be easily distinguished due to its upfield signal at δ 10.09 ppm (Figure 1B). Apart from the four structures observed for oligonucleotides with SNPs 8G > A and 22G > A, detailed analysis of imino region of 1D ^{1}H spectra revealed at least one additional species for HPV52$_{(1-5)}$. Four structures of HPV52$_{(1-5)}$ that are present for oligonucleotides with SNPs 8G > A and 22G > A most likely incorporate one of the central G-tracts in their loop regions, which results in structures with very long loops (i.e., either 7 or 11 nt). Respective thermal stabilities support this assumption, as apparent T_m values decrease for oligonucleotides with SNPs (Figure 1D and Figure S2). Clearly, melting temperature can be determined only for a two-state equilibrium, which is not the case for HPV52$_{(1-5)}$. However, apparent melting temperatures can still give a useful estimation of thermal stability of structures adopted by oligonucleotides and are used as such in our case. The highest apparent T_m decrease of 10 °C is observed for HPV52$_{(1-5)}$ 22G > A, which exhibits the longest possible loop (11 nt) within HPV52 G-rich sequence that encompasses the fourth G-tract (Figure 1A). HPV52$_{(1-5)}$, however, displays the highest apparent melting temperature, which allows for several inferences to be made. First, the most stable structure of HPV52$_{(1-5)}$ is not one of those observed for HPV52$_{(1-5)}$ 8G > A and HPV52$_{(1-5)}$ 22G > A since apparent melting temperature for HPV52$_{(1-5)}$ is the highest among the three oligonucleotides. As a consequence, HPV52$_{(1-5)}$ must contain both the second and the fourth G-tracts, which are not present in the structures of HPV52$_{(1-5)}$ 8G > A and HPV52$_{(1-5)}$ 22G > A. Second, the most stable structure of HPV52$_{(1-5)}$ has loops that are shorter than 7 nt, as structures with longer loops are expected to exhibit lower thermal stability [35], as has been observed for HPV52$_{(1-5)}$ 8G > A and HPV52$_{(1-5)}$ 22G > A. Therefore, the most stable structure must also comprise the third G-tract of HPV52$_{(1-5)}$ as a part of the G-quadruplex core. Third, thermally most stable structure is arguably the most relevant in biological context. These initial results suggested that reducing the number of G-tracts at either 5' or 3' end might be a favourable strategy for reducing polymorphism of HPV52$_{(1-5)}$, thus enabling determination of topology of the most stable and biologically relevant G-quadruplex structure. Further studies were therefore performed on shorter oligonucleotides, HPV52$_{(1-4)}$ and HPV52$_{(2-5)}$ that comprise the first to the fourth and the second to the fifth G-tract, respectively.

Titration of HPV52$_{(1-4)}$ and HPV52$_{(1-4)}$ 18C > T with aqueous solution of KCl resulted in twelve sharp signals in the region between δ 11.8 and 12.3 ppm, characteristic of a structure with three G-quartets. Position of signals in CD spectra is typical for a (3 + 1) topology (Figure 1B–C) [36]. SNPs 8G > A and 22G > A have detrimental effect on the formation of G-quadruplex structure, more so for the former (Figure 1B). In agreement, a larger decrease in apparent T_m was observed for HPV52$_{(1-4)}$ 8G > A (25 °C) than for HPV52$_{(1-4)}$ 22G > A (18 °C) compared to the apparent T_m of parent oligonucleotide HPV52$_{(1-4)}$ (Figure 1D). PAGE gel shows bands with slow(er) mobilities for HPV52$_{(1-4)}$ 8G > A and 22G > A, which are characteristic for formation of intermolecular species, presumably dimers (Figure S1).

Upon titration of HPV52$_{(2-5)}$ and HPV52$_{(2-5)}$ 18C > T with KCl solution several structures were formed (Figure 1B). CD spectra are characteristic of a (3 + 1) topology, while the apparent T_m is 60 °C for both oligonucleotides (Figure 1B–C). For HPV52$_{(2-5)}$ 8G > A eight partially overlapped signals are observed in the region from δ 11.4 and 11.8 ppm of ^{1}H-NMR spectrum, which in combination with distribution of CD signals points to the formation of an antiparallel structure with two G-quartets [36]. Similarly, for HPV52$_{(2-5)}$ 22G > A eight partially overlapped signals assigned to antiparallel fold are observed in the imino region of the ^{1}H-NMR spectrum. Several other signals of low intensity most likely correspond to non-antiparallel species, since CD spectrum of HPV52$_{(2-5)}$ 22G > A that represents a sum of CD spectra of all species exhibits characteristics for mixture of different topologies [37].

2.2. Topology of G-quadruplex Adopted by HPV52$_{(1-4)}$

Residue-specifically ^{15}N isotope labelled oligonucleotides were used to resolve ambiguity as to which guanine residues of HPV52$_{(1-4)}$ with uneven G-tract lengths (i.e., 3, 3, 4 and 3 nt) are involved in the G-quartet formation. Unexpectedly, only G1 and G2 from the first G-tract and all four residues from the third G-tract (i.e., G11, G12, G13 and G14) are incorporated in the G-quadruplex core (Figure 2A).

We were able to establish topology model of HPV52$_{(1-4)}$ through analysis of NOE contacts in the imino-imino region of 2D NOESY spectrum (Figure 2C,D).

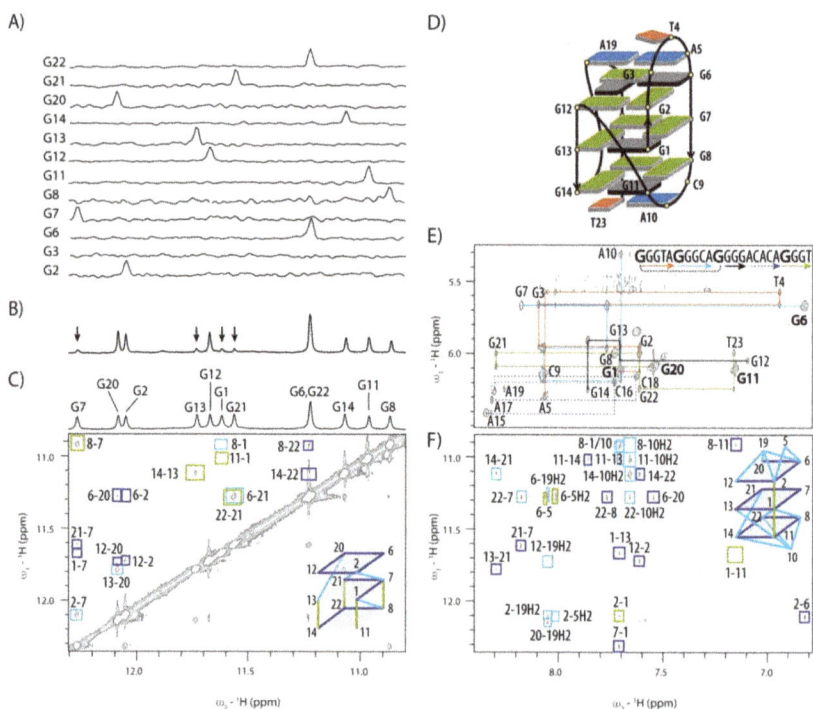

Figure 2. Topology determination of HPV52$_{(1-4)}$. (**A**) 1D ^{1}H-^{15}N HSQC spectra of site-specific partially labelled oligonucleotides for identification of guanine residues in the G-quadruplex core. (**B**) Imino region of ^{1}H-NMR spectrum 5 min after D$_2$O-H$_2$O exchange. Arrows point to the resonances of the least water accessible imino protons. (**C**) Imino-imino region of 2D NOESY spectrum (τ_m 250 ms) with assigned contacts between pairs of imino protons and schematics of correlations within G-quadruplex core. (**D**) Topology of HPV52$_{(1-4)}$, where residues with extensive contacts to G-quadruplex core are shown with rectangles. Guanine residues in *syn* and *anti*-conformation, thymine and adenine residues are shown in dark grey, green, orange and blue colours, respectively. (**E**) Anomeric-aromatic region of 2D NOESY spectrum with sequential walk along the oligonucleotide sequence. (**F**) Imino-aromatic region of 2D NOESY spectrum with assigned connectivities between H1 and H8 pairs of protons within G-quadruplex core and contacts that define position of loop residues. Spectra were recorded at 25 °C, pH 7, 50 mM [K$^+$] and c$_{oligo}$ between 1.0 and 2.7 mM. 2D NOESY was recorded with τ_m of 250 ms.

G1 is involved in the central G-quartet and is followed by G2 and G3-T4-A5 in edgewise loop orientation. G6-G7-G8 segment represents the second edge of the G-quadruplex core and adopts antiparallel orientation with respect to the first edge. Missing spot in the first edge of a G-quadruplex core defined by G1 and G2 is filled with G11, which is made possible by folding back of the DNA chain facilitated by C9 and A10 forming an edgewise loop. A no-residue V loop traverses the central G-quartet plane and connects G11 with G12-G13-G14 segment constituting the third edge. The loop consisting of A15-C16-A17-C18-A19 segment connects G12-G13-G14 and G20-G21-G22 edges of G-quadruplex core in a propeller-type orientation (Figure 2D).

Sequential connectivities in the anomeric-aromatic region of 2D NOESY spectra of HPV52$_{(1-4)}$ are broken as expected at either *anti-syn* steps or in the loop regions (Figure 2E). Four instead of five strong intra-residual H1'-H8 cross-peaks denoting *syn* conformation are observed in NOESY spectrum for residues G1, G6, G11 and G20 (marked in bold in Figure 2E and colored grey in Figure 2D). G12 would be assumed to adopt *syn* conformation considering the established 'rules' on orientation of the strands within the G-quadruplex core [38], but it displays a weak H1'-H8 cross-peak and clearly adopts an *anti*-conformation. In full support, ^{13}C-NMR chemical shifts of C8 atoms are downfield [39–41] for four guanine residues adopting predominantly *syn* conformation (Figure S3).

Several NOE contacts of imino protons of guanine residues involved in the G-quadruplex core with methyl group of T23 and H2 and H8 protons of A5, A19 and especially A10 suggest extensive nucleobase stacking of loop residues on G-quartets (Figure 2F). Altogether the observed NOE contacts indicate that the capping structures on the both sides of the G-quadruplex core formed by the two edgewise loops together with A19 and T23 add to the overall stability of the structure. Interestingly, capping structures do not increase protection of imino protons in the G-quadruplex core from exchange with bulk water as hydrogen exchange times for all residues in the two outer G-quartets are relatively short. Signals in the imino region of ^{1}H-NMR spectrum are observed already 5 minutes after change of solvent from D_2O to H_2O (Figure 2B). Signals of guanine imino protons of the central G-quartet also re-appear relatively quickly, which shows that they are relatively poorly protected from exchange with bulk water molecules (Figure 2B).

High-resolution structure of HPV52$_{(1-4)}$ (Figure 3A) was calculated with 377 NOE and 82 torsion angle restraints and is with the exception of C16–C18 region very well-defined (Table 1). Insertion of G1 in the middle of the G-quadruplex core introduces a loop extension, similar to the fold-back feature found in other G-quadruplexes. Hydrogen bond directionalities are in agreement with (3 + 1) topology and follow clockwise orientation for two G-quartets (G11→G14→G22→G8 and G1→G13→G21→G7) and anti-clockwise for one G-quartet (G2→G6→G20→G12). Stacking of G-quartets is based on 5/5-membered ring overlap between G1-G13-G21-G7 and G2-G6-G20-G12 quartets, and on 6/5-membered ring overlap between G1→G13→G21→G7 and G11→G14→G22→G8 quartets. Stacking of the loop residues onto the G-quadruplex core is especially pronounced for both capping structures. Capping structure formed by G3-T4-A5 edgewise loop is complemented by A19 from propeller loop at the opposite side of G2-G6-G20-G12 quartet (Figure 3B). On the other side of the G-quadruplex core, residues C9, A10 and T23 form capping structure that has been found to adopt two different conformations in the ensemble of calculated structures. In the first conformation that accounts for 70% of lowest energy structures, methyl group of T23 points away from G8-G11-G14-G22 quartet (Figure 3C). In the second, T23 lies in the plane with C9 and A10, while hydrogen bonds are formed between amino proton of A10 and O4 of T23 as well as between amino proton of C9 and O2 of T23. Even though cumulative length of loops for HPV52$_{(1-4)}$ quadruplex is considerable, only three (T4, C16 and C18) out of 11 residues protrude from the structure. T4, however, is stacked with G3 and is quite well defined. C16 and C18, on the other hand, represent the least defined part of the 5-residue long propeller loop, while its three adenine residues are less flexible. A15 aligns in the plane of the central G-quartet, A17 is found in different positions under A15, while A19 is involved in the capping structure and interacts with G3 and A5 of edgewise loop (Figure 3B). It must be emphasized that several NOE contacts that could lead to a well-defined A15-C16-A17-C18-A19 loop conformation were not used in structure calculations due to spectral overlap. For example, interesting sequential-like H1'-H8 NOE contacts were observed between the A15 and A17 residues, suggesting that they are most likely stacked on each other and possibly aligned in the planes of G-quartets.

Residues that display non-B-DNA ranges of sugar-backbone torsion angles cluster in the regions of sharp turns of DNA chain, most notably at A5, C9-A10 and G12-G13. Calculated structures showed that position of these residues was insufficiently defined by NOE contacts alone and that introducing torsion angles restraints importantly reduced their indeterminacy. For example, C9 is localized in the groove defined by residues G11-G1-G2 and G6-G7-G8 in several structures that were calculated without restraint for β and γ torsion angles of C9, although no NOE contacts between C9 and residues on the both sides of the groove were observed. Analysis of backbone torsion angles in those structures revealed that in-groove conformation shown to be most stable in MD simulations was not in agreement with experimentally determined β (g^+) and γ (t) values of C9. Using β and γ torsion angle restraints led to C9 being positioned below G8-G11-G14-G22 quartet (Figure 3C). G12 is the only residue of HPV52$_{(1-4)}$ that adopts the C3′-*endo* conformation, which may be attributed to the sharp turn of DNA chain and fits well with unusual torsion angles of G12 and G13.

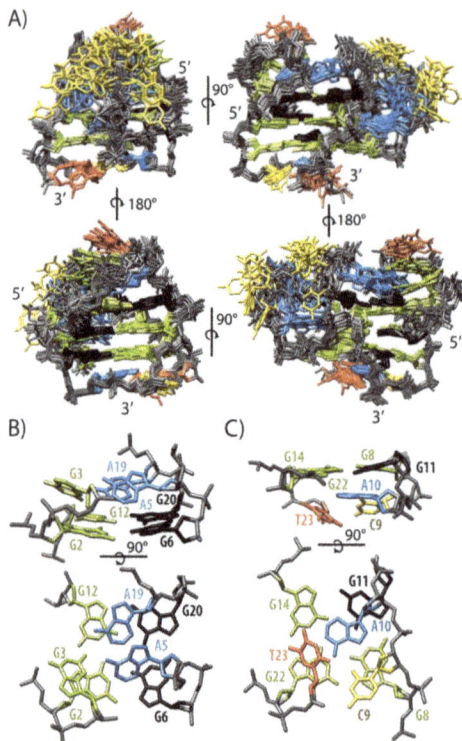

Figure 3. Structure of HPV52$_{(1-4)}$. (**A**) Superposition of 10 lowest-energy structures of HPV52$_{(1-4)}$. (**B**) Capping structure formed by G3, A5 and A19. (**C**) Capping structure formed by C9, A10 and T23. Guanine residues in *syn* and *anti*-conformation, thymine, adenine and cytosine residues are shown in black, green, orange, blue and yellow colour, respectively. DNA backbone is shown in grey.

2.3. *Conformations of Edgewise G3-T4-A5 and A No-Residue V Loop Justify Unusual Chemical Shifts*

The observed NMR chemical shifts of HPV52$_{(1-4)}$ exhibit several uncommon values which are however in perfect agreement with the calculated high-resolution structure. Most notable is the chemical shift of H4′ of T4 at δ 2.097 ppm (Figure 4A), which is shifted upfield by more than 2 ppm in comparison to the average chemical shift of H4′ of thymine residues (δ 4.14 ppm) [42]. As G3-T4-A5 edgewise loop conforms to the GNA loop sequence requirements [43–48], its distinct conformation brings T4 H4′ proton in close proximity of shielding zone of A5 (Figure 4B). Although resonance of G3 amino proton was not observed even at low temperatures, and therefore the sheared base pair between G3 and A5 that is typical for GNA loops could not be confirmed experimentally, conformation of G3 and A5 in calculated structures is very similar to a GA sheared base pair. Non-observed signal for amino group of G3 could be rationalized by the involvement of A19 in the dynamic hydrogen bonding network with G3 and A5 (Figure 3B). This could reduce the intensity of the signals corresponding to hydrogen-bonded protons of G3. Moreover, intermediate to fast exchange on NMR chemical shift time scale was observed from 0 to 40 °C for G3-T4-A5 residues formally constituting an edgewise loop (*vide infra*), which might have also precluded observation of signals corresponding to hydrogen bonded amino protons at low temperatures.

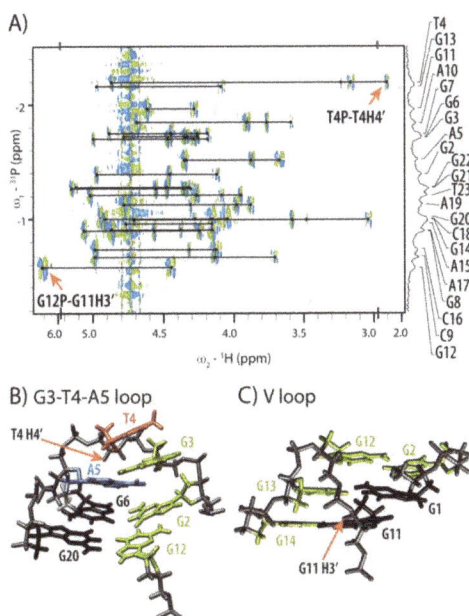

Figure 4. HP-COSY spectrum and structural details of G3-T4-A5 edgewise and no-residue V loop. (**A**) HP-COSY spectrum with assignment of phosphorus resonances in 1D ^{31}P spectrum. (**B**) Close-up of G3-T4-A5 edgewise loop shows proximity of H4′ proton of T4 residue to aromatic ring of A5. (**C**) Perusal of V loop shows position of H3′ proton of G11 residue. Colour scheme used is the same as in Figure 3.

Second atypical chemical shift has been observed for G11 H3′, which is shifted downfield to δ 6.088 ppm into the region of anomeric protons (Figure 4A). Together with unusual conformations of torsion angles β (g^+) and γ (t) of G13, α, ε and ζ torsion angles of G12 as well as C3′-*endo* puckering and *anti*-conformation of G12, atypical chemical shift of H3′ proton of G11 substantiates unusual conformation of G12-G13 part of DNA chain. Perusal of the calculated structures shows that sugar-phosphate backbone undergoes effectively a 180° turn at G12 in order to accommodate a no-residue V loop (Figure 4C). As a consequence, H3′ proton of G11 is positioned in close proximity of deshielding zone of its aromatic ring, which rationalizes its downfield shift. Furthermore, G11 H3′ proton is positioned also in the close proximity to H8 proton of G13 (3.5 Å), whose dipole-dipole interaction was indeed observed as a cross-peak in NOESY spectrum, albeit it was not used in structure calculations due to the spectral overlap.

Table 1. Structural statistics.

NMR Distance and Torsion Angle Restraints			
NOE-derived distance restraints	Non-exch.	Exch.	All
Total	322	55	377
Intra-residue	215	0	215
Inter-residue	107	55	162
Sequential	88	15	103
Long-range	19	40	59
Chemical shift derived distance restraints		4	
Hydrogen bond restraints		24	
Hydrogen bonds non-observed		3	
Torsion angle restraints		82	
G-quartet planarity restraints		36	
Structure statistics			
Violations			
Mean NOE restraint violation (Å)		0.14 ± 0.001	
Max. NOE restraint violation (Å)		0.33	
Max torsion angle restraint violation (°)		6.768	
Deviation from idealized geometry			
Bonds (Å)		0.012 ± 0.000	
Angles (°)		2.43 ± 0.03	
Pairwise heavy atom RMSD (Å)			
Overall		1.779	
G1-G14 + G20-G23		0.987	
G-quartets		0.751	

2.4. Internal Motion of G3-T4-A5 Edgewise Loop

^{1}H-NMR spectra recorded in 0 to 40 °C temperature range show that several imino and aromatic resonances of G1, G2, T4, A5, G6, G7 and G12 broaden severely and some even merge into the baseline at lower temperatures (Figure 5A). The largest changes in resonance linewidths are concentrated at A5-G6 and neighboring residues (Figure 5B,C). The largest signal broadening has been observed for A5, with its inter- and intra-residual NOESY cross-peaks involving sugar and aromatic protons practically non-observable below 15 °C. Signals for G6 also broaden dramatically, although effect on its H1 resonance could not be evaluated unambiguously due to the overlap with G22 H1. As *syn* to *anti* reorientations of G6 could be a possible cause for the observed dynamics, we prepared oligonucleotide with 8Br-dG residue at position 6. We reasoned that modification should prevent G6 from adopting *anti* conformation due to the sterically preferred orientation of large bromine atom away from the sugar moiety. Spectra of 8Br-G6-modified HPV52$_{(1-4)}$ at 25 and 5 °C showed similar line broadening for imino resonances of the residues G1, G2, G20, G6, G7 and G12, while other residues were affected minimally (Figure S4B). However, we observed that imino resonances of G2-G6-G20-G12 quartet of G6-8Br HPV52$_{(1-4)}$ were broadened at 5 and 10 mM potassium concentration (Figure S4A), which was attributed to slow formation of G2-G6-G20-G12 quartet as a result of incorporation of bulky G-8Br modification. In agreement with presumption of more open conformation of G2-G6-G20-G12 quartet, imino protons were more susceptible to exchange with water. Namely, cross-peaks of G20, G12 and G6 with water were observed for the G6-8Br HPV52$_{(1-4)}$ oligonucleotide, but not for the parent

HPV52$_{(1-4)}$. To exclude slow G-quartet formation as the cause of spectral similarities with HPV52$_{(1-4)}$ at low temperatures, 2D NOESY spectra of both oligonucleotides at 25 and 5 °C were compared. Analysis showed that 8Br-G6 modification did not prevent dynamics in the G3-T4-A5 loop, since H1'/H2'/H2''-H8 and H2'/H2''-H1' cross-peaks of A5 of G6-8Br HPV52$_{(1-4)}$ were not observed at 5 °C, while resonances of G12 and T4 were severely broadened and no additional cross-peaks appeared. As the same behavior was detected for HPV52$_{(1-4)}$ (Figure 5), *syn-anti*-reorientation of G6 is not the cause of observed dynamics. In attempt to reach slow dynamic regime to be able to identify species in conformational exchange temperature was lowered to −10 °C or 1 M choline dihydrogenphosphate was added to the sample to increase viscosity. Nevertheless, similar spectral characteristic at those conditions indicated that exchange observed was still in intermediate regime. Interestingly, structural fluctuations presumably due to the wobbling of A residue between *syn* and *anti*-position was reported for GNA minihairpin loops [47], while for (GGA)$_4$ G-quadruplex that consists of three consecutive GNA loops no reports of dynamic behavior exist [45,46].

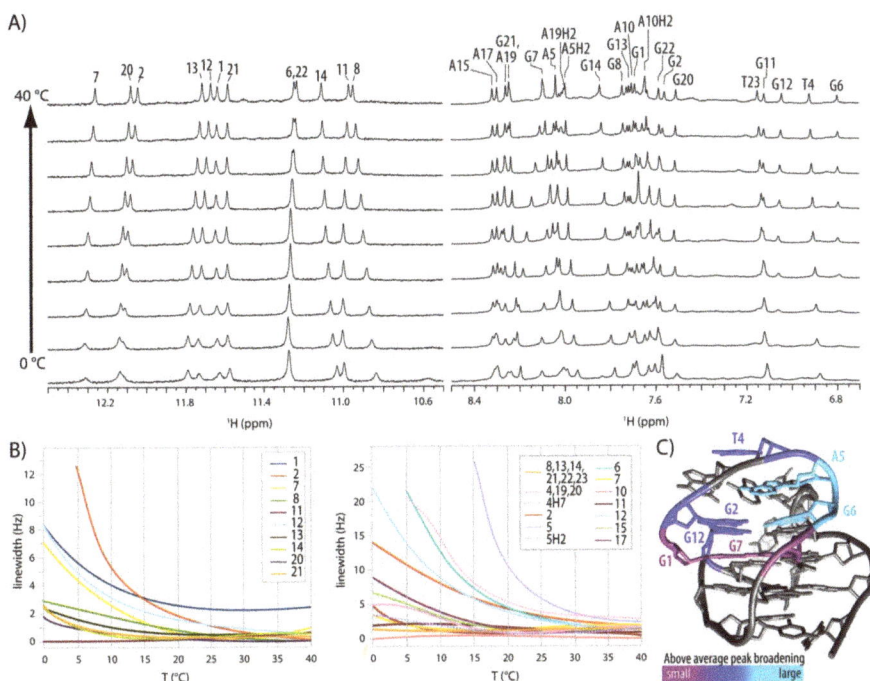

Figure 5. Spectral changes of HPV51$_{(1-4)}$ as a function of temperature. (**A**) Imino and aromatic regions of 1D ^{1}H spectra in 5 °C steps from 0 to 40 °C. (**B**) Temperature dependency of signal width at half-height of imino (left) and aromatic and methyl protons (right). To estimate contributions other than change of temperature and viscosity the minimal line broadening observed at certain temperature has been subtracted from measured values for specific residues. (**C**) Structure of HPV52$_{(1-4)}$ with coloured residues displaying line-broadening above 10 and 15 Hz for imino and aromatic protons, respectively.

2.5. GNA and Four Guanine Tract Are Crucial Structural Elements That Guide Folding of HPV52$_{(1-4)}$

G3-T4-A5 segment with its predisposition to adopt a structure of a well-described GNA trinucleotide loop could drive conformation of HPV52$_{(1-4)}$ into a preorganized state that is on the pathway for folding into a G-quadruplex, even more so since structuring of GNA loops is not [K$^+$]-dependent in a way that is critical for G-quadruplex folding. Several modifications were introduced into HPV52$_{(1-4)}$ in order to better understand sequence requirements for its structure

(Figure S5). First, 4T > A modification in HPV52$_{(1-4)}$ was used to examine effect of N residue in GNA loop on G-quadruplex stability. Yoshizawa et al. [47] have shown that the stacking capability of N residue onto the sheared GA base-pair correlates with GNA minihairpin stability with a 6 °C increase in Tm in the case of GAA compared to GTA loop. Thermal stability of HPV52(1-4) with 4T > A modification was therefore expected to increase. However, no substantial change in melting temperature of HPV52$_{(1-4)}$ 4T > A compared to HPV52$_{(1-4)}$ was observed, while NMR experiments clearly showed conservation of the fold (Figure S5). This suggests that contribution of GNA loop to the overall G-quadruplex stability is not as straightforward as in the hairpin-stem loop structures and depends on a wider structural context. Thymine residue in GTA loop in HPV52(1-4) could, for example, importantly facilitate initial stages of G-quadruplex folding if not even trigger it via molten globule-like state, as was shown for telomeric sequences [49].

Next, we examined the overall importance of 5A > T modification for conservation of HPV52$_{(1-4)}$ fold, while keeping in mind that a mutated GTT loop does not conform to GNA sequence requirements. As expected, 5A > T modification was found to abolish formation of HPV52$_{(1-4)}$ G-quadruplex and resulted in the formation of more than one structure (Figure S5B). These observations confirmed importance of GNA loop for structural integrity of G-quadruplex structure adopted by HPV52$_{(1-4)}$.

Influence of interaction of GNA loop with residues in other loops for G-quadruplex formation was tested with deletion of A19 that is included in hydrogen bonding network of GTA loop. We hypothesized that if GTA loop on its own can stabilize or lead folding of HPV52$_{(1-4)}$, deleting A19 should not affect HPV52$_{(1-4)}$ structure. Surprisingly, A19 was found to play an important part in formation of capping structure together with GNA loop, since deletion of A19 did not retain HPV52$_{(1-4)}$ G-quadruplex fold (Figure S5B).

Finally, interruption of four guanine tract with T12 insertion was designed to test if G4 tract is actually beneficial for G-quadruplex formation, or does it complement formation of G-quadruplex framework that is set up by other very stable or faster forming structural elements. Titration of the oligonucleotide with T12 insertion with aqueous KCl prevented formation of HPV52$_{(1-4)}$, G-quadruplex and resulted in several different structures (Figure S5), which leads us to conclude that G4 tract and resulting V loop are important for formation of HPV52$_{(1-4)}$ G-quadruplex.

3. Discussion

G-rich sequence from genome of HPV type 52 which is the cause of 20% of cervical cancer comprises five G-rich tracts. Their number and variation in length (3, 3, 4, 3 and 3 nt) lead to folding into several different G-quadruplex structures. We could detect at least five different monomeric folds for HPV52$_{(1-5)}$ with the help of analysis of imino fingerprint region and naturally occurring SNPs [10]. In order to unveil and possibly determine structure(s) of predominant forms involved in dynamic equilibrium we focused on oligonucleotide HPV52$_{(1-4)}$ that consists of the first four G-tracts and which demonstrated promising preliminary NMR data. High-resolution NMR structure of a G-quadruplex adopted by 23 nt HPV52$_{(1-4)}$ has several exciting structural features, in line with observation of unusual NMR parameters. G1 is found in the central G-quartet stacked between G2 and G11, which constitute one of the outer G-quartets each. Formally, G1–G11 segment adopts a circular arrangement with G11-G1-G2 and G6-G7-G8 forming edges of a G-quadruplex adopted by HPV52$_{(1-4)}$. A double fold-back of DNA chain is made possible by three (G3-T4-A5) and two (C9-A10) residue edgewise loops that span the opposite sites of the same wide groove. At the same time, G11 is in the terms of primary sequence part of the four consecutive guanine residues (i.e., G11–G14) that are all included in the three G-quartet core and are connected via a no-residue V loop. The last loop consisting of A15-C16-A17-C18-A19 connects G12-G13-G14 and G20-G21-G22 edges of G-quadruplex core in a propeller type orientation. Perusal of G-quadruplex adopted by HPV52$_{(1-4)}$ suggests that capping structures on both sides of the three G-quartet core contribute substantially to its stabilization. In particular, G3-T4-A5 edgewise loop in the GNA loop conformation interacts with A19 at the 5′-end, while C9-A10 edgewise loop interacts with T23 at the 3′-end.

The structure of HPV52$_{(1-4)}$ is similar to a G-quadruplex adopted by $5'$ intronic sequence of gene *chl1*, whose product belongs to a FANCJ helicases. The *chl1* G-quadruplex has been reported earlier when searching for sequence pattern G_3-T-G_4-AA-G_4-T-G_3T [50]. However, HPV52$_{(1-4)}$ does not adhere to G_3-N-G_4-NA-G_4-A/C/T-G_3-A/C/T sequence requirements that were at that time recognized as vital for adopting the fold. In fact, HPV52$_{(1-4)}$ has only the following few characteristics in common: (i) the $5'$-end G_3 tract of which only the first two guanine residues are involved in the G-quadruplex core, (ii) an NAG$_4$ tract that incorporates a no-residue V-loop, and (iii) a thymine residue at the $3'$-end. Updated sequence requirement for folding of HPV52$_{(1-4)}$ and *chl1* into their respective G-quadruplex structures is G_3-N_n-G_3-N_nA-G_4-N_n-G_3-A/C/T, where $n \geq 1$ and N can be any nucleotide. Furthermore, HPV52$_{(1-4)}$ and *chl1* allow us to better understand importance of specific structural elements that stabilize the fold. From comparison of the two structures it can be concluded that the length of both edgewise loops spanning the wide groove may vary and any structural elements formed within the two edgewise loops contribute to additional stabilization of the structure, but are not essential for folding. However, considering that the two-residue edgewise loops spanning wide grooves were shown to be very rare due to imposing the strain in structure [51], it is highly unlikely that two short (2 nt) loops could be accommodated in the same structure. As a consequence, the minimal cumulative length of both edgewise loops of a double fold-back circular element is presumably five residues. Interestingly, the sugar-phosphate backbone conformation of a two-residue edgewise loop bridging wide groove is the same for both HPV52$_{(1-4)}$ (C9-A10 loop) and *chl1* (G3-T4 loop). Very similar sugar-phosphate backbone conformation was observed in the structure of $d(G_4C_2)_3G_4)$, the only other known experimentally observed example of a two-residue edgewise loop (C11-C12) spanning a wide groove (PDB ID 2N2D) (Figure S6) [52]. In contrast to the experimentally determined structures with both residues of the loop positioned above a G-quartet, MD simulations have shown the first residue of a two-residue edgewise loop to reside in the wide groove [51]. It must be emphasized that in-groove conformation was observed for C9 during structure calculations of HPV52$_{(1-4)}$ when experimentally determined restrains for backbone torsion angles of C9 were excluded from structural calculations, which shows that other interactions within the loop must compensate for energetically less favorable loop conformation.

For HPV52$_{(1-4)}$ the first edgewise loop was recognized as a very stable GNA type of loop. Modification of oligonucleotide sequence, however, showed that this loop stabilized fold together with A19 residue from the propeller loop stacking on G2-G6-G20-G12 quartet. Interestingly, the second edgewise loop of *chl1* with sequence G8-A9-A10 can also fold as GNA type loop. Indeed, sheared GA base-pair was detected for *chl1* and although chemical shift of A9 H4' proton was not reported, the conformation of the loop fits to the GNA type loop. Sheared GA base-pair is involved in triple with $3'$-end residue (T19 and A19), which means that in both *chl1* and HPV52$_{(1-4)}$ structures additional interactions with other residues involve GNA type of loop in the capping structures.

The most defining part of HPV52$_{(1-4)}$ and *chl1* structures seems to be AG$_4$ tract that results in A10 residue being stacked on the outer G-quartet and thus contributing to the stabilization of a no-residue V loop. To the best of our knowledge, HPV52$_{(1-4)}$ represents the third structure with such a loop, the first one being found in the dimeric $d(G_3T_4G_4)_2$ [53]. In comparing structures of V loops it becomes clear, however, that they differ in conformation of their sugar-phosphate backbone (Figure S7). Namely, HPV52$_{(1-4)}$ is the only case in which H3' of G11 is observed at δ 6.088 ppm and in which this proton is placed in the plane and close to the aromatic ring of G11, resulting in considerable deshielding related to the decreased electron density. While structures of HPV52$_{(1-4)}$ fall into two different groups with regards to the sugar-phosphate backbone torsion angle values of G11-G12, spatial position of sugar-phosphate backbone changes minimally within the two groups and position of H3' of G11 is conserved (Figure S7). Several conformations of sugar-phosphate backbone between G11 and G12 were found also for *chl1*, but while H3' of G11 is placed close to the aromatic ring in *chl1*, it is not in plane with it, as in HPV52$_{(1-4)}$. Therefore, δ (H3') of G11 in *chl1* is somewhat, but not substantially downfield shifted (δ 5.62 ppm) [50]. For $d(G_3T_4G_4)_2$, H3' of G19 is placed far away from its aromatic ring and its chemical shift (δ 5.00 ppm) is close to the average value of H3′ chemical shifts of guanine residues (δ 4.95 ppm) [42].

Another interesting feature of V loop region of G-quadruplex adopted by HPV52$_{(1-4)}$ is that sugar ring of G12 predominantly adopts North-type conformation, while it is 80% South in d(G$_3$T$_4$G$_4$)$_2$ [53] and no data has been reported for *chl1* [50]. The difference is also in glycosidic torsion angle χ of G12, which is in *anti*-region for HPV52$_{(1-4)}$ and *chl1*, but in *high-anti* region for G20 of d(G$_3$T$_4$G$_4$)$_2$. As North conformation of sugar ring is energetically less favorable for DNA, structural flexibility must be additionally restricted for HPV52$_{(1-4)}$ in comparison to d(G$_3$T$_4$G$_4$)$_2$. In summary, while HPV52$_{(1-4)}$ shares a no-residue V loop with the two other known G-quadruplexes, structural details show existence of several distinct loop subtypes, which is rather unanticipated for such a short structural element. We hypothesize that combination of a two-residue edgewise loop that traverses wide groove and a no-residue V loop in HPV52$_{(1-4)}$ represents two consecutive strained elements that impose spatial limitations on the structure and result in the accumulation of unusual and, in a classical view, energetically less favorable torsion angles conformations.

Our study has been focused on formation of G-quadruplex structures formed by G-rich sequence of HPV type 52. Recently, increasingly large efforts have been made by G-quadruplex community to understand biological role of G-quadruplexes, while structural part of this effort is complicated by polymorphism and challenges in relating a specific (element of) structure to a specific function. If, however, G-quadruplexes are ever to be used as targets for rational drug design, structural information is of paramount importance. This knowledge is also vital for our understanding of processes that G-rich sequences found in various parts of genomes are involved in. Moreover, while number of detailed 3D structures of G-quadruplexes has been increasing steadily, we are still very far from understanding their folding or polymorphism of even quite simple G-rich sequences, such as HPV52$_{(1-4)}$. SNPs were proven useful to better understand structural polymorphism of HPV52$_{(1-4)}$, albeit G-quadruplexes with SNPs are supposedly less relevant in biological context as they form structures with lower melting temperatures and were, as expected for SNPs, found in only a very low number of isolates. While G-quadruplex structures formed by G-rich HPV52 oligonucleotides display high enough thermal stability to reduce expression levels in usual in vitro transcription experiments, the high complexity of the HPV viral life cycle precludes us from drawing any (definite) conclusions from simplified model systems. More comprehensive understanding of impact of G-quadruplex formation on gene expression of HPV52 will therefore require further and more complex studies. Nevertheless, it is tempting to speculate that formation of a certain structure would depend on the direction in which the DNA chain is unwound by DNA processing enzymes, as it would expose single stranded DNA at either 5′ or 3′ ends of G-rich sequence, corresponding to HPV52$_{(1-4)}$ and HPV52$_{(2-5)}$ oligonucleotides, respectively. Formation of a HPV52$_{(1-4)}$ structure with G1 in the central G-quartet opens a question of relevance of such structure within DNA of viral genome. However, increasing the length of HPV52$_{(1-4)}$ at both 5′ or 3′ ends does not preclude G-quadruplex formation (Figure S5), suggesting that the G-quadruplex structure described herein can form even in the context of longer DNA chain. Moreover, HPV52$_{(1-4)}$ offers several structurally distinct elements besides G-quartet planes that are common to all G-quadruplexes and are typically targeted with ligands. For example, while narrow groove that accommodates a no residue V-loop is inaccessible for HPV52$_{(1-4)}$, both medium and wide grooves are completely accessible for hydrogen bond recognition of the G-quartet edges (Figure S8). Moreover, capping structures on both sides efficiently lengthen wide and medium grooves between G20-G22 and G6-G8 tracts, while A15-C16-A17-C18-A19 loop defines a pocket in medium groove between G12-G14 and G20-G22 tracts (Figure S8) that is particularly interesting potential target.

4. Materials and Methods

4.1. Sample Preparation

Oligonucleotides were either purchased from Eurogentec (Seraing, Belgium) and Metabion (Planegg, Germany) or synthesized on a DNA/RNA Synthesizer H-8 (K&A Laborgeraete GbR, Schaafheim, Germany) using standard phosphoramidite solid-phase chemistry. Cleavage of protecting groups was carried out in 1:1 solution of methylamine and aqueous ammonia at 65 °C for 20 min. All samples were purified and desalted with the use of a Millipore Stirred Ultrafiltration Cell model 8010 (Cole-Parmer, Vernon Hills, Illinois, USA). Samples were prepared by dissolution in H_2O containing 10% of ^2H_2O. pH was adjusted to 6.8 or 7.0 with LiOH solution and held constant with 10 mM potassium phosphate buffer (pH 6.8/7.0). Aqueous KCl was titrated into the samples to the final concentration of 50 mM. For measurements at -10 °C oligonucleotide sample was dissolved in 20% deuterated aqueous methanol, while for measurements in choline dihydrogen phosphate lyophilized sample was dissolved in its 1M solution. Annealing procedures included heating of the sample to 95 °C for 3 min and slow cooling to room temperature overnight. Strand concentration in the samples was ranging from 0.26–2.7 mM and was determined by UV absorption at 260 nm using CARY-100 BIO UV-VIS spectrophotometer (Varian, Santa Clara, CA, USA) and the computer program UV WinLab. Extinction coefficients used were 2.80×10^5, 2.36×10^5 and 2.28×10^5 l mol^{-1} cm^{-1} for $HPV52_{(1-5)}$, $HPV52_{(2-5)}$ and $HPV52_{(1-4)}$, respectively, and were determined by the nearest neighbour method.

4.2. CD Spectroscopy

The CD spectra are the average of five scans and were recorded on an Chirascan CD spectrometer (Applied Photophysics, Leatherhead, Surrey, UK) at 25 °C using a 0.1 cm path length quartz cell. The wavelength was varied from 200 to 320 nm in 1 nm steps. Samples for CD measurements were prepared at 10 µM oligonucleotide concentration in 10 mM potassium phosphate buffer and 40 mM KCl. A blank containing only 10 mM potassium phosphate buffer and 40 mM KCl was used for baseline correction.

4.3. UV Spectroscopy

UV melting curves were recorded with a Varian CARY-100 BIO UV/VIS spectrophotometer equipped with Cary Win UV Thermal program in cuvettes with 1 and 0.5 cm path-length at 260, 295 and 350 nm. Temperature interval was 70 °C or 80 °C with 0.1 °C/min temperature change. Measurements started at 10 °C for thermally susceptible samples ($HPV52_{(1-4)}$ G22 > A and $HPV52_{(2-5)}$ G22 > A) and at 90 °C for all other samples and were repeated four times. Samples were covered with mineral oil and stopped to prevent evaporation at high temperatures. Stream of nitrogen was applied throughout the measurements to prevent condensation at low temperatures. Sample concentration was 10 µM in 10 mM KPi/40 mM KCl.

4.4. Native Gel Electrophoresis

Polyacrylamide gel electrophoresis was carried out in temperature-controlled vertical Protean II XI Cell with PowerPac 3000 power supply machine (BioRad, Hercules, CA, USA) at 10 °C for 22 h at 120 V. Gel concentration was 15% (19:1 monomer to bis ratio). Gel was run in 25 mM Britton-Robinson buffer, pH 7, and 50 mM KCl. Sample concentration was 0.24 mM. DNA was visualized with Stains-all (Sigma Aldrich, St. Louis, MO, USA) staining. GeneRuler Ultra Low Range DNA ladder with 12-300 base pairs (Thermo Scientific, Waltham, MA, USA) was used as a relative mobility marker. Gel was photographed with a D3200 camera (Nikon, Minato, Tokyo, Japan).

4.5. NMR Spectroscopy

NMR spectra were recorded on VNMRS 600 and 800 MHz NMR spectrometers (Agilent-Varian, Santa Clara, CA, USA) in the temperature range 0–45 °C. DPFGSE pulse sequence was used to suppress the water signal. 2D NOESY spectra acquired at τ_m of 80, 150 and 250 ms were used to determine glycosidic torsion angle conformation, to establish oligonucleotide topology and consequently to assign exchangeable and non-exchangeable proton resonances. 2D DQF-COSY and TOCSY (τ_m of 20 and 80 ms) spectra were used to cross-check assignment of 2D NOESY spectra and to estimate sugar conformations.

Spectra were processed with programs VNMRJ (Agilent Technologies, Santa Clara, CA, USA) and NMRPipe [54]. Cross-peak assignment and integration with Gaussian fit procedure was achieved using software NMRFAM-SPARKY (NMRFAM) [55,56]. NOE distance restraints for non-exchangeable protons were obtained from 2D NOESY spectra (τ_m 80, 150 and 250 ms) recorded at 25 °C in 100% ^2H_2O and 10% ^2H_2O/90% H_2O. Non-overlapping peaks only were used for the distance restraints calculations. Average volume of H7-H6 cross-peaks of T4 and T23 was used as reference distance of 3.0 Å [57,58]. Cross-peaks were classified as strong (1.8–3.6 Å), medium (2.5–5.0 Å) and weak (3.6–6.5 Å). Another 0.5 Å was added for restraints for ambiguous geminal protons (H2'/H2" or H5'/H5"), as restraint was placed on a C atom (either C2' or C5'). NOE distance restraints for exchangeable protons were obtained from 2D NOESY spectra recorded at 25 °C in 10% ^2H_2O/90% H_2O with mixing times of 80, 150 and 250 ms. Cross-peaks of medium and weak intensity that could be observed in 2D NOESY spectrum with a mixing time of 80 ms were classified as strong (1.8–4.1 Å) and medium (2.5–5.5 Å), respectively. Cross-peaks that appeared in 2D NOESY spectrum with a mixing time of 150 and 250 ms were classified as weak (3.6–7.0 Å).

Data at 25 °C only were used in structure calculations, even though spectra recorded at 0 °C displayed several additional cross-peaks with exchangeable protons. However, as part of the structure was shown to be dynamic, the intensity of NOE cross-peaks at lower temperatures was considered unreliable. Torsion angle χ was restrained to *syn* (0 ± 90) for G1, G6, G11 and G20 and to *anti* region (240 ± 70) for all other residues, except A5 and A15. High intensity of the H1'–H8 cross-peak for A15 showed this residue might be involved in *syn-anti* equilibrium and was therefore left unrestrained, while residue A5 was left unrestrained due to the dynamic nature of the T4-A5-G6 region. Backbone torsion angles were restrained to typical values of g^+/g^-, t, g^+, t and g^+/g^- for α (G2, G3, G6, G7, G21), β (G2, G3, T4, G11, G12, G14, G21, G22), γ (G2, G3, T4, G8, A10, G14, A19, G21), ε (G1, G7, G8, G9, A10, G11, G14, A15, C16, A17, C18, A19, G21, G22) and ζ (G2, G3, G6, G7, G21) based on phosphorous chemical shift (α and ζ), visible 31P-H4' cross-peak (β and γ) and strong 31P-H3' cross-peak (ε) [46,59–63]. For A5, C9, A10 and G13 strong P-H5'/H5" cross-peaks were observed, which indicate unusual rotamers of β. Unusual splitting patterns (−−++) of these residues were then compared with simulated HP-COSY cross-peaks in the Pikkemaat and Altona paper [62], which lead to limiting β to g^+ for A5, C9, G13 and g^+/t for A10. Intense H4'-H5' or H4'-H5" cross-peaks in DQF-COSY spectrum for residues A5, C9, G13 and G20 indicated that their γ torsion angle values are not in typical g^+ range. Strong intensity of H2'/H2"-H5'/H5" NOE cross-peaks and similar intensity of H3'-H5' and H3'-H5" cross-peaks in combination with intense H5"-H8 cross peaks for residues in *anti*-conformation indicated t conformation of γ torsion angle, which was determined for C9, G13 and G20. For A5, g^- conformation could not be excluded, which is why γ torsion angle of A5 was restrained to g^-/t to exclude typical g^+ values. Torsion angles that were shown to be involved in equilibria between several distinct conformations on the basis of spectral characteristics were left unrestrained.

4.6. Structure Calculations

Structure calculations were performed with CUDA version of pmemd module of AMBER 14 software [64], and parmbsc0 [65] force field with χ_{OL4} [66] and $\varepsilon\zeta_{OL1}$ [67] corrections. The initial extended single-stranded DNA structure was obtained with tleap program of AMBER14. Pairwise generalized Born implicit model was used with 0.4 fs time steps and collision frequency of 5 ps^{-1}. For each simulated annealing (SA) a random velocity was used. The cut-off for non-bonded interactions was 999 Å and the SHAKE algorithm for hydrogen atoms was used. Solution-state structure was calculated in two steps of NMR restrained SA simulations. Topology was built in the first step with the help of restraints for hydrogen bonds, G-quartet planarities and limited number of H1-H1 and H6/8-H6/8 distance restraints. 1000 final structures were then calculated in 300 ps SA with the following temperature program: temperature was raised from 300 to 1000 K in the first 5 ps, held constant at 1000 K for 65 ps and scaled down to 0 K in the next 235 ps. Restraints used in the calculation were hydrogen bond (force constant 30 kcal mol^{-1} Å^{-2}, 0–300 ps) and NOE-derived distance restraints (force constant 10 kcal mol^{-1} Å^{-2}, 100–300 ps), torsion angles χ, υ_2, α, β, γ, ε and ζ restraints (force constant 200 kcal mol^{-1} rad^{-2}, 0–300 ps) and planarity restraints for G-quartets (force constant 20 kcal mol^{-1} rad^{-2}, 50–290 ps). All restraints were linearly increased to their final value in the first 100 ps of SA. A family of ten structures was selected based on the lowest energy and the smallest restraints violations. Structures were minimized with 100,000 cycles of steepest descent minimization. No planarity restraints were used in the final stage of structure refinement.

Atomic coordinates and chemical shifts for the reported NMR structure have been deposited with the Protein Data bank under accession number 5O4D and with the Biological Magnetic Resonance Bank under accession number 34145.

Supplementary Materials: The following are available online at http://www.mdpi.com/1420-3049/24/7/1294/s1, Figure S1: HPV52 oligonucleotides resolved by PAGE electrophoresis, Figure S2: Melting profiles [68] of HPV52 oligonucleotides at 295 nm, Figure S3: C8 chemical shift differences for guanine residues, Figure S4: NMR characterization of G6-8Br modified HPV52$_{(1–4)}$, Figure S5: Extended and modified sequences of HPV52$_{(1–4)}$ and their NMR characterization, Figure S6: Comparison of 2-residue edgewise loops spanning the wide groove in HPV52$_{(1–4)}$, *chl1* and (G$_4$C$_2$)$_3$G$_4$ G-quadruplexes, Figure S7: Comparison of a no-residue V loops in HPV52$_{(1–4)}$, *chl1* and (G$_3$T$_3$G$_4$)$_2$ G-quadruplexes, Figure S8: Surface representation of grooves of HPV52$_{(1–4)}$.

Author Contributions: Conceptualization, M.M. and J.P.; Data curation, M.M.; Formal analysis, M.M. and J.P.; Investigation, M.M. and J.P.; Project administration, J.P.; Software, M.M. and J.P.; Supervision, J.P.; Validation, M.M. and J.P.; Visualization, M.M.; Writing—original draft, M.M. and J.P.; Writing—review & editing, M.M. and J.P.

Funding: This research was funded by Slovenian Research Agency—ARRS, grant numbers P1-242, J3-7245 and J7-9399.

Acknowledgments: M.M. acknowledges the support of National programme L'Oreal-UNESCO for Women in Science.

Conflicts of Interest: The authors declare no conflict of interest.

References

1. Hpvcenter—International Human Papillomavirus Reference Center. Available online: http://www.nordicehealth.se/hpvcenter/ (accessed on 24 January 2019).

2. Hong, S.; Laimins, L.A. Regulation of the life cycle of HPVs by differentiation and the DNA damage response. *Future Microbiol.* **2013**, *8*, 1547–1557. [CrossRef] [PubMed]

3. Winer, R.L.; Kiviat, N.B.; Hughes, J.P.; Adam, D.E.; Lee, S.-K.; Kuypers, J.M.; Koutsky, L.A. Development and duration of human papillomavirus lesions, after initial infection. *J. Infect. Dis.* **2005**, *191*, 731–738. [CrossRef]

4. Doorbar, J.; Quint, W.; Banks, L.; Bravo, I.G.; Stoler, M.; Broker, T.R.; Stanley, M.A. The biology and life-cycle of human papillomaviruses. *Vaccine* **2012**, *30* (Suppl. 5), F55–F70. [CrossRef]

5. Roman, A.; Munger, K. The papillomavirus E7 proteins. *Virology* **2013**, *445*, 138–168. [CrossRef] [PubMed]

6. Vande Pol, S.B.; Klingelhutz, A.J. Papillomavirus E6 oncoproteins. *Virology* **2013**, *445*, 115–137. [CrossRef]

7. Bosch, F.X.; Broker, T.R.; Forman, D.; Moscicki, A.-B.; Gillison, M.L.; Doorbar, J.; Stern, P.L.; Stanley, M.; Arbyn, M.; Poljak, M.; et al. Comprehensive Control of Human Papillomavirus Infections and Related Diseases. *Vaccine* **2013**, *31* (Suppl. 7), H1–H31. [CrossRef]

8. Doorbar, J.; Egawa, N.; Griffin, H.; Kranjec, C.; Murakami, I. Human papillomavirus molecular biology and disease association. *Rev. Med. Virol.* **2015**, *25* (Suppl. 1), 2–23. [CrossRef]

9. Burk, R.D.; Harari, A.; Chen, Z. Human papillomavirus genome variants. *Virology* **2013**, *445*, 232–243. [CrossRef] [PubMed]

10. Marušič, M.; Hošnjak, L.; Krafčikova, P.; Poljak, M.; Viglasky, V.; Plavec, J. The effect of single nucleotide polymorphisms in G-rich regions of high-risk human papillomaviruses on structural diversity of DNA. *Biochim. Biophys. Acta BBA Gen. Subj.* **2017**, *1861*, 1229–1236. [CrossRef]

11. Gellert, M.; Lipsett, M.N.; Davies, D.R. Helix formation by guanylic acid. *Proc. Natl. Acad. Sci. USA* **1962**, *48*, 2013–2018. [CrossRef] [PubMed]

12. Paeschke, K.; Bochman, M.L.; Garcia, P.D.; Cejka, P.; Friedman, K.L.; Kowalczykowski, S.C.; Zakian, V.A. Pif1 family helicases suppress genome instability at G-quadruplex motifs. *Nature* **2013**, *497*, 458–462. [CrossRef]

13. Rodriguez, R.; Miller, K.M.; Forment, J.V.; Bradshaw, C.R.; Nikan, M.; Britton, S.; Oelschlaegel, T.; Xhemalce, B.; Balasubramanian, S.; Jackson, S.P. Small-molecule–induced DNA damage identifies alternative DNA structures in human genes. *Nat. Chem. Biol.* **2012**, *8*, 301–310. [CrossRef] [PubMed]

14. Wolfe, A.L.; Singh, K.; Zhong, Y.; Drewe, P.; Rajasekhar, V.K.; Sanghvi, V.R.; Mavrakis, K.J.; Jiang, M.; Roderick, J.E.; Van der Meulen, J.; et al. RNA G-quadruplexes cause eIF4A-dependent oncogene translation in cancer. *Nature* **2014**, *513*, 65–70. [CrossRef]

15. Siddiqui-Jain, A.; Grand, C.L.; Bearss, D.J.; Hurley, L.H. Direct evidence for a G-quadruplex in a promoter region and its targeting with a small molecule to repress c-MYC transcription. *Proc. Natl. Acad. Sci. USA* **2002**, *99*, 11593–11598. [CrossRef] [PubMed]

16. Lavezzo, E.; Berselli, M.; Frasson, I.; Perrone, R.; Palù, G.; Brazzale, A.R.; Richter, S.N.; Toppo, S. G-quadruplex forming sequences in the genome of all known human viruses: A comprehensive guide. *PLoS Comput. Biol.* **2018**, *14*, e1006675. [CrossRef] [PubMed]

17. Ruggiero, E.; Richter, S.N. G-quadruplexes and G-quadruplex ligands: Targets and tools in antiviral therapy. *Nucleic Acids Res.* **2018**, *46*, 3270–3283. [CrossRef]

18. Métifiot, M.; Amrane, S.; Litvak, S.; Andreola, M.-L. G-quadruplexes in viruses: Function and potential therapeutic applications. *Nucleic Acids Res.* **2014**, *42*, 12352–12366. [CrossRef]

19. Baran, N. The SV40 large T-antigen helicase can unwind four stranded DNA structures linked by G-quartets. *Nucleic Acids Res.* **1997**, *25*, 297–303. [CrossRef]

20. Madireddy, A.; Purushothaman, P.; Loosbroock, C.P.; Robertson, E.S.; Schildkraut, C.L.; Verma, S.C. G-quadruplex-interacting compounds alter latent DNA replication and episomal persistence of KSHV. *Nucleic Acids Res.* **2016**, *44*, 3675–3694. [CrossRef]

21. Murat, P.; Zhong, J.; Lekieffre, L.; Cowieson, N.P.; Clancy, J.L.; Preiss, T.; Balasubramanian, S.; Khanna, R.; Tellam, J. G-quadruplexes regulate Epstein-Barr virus–encoded nuclear antigen 1 mRNA translation. *Nat. Chem. Biol.* **2014**, *10*, 358–364. [CrossRef]

22. Perrone, R.; Nadai, M.; Frasson, I.; Poe, J.A.; Butovskaya, E.; Smithgall, T.E.; Palumbo, M.; Palù, G.; Richter, S.N. A dynamic G-quadruplex region regulates the HIV-1 long terminal repeat promoter. *J. Med. Chem.* **2013**, *56*, 6521–6530. [CrossRef]

23. Plyler, J.; Jasheway, K.; Tuesuwan, B.; Karr, J.; Brennan, J.S.; Kerwin, S.M.; David, W.M. Real-time Investigation of SV40 Large T-antigen Helicase Activity Using Surface Plasmon Resonance. *Cell Biochem. Biophys.* **2009**, *53*, 43–52. [CrossRef] [PubMed]

24. Shen, W.; Gorelick, R.J.; Bambara, R.A. HIV-1 Nucleocapsid Protein Increases Strand Transfer Recombination by Promoting Dimeric G-quartet Formation. *J. Biol. Chem.* **2011**, *286*, 29838–29847. [CrossRef]

25. Huppert, J.L.; Balasubramanian, S. Prevalence of quadruplexes in the human genome. *Nucleic Acids Res.* **2005**, *33*, 2908–2916. [CrossRef] [PubMed]

26. Todd, A.K.; Johnston, M.; Neidle, S. Highly prevalent putative quadruplex sequence motifs in human DNA. *Nucleic Acids Res.* **2005**, *33*, 2901–2907. [CrossRef] [PubMed]

27. Chambers, V.S.; Marsico, G.; Boutell, J.M.; Di Antonio, M.; Smith, G.P.; Balasubramanian, S. High-throughput sequencing of DNA G-quadruplex structures in the human genome. *Nat. Biotechnol.* **2015**, *33*, 877–881. [CrossRef]

28. Hänsel-Hertsch, R.; Beraldi, D.; Lensing, S.V.; Marsico, G.; Zyner, K.; Parry, A.; Di Antonio, M.; Pike, J.; Kimura, H.; Narita, M.; et al. G-quadruplex structures mark human regulatory chromatin. *Nat. Genet.* **2016**, *48*, 1267–1272. [CrossRef] [PubMed]

29. Huppert, J.L. Four-stranded DNA: Cancer, gene regulation and drug development. *Philos. Trans. R. Soc. Lond. Math. Phys. Eng. Sci.* **2007**, *365*, 2969–2984. [CrossRef] [PubMed]

30. Tlučková, K.; Marušič, M.; Tóthová, P.; Bauer, L.; Šket, P.; Plavec, J.; Viglasky, V. Human Papillomavirus G-Quadruplexes. *Biochemistry* **2013**, *52*, 7207–7216. [CrossRef] [PubMed]

31. Bedrat, A.; Lacroix, L.; Mergny, J.-L. Re-evaluation of G-quadruplex propensity with G4Hunter. *Nucleic Acids Res.* **2016**, *44*, 1746–1759. [CrossRef] [PubMed]

32. Kikin, O.; D'Antonio, L.; Bagga, P.S. QGRS Mapper: A web-based server for predicting G-quadruplexes in nucleotide sequences. *Nucleic Acids Res.* **2006**, *34*, W676–W682. [CrossRef] [PubMed]

33. Chan, P.K.S.; Ho, W.C.S.; Chan, M.C.W.; Wong, M.C.S.; Yeung, A.C.M.; Chor, J.S.Y.; Hui, M. Meta-Analysis on Prevalence and Attribution of Human Papillomavirus Types 52 and 58 in Cervical Neoplasia Worldwide. *PLoS ONE* **2014**, *9*, e107573. [CrossRef]

34. Benson, D.A.; Cavanaugh, M.; Clark, K.; Karsch-Mizrachi, I.; Lipman, D.J.; Ostell, J.; Sayers, E.W. GenBank. *Nucleic Acids Res.* **2013**, *41*, D36–D42. [CrossRef]

35. Guédin, A.; Gros, J.; Alberti, P.; Mergny, J.-L. How long is too long? Effects of loop size on G-quadruplex stability. *Nucleic Acids Res.* **2010**, *38*, 7858–7868. [CrossRef]

36. Karsisiotis, A.I.; Hessari, N.M.; Novellino, E.; Spada, G.P.; Randazzo, A.; Webba da Silva, M. Topological Characterization of Nucleic Acid G-Quadruplexes by UV Absorption and Circular Dichroism. *Angew. Chem. Int. Ed.* **2011**, *50*, 10645–10648. [CrossRef]

37. Del Villar-Guerra, R.; Trent, J.O.; Chaires, J.B. G-Quadruplex Secondary Structure Obtained from Circular Dichroism Spectroscopy. *Angew. Chem. Int. Ed. Engl.* **2018**, *57*, 7171–7175. [CrossRef]

38. Webba da Silva, M. Geometric Formalism for DNA Quadruplex Folding. *Chem. Eur. J.* **2007**, *13*, 9738–9745. [CrossRef]

39. Greene, K.L.; Wang, Y.; Live, D. Influence of the glycosidic torsion angle on 13C and 15N shifts in guanosine nucleotides: Investigations of G-tetrad models with alternating syn and anti bases. *J. Biomol. NMR* **1995**, *5*, 333–338. [CrossRef] [PubMed]

40. Fonville, J.M.; Swart, M.; Vokáčová, Z.; Sychrovský, V.; Šponer, J.E.; Šponer, J.; Hilbers, C.W.; Bickelhaupt, F.M.; Wijmenga, S.S. Chemical Shifts in Nucleic Acids Studied by Density Functional Theory Calculations and Comparison with Experiment. *Chem. Eur. J.* **2012**, *18*, 12372–12387. [CrossRef] [PubMed]

41. Dickerhoff, J.; Weisz, K. Flipping a G-Tetrad in a Unimolecular Quadruplex without Affecting Its Global Fold. *Angew. Chem. Int. Ed.* **2015**, *54*, 5588–5591. [CrossRef] [PubMed]

42. Ulrich, E.L.; Akutsu, H.; Doreleijers, J.F.; Harano, Y.; Ioannidis, Y.E.; Lin, J.; Livny, M.; Mading, S.; Maziuk, D.; Miller, Z.; et al. BioMagResBank. *Nucleic Acids Res.* **2008**, *36*, D402–D408. [CrossRef]

43. Chou, S.-H.; Zhu, L.; Gao, Z.; Cheng, J.-W.; Reid, B.R. Hairpin Loops Consisting of Single Adenine Residues Closed by Sheared A·A and G·G Pairs Formed by the DNA Triplets AAA and GAG: Solution Structure of the d(GTACAAAGTAC) Hairpin. *J. Mol. Biol.* **1996**, *264*, 981–1001. [CrossRef]

44. Hirao, I.; Kawai, G.; Yoshizawa, S.; Nishimura, Y.; Ishido, Y.; Watanabe, K.; Miura, K. Most compact hairpin-turn structure exerted by a short DNA fragment, d(GCGAAGC) in solution: An extraordinarily stable structure resistant to nucleases and heat. *Nucleic Acids Res.* **1994**, *22*, 576–582. [CrossRef]

45. Kettani, A.; Gorin, A.; Majumdar, A.; Hermann, T.; Skripkin, E.; Zhao, H.; Jones, R.; Patel, D.J. A dimeric DNA interface stabilized by stacked A · (G · G · G · G) · A hexads and coordinated monovalent cations. *J. Mol. Biol.* **2000**, *297*, 627–644. [CrossRef]

46. Matsugami, A.; Ouhashi, K.; Kanagawa, M.; Liu, H.; Kanagawa, S.; Uesugi, S.; Katahira, M. An intramolecular quadruplex of (GGA)4 triplet repeat DNA with a G:G:G:G tetrad and a G(:A):G(:A):G(:A):G heptad, and its dimeric interaction. *J. Mol. Biol.* **2001**, *313*, 255–269. [CrossRef] [PubMed]

47. Yoshizawa, S.; Kawai, G.; Watanabe, K.; Miura, K.; Hirao, I. GNA Trinucleotide Loop Sequences Producing Extraordinarily Stable DNA Minihairpins. *Biochemistry* **1997**, *36*, 4761–4767. [CrossRef]

48. Zhu, L.; Chou, S.-H.; Xu, J.; Reid, B.R. Structure of a single-cytidine hairpin loop formed by the DNA triplet GCA. *Nat. Struct. Biol.* **1995**, *2*, 1012–1017. [CrossRef] [PubMed]

49. Bončina, M.; Vesnaver, G.; Chaires, J.B.; Lah, J. Unraveling the Thermodynamics of the Folding and Interconversion of Human Telomere G-Quadruplexes. *Angew. Chem. Int. Ed. Engl.* **2016**, *55*, 10340–10344. [CrossRef] [PubMed]

50. Kuryavyi, V.; Patel, D.J. Solution Structure of a Unique G-Quadruplex Scaffold Adopted by a Guanosine-Rich Human Intronic Sequence. *Structure* **2010**, *18*, 73–82. [CrossRef] [PubMed]

51. Cang, X.; Šponer, J.; Cheatham, T.E. Insight into G-DNA structural polymorphism and folding from sequence and loop connectivity through free energy analysis. *J. Am. Chem. Soc.* **2011**, *133*, 14270–14279. [CrossRef] [PubMed]

52.   Brčić, J.; Plavec, J. Solution structure of a DNA quadruplex containing ALS and FTD related GGGGCC repeat stabilized by 8-bromodeoxyguanosine substitution. *Nucleic Acids Res.* **2015**, *43*, 8590–8600. [CrossRef] [PubMed]

53.   Crnugelj, M.; Sket, P.; Plavec, J. Small change in a G-rich sequence, a dramatic change in topology: New dimeric G-quadruplex folding motif with unique loop orientations. *J. Am. Chem. Soc.* **2003**, *125*, 7866–7871. [CrossRef]

54.   Delaglio, F.; Grzesiek, S.; Vuister, G.W.; Zhu, G.; Pfeifer, J.; Bax, A. NMRPipe: A multidimensional spectral processing system based on UNIX pipes. *J. Biomol. NMR* **1995**, *6*, 277–293. [CrossRef] [PubMed]

55.   Goddard, T.D.; Kneller, D.G. *SPARKY 3*; University of California: San Francisco, CA, USA, 2008.

56.   Lee, W.; Tonelli, M.; Markley, J.L. NMRFAM-SPARKY: Enhanced software for biomolecular NMR spectroscopy. *Bioinformatics* **2015**, *31*, 1325–1327. [CrossRef]

57.   Clore, G.M.; Gronenborn, A.M. Interproton distance measurements in solution for a double-stranded DNA undecamer comprising a portion of the specific target site for the cyclic AMP receptor protein in the *gal* operon: A nuclear Overhauser enhancement study. *FEBS Lett.* **1984**, *175*, 117–123. [CrossRef]

58.   Wijmenga, S.S.; van Buuren, B.N.M. The use of NMR methods for conformational studies of nucleic acids. *Prog. Nucl. Magn. Reson. Spectrosc.* **1998**, *32*, 287–387. [CrossRef]

59.   Webba da Silva, M. Experimental Demonstration of T:(G:G:G:G):T Hexad and T:A:A:T Tetrad Alignments within a DNA Quadruplex Stem. *Biochemistry* **2005**, *44*, 3754–3764. [CrossRef] [PubMed]

60.   Nielsen, J.T.; Arar, K.; Petersen, M. NMR solution structures of LNA (locked nucleic acid) modified quadruplexes. *Nucleic Acids Res.* **2006**, *34*, 2006–2014. [CrossRef]

61.   Kim, S.-G.; Lin, L.-J.; Reid, B.R. Determination of nucleic acid backbone conformation by proton NMR. *Biochemistry* **1992**, *31*, 3564–3574. [CrossRef]

62.   Pikkemaat, J.A.; Altona, C. Fine Structure of the P–H5′ Cross-Peak in 31P–1H Correlated 2D NMR Spectroscopy. An Efficient Probe for the Backbone Torsion Angles β and γ in Nucleic Acids. *Magn. Reson. Chem.* **1996**, *34*, S33–S39. [CrossRef]

63.   Roongta, V.A.; Jones, C.R.; Gorenstein, D.G. Effect of distortions in the deoxyribose phosphate backbone conformation of duplex oligodeoxyribonucleotide dodecamers containing GT, GG, GA, AC, and GU base-pair mismatches on 31P NMR spectra. *Biochemistry* **1990**, *29*, 5245–5258. [CrossRef]

64.   Case, D.A.; Babin, V.; Berryman, J.T.; Betz, R.M.; Cai, Q.; Cerutti, D.S.; Cheatham, T.E.; Darden, T.A.; Duke, R.E.; Gohlke, H.; et al. *AMBER 14*; University of California: San Francisco, CA, USA, 2014.

65.   Aduri, R.; Psciuk, B.T.; Saro, P.; Taniga, H.; Schlegel, H.B.; SantaLucia, J. AMBER Force Field Parameters for the Naturally Occurring Modified Nucleosides in RNA. *J. Chem. Theory Comput.* **2007**, *3*, 1464–1475. [CrossRef]

66.   Krepl, M.; Zgarbová, M.; Stadlbauer, P.; Otyepka, M.; Banáš, P.; Koča, J.; Cheatham, T.E.; Jurečka, P.; Sponer, J. Reference simulations of noncanonical nucleic acids with different χ variants of the AMBER force field: Quadruplex DNA, quadruplex RNA and Z-DNA. *J. Chem. Theory Comput.* **2012**, *8*, 2506–2520. [CrossRef] [PubMed]

67.   Zgarbová, M.; Luque, F.J.; Šponer, J.; Cheatham, T.E.; Otyepka, M.; Jurečka, P. Toward Improved Description of DNA Backbone: Revisiting Epsilon and Zeta Torsion Force Field Parameters. *J. Chem. Theory Comput.* **2013**, *9*, 2339–2354. [CrossRef] [PubMed]

68.   Zhang, Y.; Chen, J.; Ju, H.; Zhou, J. Thermal denaturation profile: A straightforward signature to characterize parallel G-quadruplexes. *Biochimie* **2019**, *157*, 22–25. [CrossRef] [PubMed]

Sample Availability: Samples of the compounds are not available from the authors.

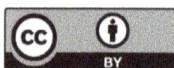

molecules

MDPI

Article

Relationship Between G-Quadruplex Sequence Composition in Viruses and Their Hosts

Emilia Puig Lombardi, Arturo Londoño-Vallejo * and Alain Nicolas *

Institut Curie, PSL Research University, UMR3244 CNRS, 75248 Paris CEDEX 05, France;
maria-emilia.puig-lombardi@curie.fr
* Correspondence: Arturo.Londono@curie.fr (A.L.-V.); alain.nicolas@curie.fr (A.N.)

Academic Editor: Sara N. Richter
Received: 2 May 2019; Accepted: 16 May 2019; Published: 20 May 2019

Abstract: A subset of guanine-rich nucleic acid sequences has the potential to fold into G-quadruplex (G4) secondary structures, which are functionally important for several biological processes, including genome stability and regulation of gene expression. Putative quadruplex sequences (PQSs) $G_{3+}N_{1-7}G_{3+}N_{1-7}G_{3+}N_{1-7}G_{3+}$ are widely found in eukaryotic and prokaryotic genomes, but the base composition of the N_{1-7} loops is biased across species. Since the viruses partially hijack their hosts' cellular machinery for proliferation, we examined the PQS motif size, loop length, and nucleotide compositions of 7370 viral genome assemblies and compared viral and host PQS motifs. We studied seven viral taxa infecting five distant eukaryotic hosts and created a resource providing a comprehensive view of the viral quadruplex motifs. Overall, short-looped PQSs are predominant and with a similar composition across viral taxonomic groups, albeit subtle trends emerge upon classification by hosts. Specifically, there is a higher frequency of pyrimidine loops in viruses infecting animals irrespective of the viruses' genome type. This observation is confirmed by an in-depth analysis of the Herpesviridae family of viruses, which showed a distinctive accumulation of thermally stable C-looped quadruplexes in viruses infecting high-order vertebrates. The occurrence of viral C-looped G4s, which carry binding sites for host transcription factors, as well as the high prevalence of viral TTA-looped G4s, which are identical to vertebrate telomeric motifs, provide concrete examples of how PQSs may help viruses impinge upon, and benefit from, host functions. More generally, these observations suggest a co-evolution of virus and host PQSs, thus underscoring the potential functional significance of G4s.

Keywords: G-quadruplex; virus; eukaryotic hosts; Herpesviridae; genome evolution

---

1. Introduction

G-quadruplexes (G4s) are alternative DNA or RNA secondary structures formed by the stacking of planar arrangements of guanine residues, further stabilized by monovalent cations [1]. The importance of quadruplex-forming sequences as regulatory elements has been supported by extensive evidence in eukaryotic cells [2–4]. Putative quadruplex-forming sequences (PQSs) are prevalent in numerous genomes [5,6] and have been implicated in key genomic functions, such as transcription regulation, replication, repair, and telomere maintenance reviewed in [7–9]. Typically, the consensus sequence motif $G_{3+}N_{1-7}G_{3+}N_{1-7}G_{3+}N_{1-7}G_{3+}$ has been used to identify potential PQSs [5,10]. This has led to an estimate of over 400,000 PQSs in the human reference genome, with a median density of 0.5 motif per kbp. In other eukaryotes and in bacteria, the density of G4 motifs is highly variable (2.5 to >0.1 motifs per kbp) [6].

PQSs are also present in viral genomes [11,12], and emerging evidence suggests that they can be implicated in viral replication and recombination, in the regulation of virulence via gene expression control [13,14], and in key steps in the viral cycles [15]. The presence of putative G4 sequences has been reported in various viral genomes, such as the human immunodeficiency virus (HIV-1) [16–20], the Epstein–Barr virus (EBV) [21,22], or papillomaviruses (HPV) [23–25]. In particular, the Epstein–Barr virus encodes the genome replication and maintenance protein EBNA1 that binds G-rich sequences to recruit the replication complex [21]. The herpes simplex virus 1 (HSV-1) genome displays multiple clusters of repeated sequences forming very stable quadruplexes that are involved in viral DNA replication [26]. The HIV-1 promoter contains a highly conserved G-rich region able to fold into a G4 structure [19] and is involved in the regulation of viral replication [18]. The presence of highly conserved PQSs able to potentially form intermolecular G4s has been reported in several human herpesvirus packaging signals [27], as well as in HIV-1 [28], further highlighting the biological role of viral G4s. In addition, several DNA aptamers (short synthetic single-stranded oligonucleotides that specifically bind to various molecular targets) containing G4-forming sequences were found to have antiviral activity [29,30] and have been used as diagnostic tools to detect viruses [11].

Within a quadruplex, the length of the G-tracts as well as the length and the base composition of the loops are critical to determine the conformation of the G4s and their stability [31–36]. Remarkably, it has been observed that most quadruplex-forming sequences found in gene promoters contain at least one single-nucleotide loop [37–41]. Genome-wide, our analyses across numerous eukaryotes outlined a striking enrichment of single-nucleotide loop G4s and further revealed a prominent trend favoring pyrimidine nucleotides in these loops as well as the accumulation of G_{15+} sequences in plants and invertebrates [36]. Whether these divergent evolutionary trends reflect differential biases in mutagenesis and DNA repair mechanisms from species to species and/or are the result of functional selection remains an open question.

Given that viruses utilize the hosts' cellular machineries for replication and transcription, especially in large DNA viruses [42], we wished to examine whether the composition of G4 motifs in the viral genomes could be correlated to that of their hosts. To address this question, we identified and analyzed all G4 motifs (size, loop length, and nucleotide compositions) present in the currently available 7370 viral genome assemblies, which include seven viral taxa infecting five evolutionary distant groups of eukaryotic hosts: vertebrates (including *Homo sapiens*), invertebrates, protozoa, fungi, and plants. Here, we provide a large comparative view of the quadruplex motif loop content at nucleotide-level resolution, with particular focus on the Herpesviridae family, ubiquitous large dsDNA (linear double-stranded DNA) viruses that are amongst the best characterized host-adapted viruses.

2. Results and Discussion

2.1. G-Quadruplex Metrics in Viral Genomes

To analyze the G4 motifs in a large panel of viruses, we retrieved the 7370 viral genome assemblies from the viruSITE [43] database. This database comprises all curated virus genomes available in the NCBI Reference Sequence Database (RefSeq), categorized into seven viral taxa: dsDNA, ssDNA, dsRNA, ssRNA, satellites, as well as retro-transcribing or unclassified viruses (Figure 1, panels A,B). These viruses infect a broad range of eukaryotic hosts (Figure 1C).

First, we analyzed several viral genome metrics: genome size (kilo base pairs, kbp), which varies from 0.2 kbp to over 2400 kbp; GC content (%), which varies from 17.8% to 76.1%; and PQS densities (PQS/kbp), that allow to compare the quadruplex content of each assembly independently of the genome lengths, as well as their presence on the positive (G-rich) or negative (C-rich) strand (Materials and Methods). To identify the G4 motifs, we searched the canonical $G_{3+}N_{1-7}G_{3+}N_{1-7}G_{3+}N_{1-7}G_{3+}$ sequences by regular expression matching (Materials and Methods), as previously described for eukaryotic genomes [5,10,36]. All the identified quadruplex sequences are individually reported along with their coordinates in Table S1 (Supplementary Materials), which we propose as a resource. Finally, we performed virus–host analyses, classifying the eukaryote hosts into vertebrate or invertebrate animals, protozoa, plants, and fungi species. Unless otherwise mentioned, the group of vertebrates includes *Homo sapiens*.

The overall viral PQS metrics, classified by viral taxa or host group, are summarized in Tables 1 and 2, respectively. Not surprisingly, the total number of quadruplexes depends on the viral genome size, albeit it displays an uneven density and moderate correlation (Spearman's *rho* = 0.38, non-parametric test for association between paired samples $p < 2.2 \times 10^{-16}$; Figure 1A). Of note, the dsDNA viruses, which greatly vary in genome size, show the highest densities of G4 sequences in the retrieved viral genomes (with an average of 0.08 ± 0.79 PQS/kbp; Table 1). Among them, the Herpesviridae family, further analyzed hereafter, exhibits the highest PQS content: we found a total of 6735 motifs, with an average density of 0.45 ± 0.60 PQS/kbp and up to 2.8 PQS/kbp in the Papiine alpha herpesvirus 2 (Table S2). In the remaining viral taxa, that include fewer G4 motifs and shorter viral genomes, the density of PQSs is not negligible since ssDNA, ssRNA, and retro-transcribing (RT) viruses carry 0.04 ± 0.18 to 0.07 ± 0.16 PQS/kbp (Table 1). However, as previously observed for human viruses [12], the viral genomes are in general relatively G4-poor, with a PQS density of <0.1 motif per kbp (Figure 1A). Nevertheless, PQSs are not less frequent than in zebrafish (0.019 G4/kbp), lower-order groupings of eukaryotes (e.g., 0.02 G4/kbp in *Caenorhabditis elegans*, 0.002 G4/kbp in *Plasmodium*), or bacteria (0.001 to 0.02 G4/kbp) (Table 3).

Table 1. Genome metrics and quadruplex sequences in seven viral taxa.

Taxon	Assemblies	Median % GC	Median Genome Size (Base Pairs)	Total PQS Count	Mean PQS Density [1]
dsDNA	2758	44.5	45,531	11,315	0.083
dsRNA	301	44.5	2178	11	0.018
RT [2]	153	43.6	7743	85	0.074
Satellites	227	41.0	1348	2	0.011
ssDNA	988	44.0	2707	102	0.058
ssRNA	1784	43.4	6944	553	0.036
Unclassified	1158	44.6	4492	206	0.024

[1] Number of PQSs per kilo base pair (PQS/kbp); [2] RT: retro-transcribing viruses.

Table 2. Genome metrics and quadruplex sequences in various organisms.

Organism	Median % GC	Genome Size (Mb)	Total PQS Count [1]	Mean PQS Density [2]
Human	37.8	3095.69	434,272	0.140
Mouse	42.6	2730.87	327,452	0.120
Zebrafish	36.8	1371.72	25,677	0.019
Drosophila melanogaster	42.1	143.73	5262	0.037
Caenorhabditis elegans	35.4	100.29	1561	0.016
Saccharomyces cerevisiae	38.4	12.16	7	0.001
Leishmania major	59.6	32.86	7913	0.241
Trypanosoma brucei	46.8	35.83	635	0.018
Plasmodium falciparum	19.6	23.33	51	0.002
Arabidopsis thaliana	36.1	119.67	338	0.003
Rhodobacter sphaeroides	68.8	4.64	5	0.001
E. coli	50.8	4.6	109	0.024

[1] PQS counts retrieved from Marsico et al. 2019 [44]; [2] Number of PQSs per kilo base pair (PQS/kbp).

We observed that giant viruses infecting protozoan hosts are relatively enriched for G4 sequences, reaching 181 PQSs in the 2,473,870 bp (0.07 PQS/kb) *Pandoravirus salinus* genome. Intriguingly, the Mimiviridae viruses, which exhibit a low GC content (≈28%), are exceptionally G4-poor with only three G4 motifs found in the Mimivirus terra2 assembly (1,168,989 bp; 0.003 PQS/kbp). Globally, there is a significant positive correlation between the PQS and GC content, although the relationship is weak (Spearman's *rho* = 0.28, non-parametric test for association between paired samples $P < 2.2 \times 10^{-16}$; Figure 1B) and the median GC content of the various viral taxa are rather similar (44% ± 8), albeit with large variations within each taxon (Figure 1B). Thus, the impact of the GC content on the probability to create a G4 motif is not strong, suggesting that at least a fraction of these quadruplex sequences may be maintained under positive selection.

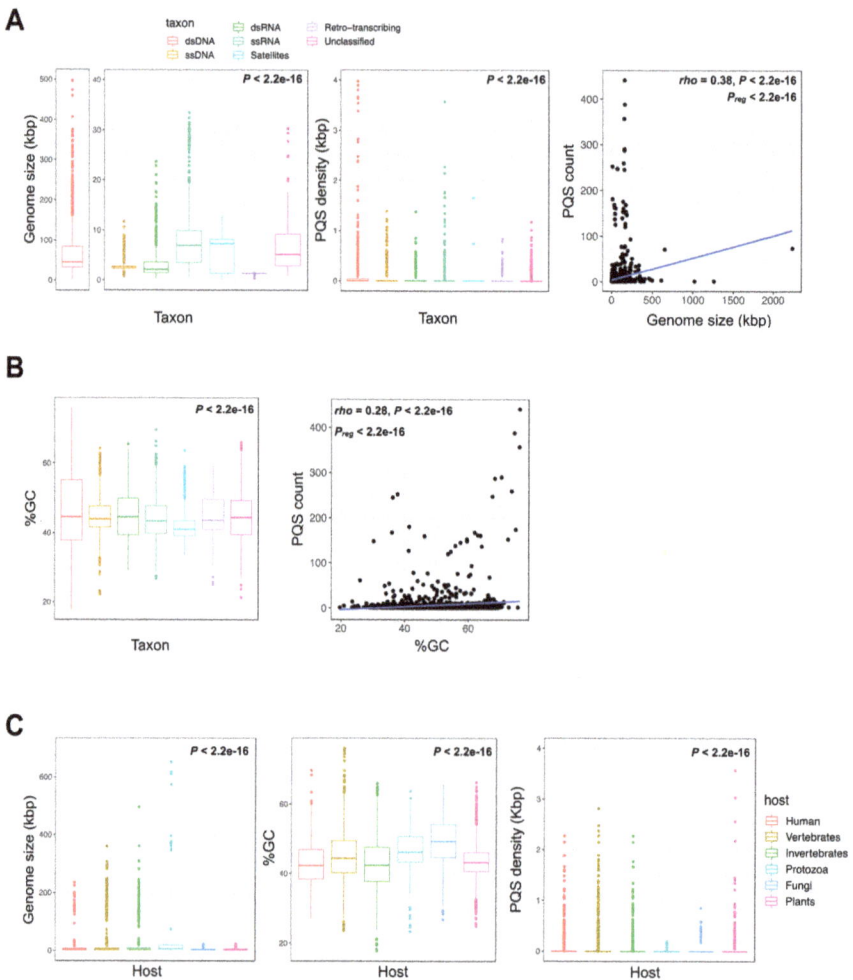

Figure 1. Genome metrics and quadruplex motif content of viral genomes. (**A**) From left to right, genome size (in kilo base pairs, kbp), putative quadruplex sequence (PQS) density (number of motifs found per kbp), and relationship between PQS content and genome size for different viral taxa. (**B**) GC content and relationship between PQS content and GC content for different viral taxa. (**C**) From left to right, genome size, GC content, and PQS density for different eukaryote host groups. For panels A through C, differences in average size, GC, and density values were assessed using Kruskal–Wallis rank sum tests and pairwise Wilcoxon rank-sum tests. Spearman correlation coefficients and their statistical significance are provided at the top of the scatterplots. Regression lines are shown in blue (P_{reg}, linear regression significance).

Finally, in our broad viral set, we detected a significant enrichment for PQSs in the negative (C-rich) strand of dsDNA, ssRNA, RT, and unclassified viruses but not for the ssDNA virus (Figure S1A, Supplementary Materials). The overall significance of this strand bias is likely diverse and complex.

Two recent functional studies suggested different and non-exclusive explanations. On one hand, Jaubert and colleagues showed that the formation of quadruplexes in the negative RNA strand of the hepatitis C virus is associated with impaired RNA synthesis [45]. On the other hand, Ding and colleagues outlined the strong bias for quadruplex sequences in the negative strand flanking the transcription start sites (TSS) in microorganisms (*Deinococcales* and *Thermales* bacterial orders), and correlated it with oxidation-dependent regulation of transcription [46].

The distribution of genome size, PQS density, GC content, and strand biases of the viruses with respect to their various hosts are reported in Figure 1C. Table 2 shows a balanced representation of the various host groups, after assessing an equivalent number of assemblies for vertebrate (2769), invertebrate (2930), and plant (2484) hosts. Within these large groups, several species are well represented. For example, in the large vertebrate group, there are numerous viruses infecting Cercopithecidae (58), Suidae (120), Bovidae (112), Pteropodidae (158), and rats (289), and over 40 avian viruses (Table S1, Supplementary Materials). Although the data were scarcer for protozoa and fungi (61 and 262 viruses, respectively), the viral genome sizes are longer in protozoa and very short in fungi and plants (Figure 1C). The PQS density is 2- to 3-fold higher in viruses infecting vertebrate hosts than any other host (Table 3). Viruses infecting plants seem particularly G4-poor (only 261 PQSs found in over 2000 genomes), with the exception of many mosaic viruses (the okra, grapevine, and chayote mosaic viruses carry over five PQSs in ≈6 kbp genomes; Table S1, Supplementary Materials). When PQSs are examined versus the host taxa, a significant excess of PQSs is again observed on the viral negative (C-rich) strand for all viruses (Figure S1B, Supplementary Materials).

Table 3. Genome metrics and quadruplex sequences classified by host group.

Host	Assemblies	Median % GC	Median Genome Size (bp)	Total PQS Count	Mean PQS Density [1]
Vertebrates	2769	44.4	5079	7945	0.082
Human [2]	1144	42.3	4325	1410	0.076
Invertebrates	2930	42.4	4534	442	0.024
Protozoa	61	46.1	6038	618	0.024
Fungi	292	49.2	3147	41	0.039
Plants	2484	43.2	2759	262	0.027

[1] Number of PQSs per kilo base pair (PQS/kbp); [2] Host group included in the Vertebrates group.

2.2. Thermodynamically Stable G4 Motifs are Enriched in Viral Genomes

To examine in more detail the nature of the quadruplex motifs, we inspected loop lengths and nucleotide compositions (irrespective of their position) for the dsDNA (11,315 PQSs), ssDNA (102 PQSs), ssRNA (553 PQSs), RT (85 PQSs), and bulk unclassified (206 PQSs) viruses. Unfortunately, the few PQSs identified in the dsRNA and satellite viruses were insufficient to pursue such in-depth analyses. As shown in Figure 2A,B, the PQS loop features differ. In the most represented vertebrate-infecting viruses, we counted 2555 different loop sequences, but 393 in the invertebrates, 648 in the protozoa, and only 66 and 52 in the fungus- and plant-infecting viruses, respectively. The median loop size is 3 nucleotides across all viral taxa, with the exception of retro-transcribing (RT) viruses which carry slightly larger loops (4 nt, all pairwise Wilcoxon rank-sum tests adj$P$ < 0.01; upper panel Figure 2A). Fungus and plants viruses also bear significantly larger loop size, frequently reaching 6–7 nt (Figure 2A), with a median value of 4 nt (all pairwise Wilcoxon rank-sum tests adj$P$ < 0.01 except Fungi-Plants adj$P$ = 0.542; lower panel Figure 2A). Furthermore, these analyses indicated that retro-transcribing, plant-infecting, and fungus-infecting viruses also show more heterogenous loop distributions than other groups (Figure 2B). Intriguingly, as previously observed in a large spectrum of eukaryotic species [36], quadruplex motifs with single-nucleotide loops are predominant both when scanned by viral taxon (upper panel, Figure 2B) or host group (lower panel, Figure 2B). Quantitatively, the single

A/T/C or G loops account for 34% of all loops when scanning by viral taxon (median value; Figure 2C) or 31% when searching the hosts genomes (median value; Figure 2C).

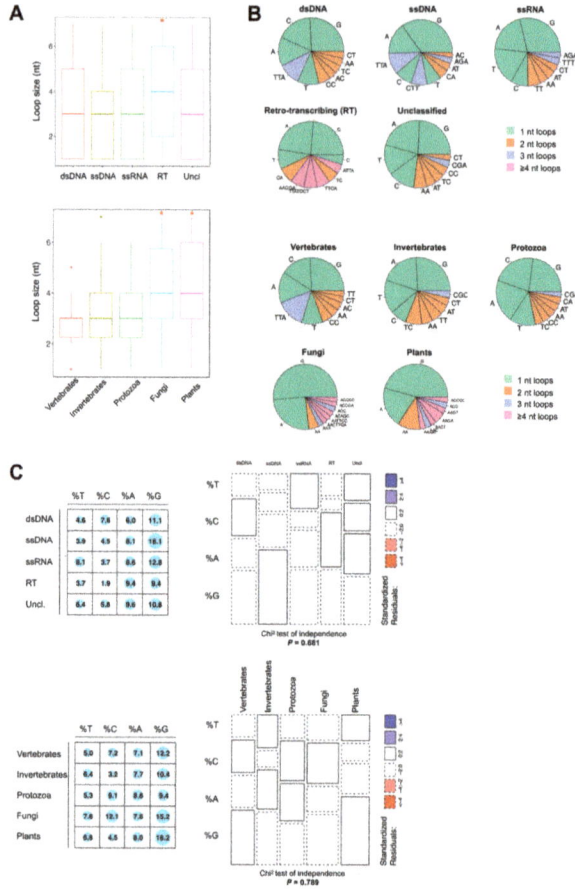

Figure 2. Quadruplex loop composition in viral genomes. (**A**) Boxplots show G-quadruplex (G4) motif loop size (in nucleotides) for each group. Top panel, for different viral taxa; bottom panel, for different host groups. Kruskal–Wallis rank sum test $P = 0.0001$ and $P = 8.19 \times 10^{-6}$ respectively; *, all pairwise Wilcoxon rank-sum tests adj$P < 0.01$. (**B**) Frequencies of 1–7 nucleotide loops, irrespective of their position within the G4 motif. Top panel, five taxa in which a significant number of G4 sequences were found: dsDNA viruses (n = 2758 assemblies, 11,315 PQSs), ssDNA viruses (n = 988 assemblies, 102 PQSs), ssRNA viruses (n = 1784 assemblies, 553 PQSs), Retro-transcribing viruses (n = 153 assemblies, 85 PQSs), and Unclassified viruses (n = 1217 assemblies, 253 PQSs). Bottom panel, five eukaryotic host taxa used in the analyses: vertebrates (n = 2,769 assemblies, 7945 PQSs), invertebrates (n = 2930 assemblies, 1410 PQSs), protozoa (n = 61 assemblies, 618 PQSs), fungi (n = 292 assemblies, 41 PQSs), and plants (n = 2484 assemblies, 261 PQSs). (**C**) Top panel and from left to right, graphical matrix where each cell contains a dot whose size reflects the relative magnitude of nucleotide proportions by viral taxa and mosaic plot of the contingency table used to perform a chi-square independence test (non-significant, $P = 0.681$); bottom panel and for left panel to right, similar for each host group (chi-square independence test non-significant, $P = 0.789$).

Thus, based on the rather short length of the loops, there is an overall bias for the most thermodynamically stable G4 motifs in viral genomes, similar to other genomes [31,34–36]. However, considering this large classification level, there is no significant difference in the distribution of single-nucleotide loop motifs between viral taxa (chi-square independence test non-significant, $P = 0.681$; upper panel Figure 2C) nor host group (chi-square independence test non-significant, $P = 0.789$; lower panel Figure 2C). Nevertheless, there is a striking resemblance in the distribution and frequency of the loop nucleotides when comparing dsDNA viruses and their vertebrate hosts: 9 out of the 10 most frequent loops are the same in both sets (G, C, A, TTA, T, CC, AA, AC, and CT loops), and are distributed in similar proportions (Figure 2B). Among dsDNA viruses, herpesviruses are particularly enriched for short-looped quadruplex motifs, which account for 35% of all PQSs (2,355 G4-L1-3 motifs, that is, the loop size is comprised between 1 and 3 nt (Table S2, Supplementary Materials).

2.3. The PQS Loop Composition Within the Herpesviridae Family of Viruses and Their Host are Correlated

Since herpesviruses infect different animal hosts, including mammals, birds, reptiles, fish, amphibians, and invertebrate animals [47], we examined in more detail the relationship between the viral and host PQSs. For this purpose, we retrieved all the available herpesvirus assemblies (n = 93 genomes). These include viruses in 65 mammals, 11 birds or reptiles, 6 fish, 4 amphibians, and 7 invertebrates (Table S2, Supplementary Materials). The PQS genome metrics for these 93 assemblies are reported in Figure S3A (Supplementary Materials). While the PQS occurrence and GC content remain strongly correlated (Spearman's *rho* = 0.73, non-parametric test for association between paired samples $P = 1.2 \times 10^{-15}$; Figure S3B, Supplementary Materials), we found no linear relationship between PQS content and genome size within this subset of viruses (Spearman's *rho* = 0.10, $P = 0.38$; Figure S3B, Supplementary Materials). However, there are significant differences in the nucleotide loop composition depending on the animal host (Figure 3A). Furthermore, single-nucleotide loops are unevenly distributed when looking at different host species (chi-square independence test $P = 0.00619$; Figure 3B). Single G loops are largely prevalent in herpesviruses infecting fish, amphibians, and invertebrates (50%, 56%, and 63% of all single-nucleotide loops, respectively). In addition, single C loops were undetected in the latter, and was marginal in the first two groups (9% in fish hosts and 3% in amphibian hosts). To a lesser extent, single T loops are more frequent in viruses infecting vertebrate hosts (on average 16% of all single-nucleotide loops) than invertebrates (8% of all single-nucleotide loops). Interestingly, the observed trends recapitulate the same existent biases in the host species (Figure 3, panels C,D): for instance, the analysis of the loop composition of short-looped G4 motifs in 52 eukaryote genomes (see Materials and Methods; Figure S4, Supplementary Materials) shows an enrichment for single G loops in amphibians and invertebrates as well as an accumulation of single T and C loops in mammals, birds, and reptiles, with the frequency of C-rich loops reaching its highest levels in viruses infecting mammals. Overall, we observed an excess of the frequency of PQSs with single pyrimidine loops in herpesviruses infecting vertebrate hosts. Interestingly, in vitro, these motifs fold into the most stable G4 structures [35,36].

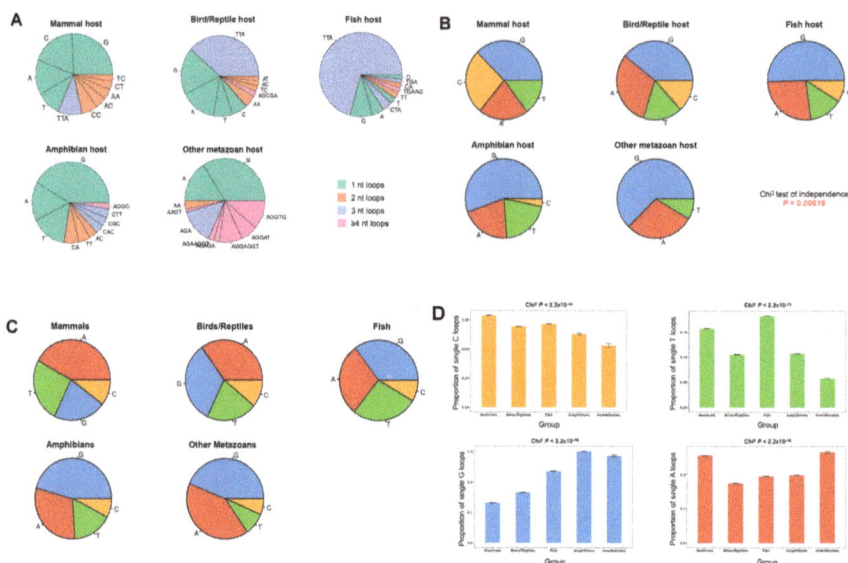

Figure 3. PQS loop content in Herpesviridae viruses and in various host animal genomes. (**A**) Most frequent N_{1-7} loops by host group. Mammals, n = 65 viruses; Birds/Reptiles, n = 11 viruses; Fish, n = 6 viruses; Amphibians, n = 4 viruses; and Invertebrates, n = 7 viruses. (**B**) Single-nucleotide loop frequencies by host group. Blue, G loops; red, A loops; orange, C loops; and green, T loops, irrespective of their positions with the G4 sequence. Chi-square independence tests were used to evaluate the significance of the association between loop proportions and host group. (**C**) Single-nucleotide loop frequencies in 52 eukaryote genomes. Mammals, n = 18 genomes; Birds/Reptiles, n = 9 genomes; Fish, n = 8 genomes; Amphibians, n = 3 genomes; and Invertebrates, n = 9 genomes. (**D**) Proportion of single C (orange, top panel), T (green, top panel), G (blue, bottom panel), or A (red, bottom panel) loops by eukaryote groups. Bars indicate the upper and lower bounds of the 95% confidence intervals. Chi-square independence tests were used to evaluate the significance of the association between loop proportions and group. All pairwise nominal independence adjusted *P*-values <0.05.

To further analyze this particular trend, we next performed an unsupervised classification, by principal component analysis, of herpesvirus assemblies based on loop composition information (Figure 4A; Materials and Methods). The first two principal components account for a restricted fraction of the sample's variance ($\approx$58%); however, quadruplex loop composition information allowed to discriminate between viruses infecting higher-order vertebrate or invertebrate hosts, mainly driven by differences in PQS^C content (Figure 4A). Indeed, we clearly observe two opposite trends in single-nucleotide loop distributions, with a significantly higher amount of single C loops in mammal-infecting viruses and, conversely, significantly more polyG sequences in invertebrate animals and amphibians (Figure 4B). These trends can be extended to the comparison of quadruplexes carrying identical loops of any size, as there is a negative correlation between G_{1-7} loop content and C_{1-7} loop content (Pearson's $r = -0.36$; Figure 4C).

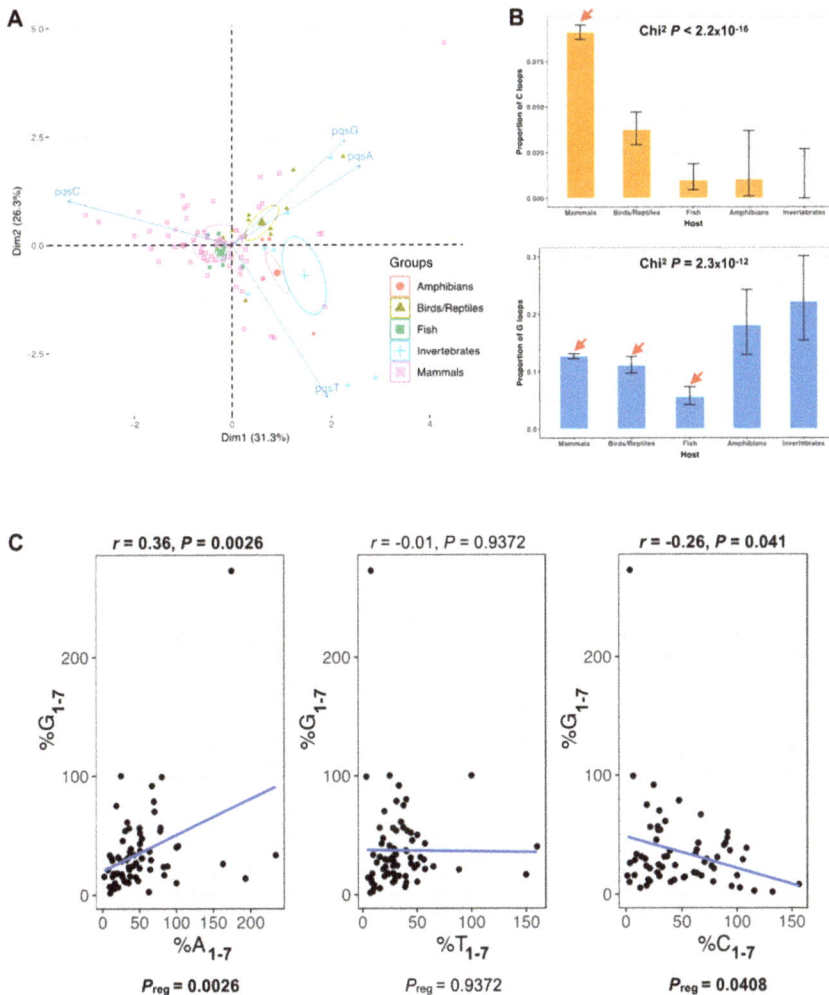

Figure 4. Herpesviridae viruses infecting mammalian hosts carry preferentially C-looped motifs. (**A**) Principal component analysis (PCA) performed on loop composition information (variables: PQS^A, PQS^T, PQS^C, PQS^G) for 93 herpesviruses, without using host group information. Ellipses indicate barycenters (weighted center of mass) for each host group. (**B**) Proportion of single C (orange, top panel) or G (blue, bottom panel) loops by host group. Bars indicate the upper and lower bounds of the 95% confidence intervals. Chi-square independence tests were used to evaluate the significance of the association between loop proportions and host group. Red arrows indicate groups with pairwise nominal independence adjusted *P*-values <0.05. (**C**) Relationship between PQS^A (PQS^T or PQS^C) motif and PQS^G motif contents. Pearson correlation coefficients are reported on each graph. Blue lines show linear regressions (P_{reg}, linear regression significance).

2.4. G4 Motifs in Viral Genomes Overlap Hosts' Transcription Factor Binding Sites

The prevalence of C-rich PQSs found in mammalian herpesviruses raises the question whether their functional role(s) are related to their potential to form a G4 structure, to the fact that they constitute a one-dimension target sequence for the binding of host's transcription factors, or to both.

Consistent with this view, we observed that 6 of the 10 most common viral PQS motifs matched several vertebrate transcription factor sites, notably SP1 and SP3 (Figure 5). Although C-rich loops appear relatively depleted in mammalian genomes, the annotation of G4 motifs, especially in humans, shows that quadruplexes with C-rich loops (and particularly single C loops) are highly enriched at gene promoters (Figure S5, Supplementary Materials). In silico analyses of the human genome have already revealed that G4 motifs often overlap with zinc-finger transcription factor binding sites (Figure S5, Supplementary Materials), such as SP1 [48]. This observation, together with the high frequency of C-rich loops in herpesviruses infecting mammals, supports the view that the herpesviruses hijack host transcription factors during the virus life cycle. Interestingly, human transcription factors that bind to these motifs also play roles in viral infection processes (SP factors [49]; EGR2 [50]). Moreover, it has been suggested that virus-associated PQSs can be recognized by human G4-binding proteins [51], which can participate in replication associated processes.

Motif search in PQS sequences found in Herpesviridae infecting Mammals	Sites found	Top hits found in the JASPAR CORE non-redundant vertebrate TF database
GGGTTAGGGTTAGGG e-value = 3.2e-274	852	No matches found
GSGGGCGCGGGSG e-value = 9.3e-23	511	Best match: **SP3** (Pearson correlation = 0.756)
GGGGGACGGGGRD e-value = 2.1e-32	411	Best matches: **SP1** (Pearson correlation = 0.760); **MZF1** (Pearson correlation = 0.902)
RSGGGGCCGGGGMK e-value = 1.3e-56	373	Best matches: **SP1** (Pearson correlation = 0.781); **SP2** (Pearson correlation = 0.761)
GCGTGGCCGGG e-value = 3.9e-2	178	Best matches: **EGR2** (Pearson correlation = 0.848); **EGR1** (Pearson correlation = 0.802); **GLI2** (Pearson correlation = 0.783);
GGGGAGGTCGCG e-value = 3.4e-4	155	Best matches: **ZBTB7B** (Pearson correlation = 0.750); **ZNF740** (Pearson correlation = 0.818)
TGGGCCTGGSS e-value = 6e-53	147	Best matches: **SP3** (Pearson correlation = 0.843); **KLF16** (Pearson correlation = 0.819); **KLF14** (Pearson correlation = 0.821);

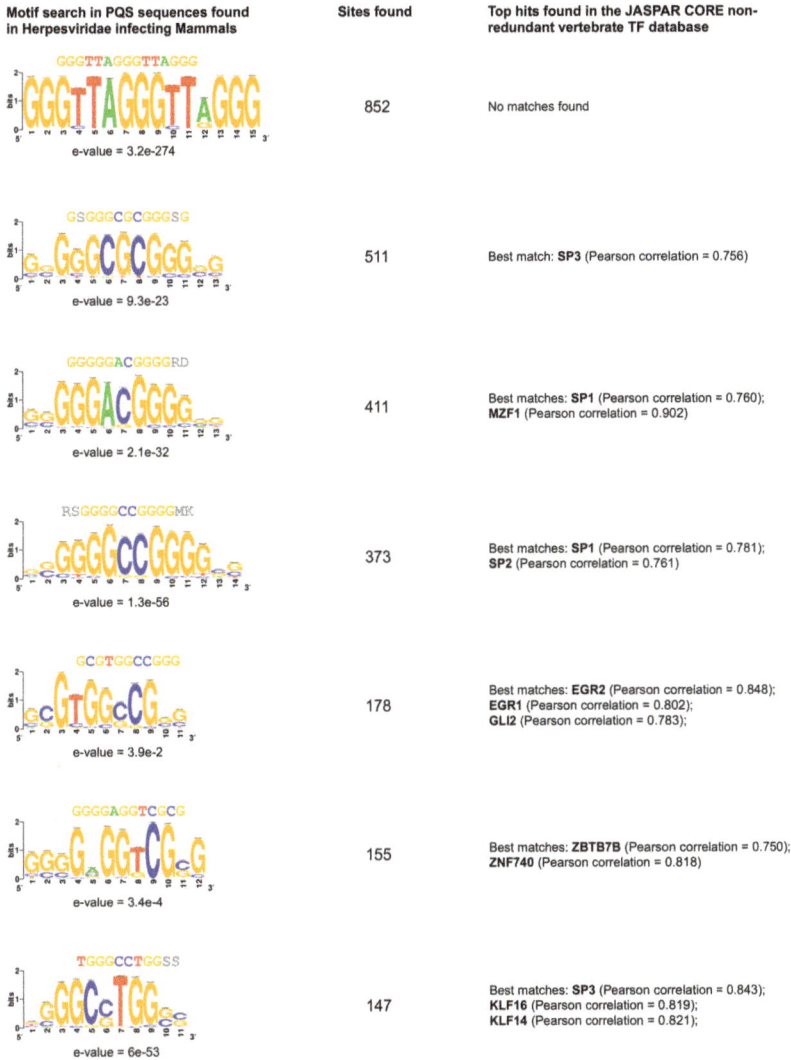

Figure 5. Consensus motif discovery in the quadruplex sequences found in mammalian herpesviruses. Top motifs found within the 5767 PQSs present in the 65 assemblies of herpesviruses infecting mammalian hosts. E-values are specified next to each sequence logo (the relative sizes of the letters indicate their frequency in the sequences and the total height of the letters depicts the information content of the position, in bits). The "Sites found" column indicates the number of times each particular motif was found in all the sequences.

2.5. High Prevalence of Telomere-Like PQSs across Herpesviridae Infecting Vertebrates

Another remarkable feature of the most frequent PQS loop composition is the excess of TTA loops that are frequent in viruses infecting mammals, birds, reptiles, and fish (Figure 3A), a loop composition that is also frequent in their hosts (Figure S4, Supplementary Materials). Of note, the TTA triplet is part of the TTAGGG telomere sequence in all vertebrates, able to form telomeric DNA G-quadruplexes [52]. It is also remarkable that the human herpesvirus 6A and 6B can integrate their linear genome into the telomeres of infected cells [53,54]. Thus, the presence/enrichment of these TTA-looped G4 sequences close to the viral genome extremities, their requirement for efficient virus integration [55], and the observation that G4 ligands can interfere with virus integration [54] point to the role played by these sequences in this crucial process that ensures virus maintenance in latently infected human cells. This potential for telomere integration is not exclusive to human herpesviruses, since it has been also described in the oncogenic Marek's disease alpha-herpesvirus, which infects chicken lymphocytes [56]. This particular virus also carries TTA-looped G4 repeats at the ends of its linear genome, and its pathogenicity partially depends on the efficiency of telomere integration [56]. Altogether, these observations suggest that the broad presence of viral TTA-looped quadruplex sequences might be functionally and evolutionary related to the telomere biology of the hosts. If so, the presence of viral G4s with TTA loops may help predict their integration potential.

3. Materials and Methods

3.1. Genome Assembly Retrieval

The full-length sequences were retrieved from the viruSITE resource [43]. A total of 7370 sequences were analyzed, including exclusively curated assemblies extracted from numerous resources (NCBI RefSeq, UniProtKB, GO, ViralZone, PubMed). Assemblies were classified either by virus taxonomy (dsDNA viruses, dsRNA viruses, retro-transcribing viruses, satellites, ssDNA viruses, ssRNA viruses, unclassified viruses, virus-associated RNAs) or by host group (Vertebrates, Invertebrates, Protozoa, Fungi, Plants). Classification by host group was refined using the Virus-Host DB [57] resource information.

3.2. Genome Metrics

For each of the 7370 assemblies, genome size (in base pairs, bp) and total GC content (GC content was defined as the sum of G and C nucleotides in the respective assembly) were evaluated using bash and Perl scripts. Spearman's rank correlation tests were used to assess correlations between the different variables.

3.3. G-Quadruplex Motif Identification and Loop Composition Analysis

We define a G-quadruplex motif as a sequence with at least four runs of 3+ guanines, separated by loop sequences containing one to seven nucleotides, that may themselves be guanines. Terminal guanines were excepted as loop sequences (i.e., the motif -GGGGGATCGCTGGGG- was evaluated has having an ATCGCT loop sequence flanked by GGGGG/GGGG runs and not GATCGCTG flanked by GGGG/GGG runs). Nevertheless, single G loops were allowed in the search. We searched, by regular expression matching, for the motifs previously defined -(G{3,}[ATGC]{1,7}){3,}G{3,}- in the *fasta* file of each of the retrieved assemblies, in both DNA/RNA strands, as originally described by Huppert and Balasubramanian [5]. Then, the obtained G4 sequences were imported into the R environment [58] for further processing: PQS density was defined as the number of G4 motifs per kilo base pair (kbp), we then assessed motif strandness (present in the G-rich or in the C-rich strand), split motifs into G-runs and loop sequences, and created loop repertoires (nucleotide composition, length, number of occurrences within a given genome) by host species or by virus taxon. Chi-square independence tests were used to evaluate the significance of the association between loop proportions and host group/viral taxa, followed by pairwise nominal independence tests and Pearson's standardized residuals calculation.

3.4. Putative Quadruplex Sequence Analysis in Eukaryote Genomes

We also retrieved 52 eukaryote genome assemblies from the UCSC Genome Browser portal. These included:

- 18 mammals (Minke whale *balAcu1*, Marmoset *calJac3*, Dog *canFam3*, Green monkey *chlSab2*, Kangaroo rat *dipOrd1*, Wallaby *macEug2*, Crab-eating macaque *macFas5*, Mouse lemur *micMur2*, Mouse *mm10*, Gibbon *nomLeu3*, Bushbaby *otoGar3*, Baboon *papAnu2*, Orangutan *ponAbe2*, Rhesus macaque *rheMac8*, Golden snub-nosed monkey *rhiRox1*, Squirrel monkey *saiBol1*, Tarsier *tarSyr2*, Tree shrew *tupBel1*);
- 9 birds/reptiles (American alligator *allMis1*, Chicken *galGal5*, Painted turtle *chrPic1*, Garter snake *thaSir1*, Lizard *anoCar2*, Zebra finch *taeGut2*, Medium ground finch *geoFor1*, Turkey *melGal5*, Budgerigar *melUnd1*);
- 8 fish (Elephant shark *calMil1*, Zebrafish *danRer11*, Fugu *fr3*, Stickleback *gasAcu1*, Coelacanth *latCha1*, Medaka *oryLat2*, Lamprey *petMar2*, Tetraodon *tetNig2*);
- 3 amphibians (Tibetan frog *nanPar1*, African clawed frog *xenLae2*, *Xenopus tropicalis xenTro7*);
- 9 invertebrates (Apis mellifera apiMel3, Caenorhabditis elegans ce11, Caenorhabditis japonica caeJap1, Caenorhabditis brenneri caePb2, Caenorhabditis remanei caeRem3, Caenorhabditis briggsae cb3, Ciona intestinalis ci3, Drosophila melanogaster dm6, Pristionchus pacificus priPac1).

We searched for short-looped quadruplex sequences, by regular expression matching, -(G{3,}[ATGC]{1,3}){3,}G{3,}-, in the *fasta* file of each of the retrieved assemblies. We performed the same subsequent analyses as described for viral sequences. Canonical PQS content (-(G{3,}[ATGC]{1,7}){3,}G{3,}-) for the 12 species reported in Table 3 was retrieved from Marsico et al. [44] and densities were calculated, as before, counting the number of PQSs per kilo base pair.

3.5. Loop Composition Analysis in Herpesviruses

Principal component analysis (PCA) was implemented using the FactoMineR and factoextra packages in the R environment. The analysis was performed on loop composition information (variables: PQS^A, PQS^T, PQS^C, PQS^G; where PQS^X is a quadruplex motif containing at least one X_{1-7} loop, X = {A,T,C, or G}), after normalizing the data matrix (variables were centered and reduced). Correlation between PQS^A (PQS^T or PQS^C) loop content and PQS^G loop content was estimated by calculating Pearson correlation coefficients. Finally, pattern discovery within the quadruplex sequences found in mammalian herpesviruses or in promoter regions of the human reference genome *hg38* was performed using the RSAT software suite [59] with default settings. The set of significant motifs discovered (e-value <0.05) was compared to the JASPAR database of vertebrate non-redundant transcription factor binding motifs [60].

3.6. Statistics

All statistical analyses were performed in R 3.4.3 for Mac OS X [58], using the built-in stats library, and the additional pwr, rcompanion, FactoMineR and factoextra packages.

4. Conclusions

Here, we report the analyses of the putative G-quadruplex-forming sequence present in 7370 virus genome assemblies. We have used this exhaustive resource to examine the potential correlations with the G4 motifs of their biological host(s), taking into account the number of motifs per genome, the length of the nucleotide loops separating the G-tracks and their base composition. Remarkably, there is a predominance of single-nucleotide loop motifs in the paired viruses and animal host genomes. These G4s are the most thermodynamically stable quadruplexes, suggesting a high folding potential and stabilization in cells. We had previously observed a strong compositional bias in these sequences in eukaryotic genomes, disfavoring pyrimidine loops while resulting in the accumulation of less stable structures (carrying single A or G loops) [36]. Here, using the G4-rich Herpesviridae family of dsDNA viruses as a case study (6735 PQSs, representing 55% of all motifs found in the >7000 viral genomes), we demonstrate a correlation between G-quadruplex sequence composition in viruses and their hosts. Indeed, herpesviruses that infect mammals, birds, or fish frequently carry TTA-looped G4 sequences, the signature of telomeric G-quadruplexes in vertebrates, which can be associated with viral integration into the hosts' genomes [55]. Although telomeric integration of herpesviruses has been shown to occur in two vertebrate hosts, the high prevalence of TTA-looped G4 in the vertebrate-related Herpesviridae family suggests that this phenomenon could occur more frequently than anticipated. Likewise, there is an accumulation of C-looped quadruplexes in viruses infecting mammals, which in turn carry significantly more such sequences than other animals. In humans, PQSs having C-rich loops, while globally depleted throughout the genome, are exceptionally enriched in promoters, where they may provide transcription factor binding sites (e.g., SP1, SP2, and other zinc-finger TFs) [48] or else promote a defined structural fold having a defined impact in transcription [61]. Thus, viral genomes are enriched with PQSs of similar loop composition to those associated with functionally relevant regions in their host species. We do not actually know if specific viral nucleotide loop patterns could have been acquired accidentally from the host as a consequence of infection, or if there are long-term virus–host co-evolution processes that influence the emergence and maintenance of particular quadruplex sequences. If so, these sequences could regulate crucial steps in the viral cycle and could represent relevant druggable structures for new anti-viral therapeutic approaches. However, pursuing further analysis of the co-evolutionary aspects hinted in this study will demand additional virus identification and sequencing, especially those infecting protozoa or plants.

Supplementary Materials: The following are available online at http://www.mdpi.com/1420-3049/24/10/1942/s1, Figure S1: Quadruplex motifs found by viral genome classification and by strand, Figure S2: Quadruplex motifs found in eukaryotes, by strand, Figure S3: Genome metrics and PQS content in the Herpesviridae family of dsDNA viruses, Figure S4: G4 motif loop content in various eukaryotes, Figure S5: Consensus motif discovery in the quadruplex sequences found in promoter regions of the human genome, Table S1: G-quadruplex sequences (and coordinates) found in seven viral taxa, Table S2: Genome metrics and quadruplex sequences for 93 herpesvirus genomes.

Author Contributions: Conceptualization, E.P.L., A.L.-V., and A.N.; Methodology and investigation, E.P.L.; Data curation, E.P.L.; Formal analysis, E.P.L.; Validation, E.P.L., A.L.-V., and A.N.; Visualization, E.P.L.; Writing—Original Draft Preparation, E.P.L.; Writing—Review and Editing, E.P.L., A.L.-V., and A.N.; Supervision, A.L.-V. and A.N.; Funding Acquisition, A.L.-V. and A.N.

Funding: This work received funding from the Agence Nationale de la Recherche (ANR 14-CE35-0003-02 to A.N.) and the PIC3i program from the Institut Curie (n° 91730 "Prospects of Anticancer" to A.L.V. and A.N.). E.P.L. is a recipient of a doctoral fellowship from the French Ministry of Education, Research and Technology.

Conflicts of Interest: The authors declare no conflict of interest.

References

1. Gellert, M.; Lipsett, M.N.; Davies, DR. Helix formation by guanylic acid. *Proc. Natl. Acad. Sci. USA* **1962**, *48*, 2013–2018. [CrossRef] [PubMed]
2. Verma, A.; Halder, K.; Halder, R.; Yadav, V.K.; Rawal, P.; Thakur, R.K.; Mohd, F.; Sharma, A.; Chowdhury, S. Genome-wide computational and expression analyses reveal G-quadruplex DNA motifs as conserved cis-regulatory elements in human and related species. *J. Med. Chem.* **2008**, *51*, 5641–5649. [CrossRef]
3. Du, Z.; Zhao, Y.; Li, N. Genome-wide analysis reveals regulatory role of G4 DNA in gene transcription. *Genome Res.* **2008**, *18*, 233–241. [CrossRef] [PubMed]
4. Bugaut, A.; Balasubramanian, S. 5′-UTR RNA G-quadruplexes: Translation regulation and targeting. *Nucleic Acids Res.* **2012**, *40*, 4727–4741. [CrossRef]
5. Huppert, J.L.; Balasubramanian, S. Prevalence of quadruplexes in the human genome. *Nucleic Acids Res.* **2005**, *33*, 2908–2916. [CrossRef] [PubMed]
6. Bedrat, A.; Lacroix, L.; Mergny, J.L. Re-evaluation of G-quadruplex propensity with G4Hunter. *Nucleic Acids Res.* **2016**, *44*, 1746–1759. [CrossRef]
7. Maizels, N.; Gray, L.T. The G4 genome. *PLoS Genet.* **2013**, *9*, e1003468. [CrossRef] [PubMed]
8. Rhodes, D.; Lipps, H.J. G-quadruplexes and their regulatory roles in biology. *Nucleic Acids Res.* **2015**, *43*, 8627–8637. [CrossRef] [PubMed]
9. Kwok, C.K.; Merrick, C.J. G-Quadruplexes: Prediction, Characterization, and Biological Application. *Trends Biotechnol.* **2017**, *35*, 997–1013. [CrossRef] [PubMed]

10. Todd, A.K.; Johnston, M.; Neidle, S. Highly prevalent putative quadruplex sequence motifs in human DNA. *Nucleic Acids Res.* **2005**, *33*, 2901–2907. [CrossRef] [PubMed]
11. Métifiot, M.; Amrane, S.; Litvak, S.; Andreola, M.-L. G-quadruplexes in viruses: Function and potential therapeutic applications. *Nucleic Acids Res.* **2014**, *42*, 12352–12366. [CrossRef]
12. Lavezzo, E.; Berselli, M.; Frasson, I.; Perrone, R.; Palu, G.; Brazzale, A.R.; Richter, S.N.; Toppo, S. G-quadruplex forming sequences in the genome of all known human viruses: A comprehensive guide. *PLoS Comput Biol.* **2018**, *14*, e1006675. [CrossRef]
13. Harris, L.M.; Merrick, C.J. G-quadruplexes in pathogens: A common route to virulence control? *PLoS Pathog.* **2015**, *11*, e1004562. [CrossRef]
14. Ravichandran, S.; Kim, Y.E.; Bansal, V.; Ghosh, A.; Hur, J.; Subramani, V.K.; Pradhan, S.; Lee, M.K.; Kim, K.K.; Ahn, J.H. Genome-wide analysis of regulatory G-quadruplexes affecting gene expression in human cytomegalovirus. *PLoS Pathog.* **2018**, *14*, e1007334. [CrossRef] [PubMed]
15. Ruggiero, E.; Richter, S.N. G-quadruplexes and G-quadruplex ligands: targets and tools in antiviral therapy. *Nucleic Acids Res.* **2018**, *46*, 3270–3283. [CrossRef]
16. Sundquist, W.I.; Heaphy, S. Evidence for interstrand quadruplex formation in the dimerization of human immunodeficiency virus 1 genomic RNA. *Proc. Natl. Acad. Sci. USA* **1993**, *90*, 3393–3397. [CrossRef] [PubMed]
17. Perrone, R.; Nadai, M.; Poe, J.A.; Frasson, I.; Palumbo, M.; Palù, G.; Smithgall, T.E.; Richter, S.N. Formation of a unique cluster of G-quadruplex structures in the HIV-1 Nef coding region: Implications for antiviral activity. *PLoS ONE* **2013**, *8*, e73121. [CrossRef]
18. Perrone, R.; Nadai, M.; Frasson, I.; Poe, J.A.; Butovskaya, E.; Smithgall, T.E.; Palumbo, M.; Palù, G.; Richter, S.N. A dynamic G-quadruplex region regulates the HIV-1 long terminal repeat promoter. *J. Med. Chem.* **2013**, *56*, 6521–6530. [CrossRef]
19. Amrane, S.; Kerkour, A.; Bedrat, A.; Vialet, B.; Andreola, M.L.; Mergny, J.L. Topology of a DNA G-quadruplex structure formed in the HIV-1 promoter: A potential target for anti-HIV drug development. *J. Am. Chem Soc.* **2014**, *136*, 5249–5252. [CrossRef] [PubMed]
20. Krafčíková, P.; Demkovičová, E.; Halaganová, A.; Víglaský, V. Putative HIV and SIV G-Quadruplex Sequences in Coding and Noncoding Regions Can Form G-Quadruplexes. *J. Nucleic Acids.* **2017**, *2017*, 6513720. [CrossRef]
21. Norseen, J.; Johnson, F.B.; Lieberman, P.M. Role for G-quadruplex RNA binding by Epstein-Barr virus nuclear antigen 1 in DNA replication and metaphase chromosome attachment. *J. Virol.* **2009**, *83*, 10336–10346. [CrossRef] [PubMed]
22. Murat, P.; Zhong, J.; Lekieffre, L.; Cowieson, N.P.; Clancy, J.L.; Preiss, T.; Balasubramanian, S.; Khanna, R.; Tellam, J. G-quadruplexes regulate Epstein-Barr virus-encoded nuclear antigen 1 mRNA translation. *Nat. Chem. Biol.* **2014**, *10*, 5358–6410. [CrossRef] [PubMed]
23. Tluckova, K.; Marusic, M.; Tothova, P.; Bauer, L.; Sket, P.; Plavec, J.; Viglasky, V. Human papillomavirus G-quadruplexes. *Biochemistry* **2013**, *52*, 7207–7216. [CrossRef] [PubMed]
24. Marušič, M.; Hošnjak, L.; Krafčikova, P.; Poljak, M.; Viglasky, V.; Plavec, J. The effect of single nucleotide polymorphisms in G-rich regions of high-risk human papillomaviruses on structural diversity of DNA. *Biochim. Biophys. Acta Gen. Subj.* **2017**, *1861*, 1229–1236. [CrossRef] [PubMed]
25. Zahin, M.; Dean, W.L.; Ghim, S.J.; Joh, J.; Gray, R.D.; Khanal, S.; Bossart, G.D.; Mignucci-Giannoni, A.A.; Rouchka, E.C.; Jenson, A.B. Identification of G-quadruplex forming sequences in three manatee papillomaviruses. *PLoS ONE* **2018**, *13*, e0195625. [CrossRef] [PubMed]
26. Artusi, S.; Nadai, M.; Perrone, R.; Biasolo, M.A.; Palù, G.; Flamand, L.; Calistri, A.; Richter, S.N. The Herpes Simplex Virus-1 genome contains multiple clusters of repeated G-quadruplex: Implications for the antiviral activity of a G-quadruplex ligand. *Antiviral Res.* **2015**, *118*, 123–131. [CrossRef] [PubMed]
27. Biswas, B.; Kumari, P.; Vivekanandan, P. Pac1 Signals of Human Herpesviruses Contain a Highly Conserved G-Quadruplex Motif. *ACS Infect. Dis.* **2018**, *4*, 744–751. [CrossRef] [PubMed]
28. Lyonnais, S.; Gorelick, R.J.; Mergny, J.L.; Le Cam, E.; Mirambeau, G. G-quartets direct assembly of HIV-1 nucleocapsid protein along single-stranded DNA. *Nucleic Acids Res.* **2003**, *31*, 5754–5763. [CrossRef]
29. Musumeci, D.; Riccardi, C.; Montesarchio, D. G-Quadruplex Forming Oligonucleotides as Anti-HIV Agents. *Molecules* **2015**, *20*, 17511–17532. [CrossRef] [PubMed]

30. González, V.M.; Martín, M.E.; Fernández, G.; García-Sacristán, A. Use of Aptamers as Diagnostics Tools and Antiviral Agents for Human Viruses. *Pharmaceuticals (Basel)* **2016**, *9*, 78. [CrossRef]

31. Risitano, A.; Fox, K.R. Influence of loop size on the stability of intramolecular DNA quadruplexes. *Nucleic Acids Res.* **2004**, *32*, 2598–2606. [CrossRef] [PubMed]

32. Rachwal, P.A.; Brown, T.; Fox, K.R. Effect of G-tract length on the topology and stability of intramolecular DNA quadruplexes. *Biochimie* **2008**, *90*, 686–696. [CrossRef]

33. Guédin, A.; De Cian, A.; Gros, J.; Lacroix, L.; Mergny, J.L. Sequence effects in single-base loops for quadruplexes. *Biochemistry* **2007**, *46*, 3036–3044. [CrossRef] [PubMed]

34. Guédin, A.; Gros, J.; Alberti, P.; Mergny, J.L. How long is too long? Effects of loop size on G-quadruplex stability. *Nucleic Acids Res.* **2010**, *38*, 7858–7868. [CrossRef]

35. Piazza, A.; Adrian, M.; Samazan, F.; Heddi, B.; Hamon, F.; Serero, A.; Lopes, J.; Teulade-Fichou, M.P.; Phan, A.T.; Nicolas, A. Short loop length and high thermal stability determine genomic instability induced by G-quadruplex-forming minisatellites. *EMBO J.* **2015**, *34*, 1718–1734. [CrossRef]

36. Puig Lombardi, E.; Holmes, A.; Verga, D.; Teulade-Fichou, M.P.; Nicolas, A.; Londoño-Vallejo, A. Thermodynamically stable and genetically unstable G-quadruplexes are depleted in genomes across species. *Nucleic Acids Res.* **2019**. [accepted].

37. Siddiqui-Jain, A.; Grand, C.L.; Bearss, D.J.; Hurley, L.H. Direct evidence for a G-quadruplex in a promoter region and its targeting with a small molecule to repress c-MYC transcription. *Proc. Natl. Acad. Sci. USA* **2002**, *99*, 11593–11598. [CrossRef]

38. Sun, D.; Guo, K.; Rusche, J.J.; Hurley, L.H. Facilitation of a structural transition in the polypurine/polypyrimidine tract within the proximal promoter region of the human VEGF gene by the presence of potassium and G-quadruplex-interactive agents. *Nucleic Acids Res.* **2005**, *33*, 6070–6080. [CrossRef]

39. De Armond, R.; Wood, S.; Sun, D.; Hurley, L.H.; Ebbinghaus, S.W. Evidence for the presence of a guanine quadruplex forming region within a polypurine tract of the hypoxia inducible factor 1alpha promoter. *Biochemistry* **2005**, *44*, 16341–16350. [CrossRef] [PubMed]

40. Dai, J.; Dexheimer, T.S.; Chen, D.; Carver, M.; Ambrus, A.; Jones, R.A.; Yang, D. An intramolecular G-quadruplex structure with mixed parallel/antiparallel G-strands formed in the human BCL-2 promoter region in solution. *J. Am. Chem. Soc.* **2006**, *128*, 1096–1098. [CrossRef]

41. Fernando, H.; Reszka, A.P.; Huppert, J.; Ladame, S.; Rankin, S.; Venkitaraman, A.R.; Neidle, S.; Balasubramanian, S. A conserved quadruplex motif located in a transcription activation site of the human c-kit oncogene. *Biochemistry* **2006**, *45*, 7854–7860. [CrossRef] [PubMed]

42. Kropp, K.A.; Angulo, A.; Ghazal, P. Viral enhancer mimicry of host innate-immune promoters. *PLoS Pathog.* **2014**, *10*, e1003804. [CrossRef]

43. Stano, M.; Beke, G.; Klucar, L. viruSITE-integrated database for viral genomics. *Database (Oxford)* **2016**, *2016*, baw162. [CrossRef]

44. Marsico, G.; Chambers, V.S.; Sahakyan, A.B.; McCauley, P.; Boutell, J.M.; Di Antonio, M.; Balasubramanian, S. Whole genome experimental maps of DNA G-quadruplexes in multiple species. *Nucleic Acids Res.* **2019**, *47*, 3862–3874. [CrossRef] [PubMed]

45. Jaubert, C.; Bedrat, A.; Bartolucci, L.; Di Primo, C.; Ventura, M.; Mergny, J.L.; Amrane, S.; Andreola, M.L. RNA synthesis is modulated by G-quadruplex formation in Hepatitis C virus negative RNA strand. *Sci. Rep.* **2018**, *8*, 8120.

46. Ding, Y.; Fleming, A.M.; Burrows, C.J. Case studies on potential G-quadruplex-forming sequences from the bacterial orders *Deinococcales* and *Thermales* derived from a survey of published genomes. *Sci Rep.* **2018**, *8*, 15679. [CrossRef]

47. Davison, A.J.; Eberle, R.; Ehlers, B.; Hayward, G.S.; McGeoch, D.J.; Minson, A.C.; Pellett, P.E.; Roizman, B.; Studdert, M.J.; Thiry, E. The Order *Herpesvirales*. *Arch. Virol.* **2009**, *154*, 171–177. [CrossRef]

48. Todd, A.K.; Neidle, S. The relationship of potential G-quadruplex sequences in cis-upstream regions of the human genome to SP1-binding elements. *Nucleic Acids Res.* **2008**, *36*, 2700–2704. [CrossRef]

49. Khalil, M.I.; Ruyechan, W.T.; Hay, J.; Arvin, A. Differential effects of Sp cellular transcription factors on viral promoter activation by varicella-zoster virus (VZV) IE62 protein. *Virology* **2015**, *485*, 47–57. [CrossRef] [PubMed]

50. Tatarowicz, W.A.; Martin, C.E.; Pekosz, A.S.; Madden, S.L.; Rauscher, F.J., 3rd.; Chiang, S.Y.; Beerman, T.A.; Fraser, N.W. Repression of the HSV-1 latency-associated transcript (LAT) promoter by the early growth response (EGR) proteins: Involvement of a binding site immediately downstream of the TATA box. *J. Neurovirol.* **1997**, *3*, 212–224. [CrossRef] [PubMed]

51. Satkunanathan, S.; Thorpe, R.; Zhao, Y. The function of DNA binding protein nucleophosmin in AAV replication. *Virology* **2017**, *510*, 46–54. [CrossRef]

52. Parkinson, G.N.; Lee, M.P.; Neidle, S. Crystal structure of parallel quadruplexes from human telomeric DNA. *Nature* **2002**, *417*, 876–880. [CrossRef]

53. Pantry, S.N.; Medveczky, P.G. Latency, Integration, and Reactivation of Human Herpesvirus-6. *Viruses* **2017**, *9*, 194. [CrossRef]

54. Gilbert-Girard, S.; Gravel, A.; Artusi, S.; Richter, S.N.; Wallaschek, N.; Kaufer, B.B.; Flamand, L. Stabilization of telomere G-quadruplexes interferes with human herpesvirus 6A chromosomal integration. *J. Virol.* **2017**, *91*, e402–e417. [CrossRef] [PubMed]

55. Wallaschek, N.; Sanyal, A.; Pirzer, F.; Gravel, A.; Mori, Y.; Flamand, L.; Kaufer, B.B. The Telomeric Repeats of Human Herpesvirus 6A (HHV-6A) Are Required for Efficient Virus Integration. *PLoS Pathog.* **2016**, *12*, e1005666. [CrossRef]

56. McPherson, M.C.; Cheng, H.H.; Smith, J.M.; Delany, M.E. Vaccination and Host Marek's Disease-Resistance Genotype Significantly Reduce Oncogenic Gallid alphaherpesvirus 2 Telomere Integration in Host Birds. *Cytogenet Genome Res.* **2018**, *156*, 204–214. [CrossRef] [PubMed]

57. Mihara, T.; Nishimura, Y.; Shimizu, Y.; Nishiyama, H.; Yoshikawa, G.; Uehara, H.; Hingamp, P.; Goto, S.; Ogata, H. Linking virus genomes with host taxonomy. *Viruses* **2016**, *8*, 66. [CrossRef] [PubMed]

58. R Core Team. *R: A Language and Environment for Statistical Computing*; R Foundation for Statistical Computing: Vienna, Austria, 2018.

59. Thomas-Chollier, M.; Sand, O.; Turatsinze, J.V.; Janky, R.; Defrance, M.; Vervisch, E.; Brohée, S.; van Helden, J. RSAT: Regulatory sequence analysis tools. *Nucleic Acids Res.* **2008**, *36*, W119–W127. [CrossRef]

60. Khan, A.; Fornes, O.; Stigliani, A.; Gheorghe, M.; Castro-Mondragon, J.A.; van der Lee, R.; Bessy, A.; Chèneby, J.; Kulkarni, S.R.; Tan, G. JASPAR 2018: Update of the open-access database of transcription factor binding profiles and its web framework. *Nucleic Acids Res.* **2018**, *46*, D260–D266. [CrossRef]

61. Huppert, J.L.; Balasubramanian, S. G-quadruplexes in promoters throughout the human genome. *Nucleic Acids Res.* **2007**, *35*, 406–413. [CrossRef]

Sample Availability: Samples of the compounds are not available from the authors.

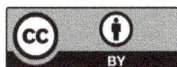

Communication

In Cellulo Protein-mRNA Interaction Assay to Determine the Action of G-Quadruplex-Binding Molecules

Rodrigo Prado Martins [1], Sarah Findakly [1], Chrysoula Daskalogianni [1,2],
Marie-Paule Teulade-Fichou [3], Marc Blondel [4,*] and Robin Fåhraeus [1,2,5,6,*]

[1] Université Paris 7, Inserm, UMR 1162, 75013 Paris, France; rodrigo.prado-martins@inserm.fr (R.P.M.); sarah.findakly@inserm.fr (S.F.); chrysoula.daskalogianni@inserm.fr (C.D.)

[2] ICCVS, University of Gdańsk, Science, ul. Wita Stwosza 63, 80-308 Gdańsk, Poland

[3] Chemistry, Modelling and Imaging for Biology, CNRS UMR9187-Inserm U1196, Institut Curie, Université Paris-Sud, F-91405, Orsay, France; mp.teulade-fichou@curie.fr

[4] GGB, Université de Brest, Inserm, CHRU Brest, EFS, UMR 1078, F-29200 Brest, France

[5] Department of Medical Biosciences, Umeå University, 90187 Umeå, Sweden

[6] RECAMO, Masaryk Memorial Cancer Institute, Zluty kopec 7, 65653 Brno, Czech Republic

* Correspondence: marc.blondel@univ-brest.fr (M.B.); robin.fahraeus@inserm.fr (R.F.); Tel.: +33-142-499-269 (R.F.)

Academic Editor: Sara N. Richter
Received: 8 November 2018; Accepted: 26 November 2018; Published: 29 November 2018

Abstract: Protein-RNA interactions (PRIs) control pivotal steps in RNA biogenesis, regulate multiple physiological and pathological cellular networks, and are emerging as important drug targets. However, targeting of specific protein-RNA interactions for therapeutic developments is still poorly advanced. Studies and manipulation of these interactions are technically challenging and in vitro drug screening assays are often hampered due to the complexity of RNA structures. The binding of nucleolin (NCL) to a G-quadruplex (G4) structure in the messenger RNA (mRNA) of the Epstein-Barr virus (EBV)-encoded EBNA1 has emerged as an interesting therapeutic target to interfere with immune evasion of EBV-associated cancers. Using the NCL-EBNA1 mRNA interaction as a model, we describe a quantitative proximity ligation assay (PLA)-based in cellulo approach to determine the structure activity relationship of small chemical G4 ligands. Our results show how different G4 ligands have different effects on NCL binding to G4 of the *EBNA1* mRNA and highlight the importance of in-cellulo screening assays for targeting RNA structure-dependent interactions.

Keywords: structure-activity relationship; protein-mRNA interactions; G-quadruplexes; PhenDC3; pyridostatin; EBNA1; Epstein-Barr virus (EBV)

1. Introduction

Accumulating evidence indicates an ever-expanding role for RNAs in regulating most aspects of cell biology that range from small non-coding RNAs to messenger RNAs (mRNAs). The more traditional role of mRNAs as "only messengers" is changing and new knowledge is emerging showing how the encoding sequences are taking on more diverse functions and can influence the activity of the encoded proteins. Most, if not all aspects of mRNAs, and this is presumably true also for non-coding RNAs, are governed by interactions with cellular proteins. These ribonucleoproteins (RNP) complexes control RNA metabolism and form scaffolds to orchestrate and organize protein networks and complex functional units [1]. Thus, interfering with specific protein-RNA complexes holds promise for new therapeutic developments as well as furthering our understanding of cell biological process. However, it is challenging to specifically target protein-RNA interactions (PRIs) for several reasons. One reason is that the interactions between proteins and RNAs, in particular mRNAs, are often dependent on RNA structures. However, the folding of RNAs, the chaperones involved, and how RNA-binding protein (RBP) specifically recognize certain RNA structures are still relatively unknown. New evidence that follows technical developments together with studies on disease-related single synonymous mutations have highlighted that folding of RNAs into 3D structures that serve as a protein-binding platform is a regulated and dynamic process encompassing relatively large sequences [2–6]. Thus, RNA structures from the same RNA sequence can be different in vitro as compared to in vivo, making it difficult to set up in vitro-based drug screening assays to identify compounds that interfere with specific PRIs.

G-quadruplexes (G4) are non-canonical nucleic acid structures based on the stacking of several G-quartets, further stabilized by cations positioned in the central channel of the G4 helix [7,8]. These structures are frequently found in eukaryotic transcripts [8] and their formation has been implicated in several steps of gene expression. Indeed, a relevant number of disease-related genes have been shown to be regulated by G4 structures and their RBP [9]. We have recently reported that nucleolin (NCL) directly binds G4 formed in the GAr-encoding sequence of the Epstein Barr virus (EBV) *EBNA1* mRNA (Figure 1A,B, see also Reference [10]). This interaction is critical for minimizing *EBNA1* mRNA translation and thereby the production of EBNA1-derived antigenic peptides for the major histocompatibility (MHC) class I pathway, allowing EBV-infected cells to evade the immune system [11]. As EBV is associated with several human cancers and as all EBV-infected cells express EBNA1, the *EBNA1* mRNA-NCL interaction represents an interesting target for developing drugs that aim to induce an immune response against EBV-related diseases. It also serves as a broader model for developing techniques required to study structured RNA-protein interactions. Here, we use the NCL-*EBNA1* mRNA interaction to illustrate how different compounds binding to the same G4 have specific effects on the interaction with NCL in cellulo. This illustrates a so far unknown role of G4 structures in mediating specific interactions with proteins, indicating that particular G4-protein interactions can be targeted specifically. We also report how to generate quantitative data using proximity ligation to verify the capacity of different G4 ligands to prevent NCL-*EBNA1* mRNA interactions and their role in controlling *EBNA1* mRNA translation.

2. Materials and Methods

2.1. Cell Culture, Transfection, and Drug Treatments

The human lung carcinoma cell line H1299 and the EBV-producing marmoset B-cell line B95-8 were cultured in RPMI-1640 supplemented with 10% fetal bovine serum (FBS), 2 mM L-glutamine, 100 U/mL penicillin, and 100 µg/mL streptomycin. H1299 transient transfections were performed using Genejuice reagent (Merck Bioscience, Darmstadt, Germany) according to manufacturer's protocol. All cells were cultured at 37 °C with 5% CO_2. For drug treatments, 10^5 B95-8 cells were incubated with 5 µM of PhenDC3 [12] or pyridostatin (PDS, Sigma-Aldrich (now Merck), Darmstadt, Germany) for 36 h. Drug stock solutions were prepared in DMSO (Euromedex, Strasbourg, France).

2.2. RNA In Situ Hybridization-Immunofluorescence (rISH-IF) and Immunofluorescence (IF)

H1299 cells were plated on 12-mm-diameter coverslips in 24-well plates and transfected with 200 ng of EBNA1 construct [13]. At 24 h post-transfection, cells were fixed with PBS 4% paraformaldehyde for 20 min and then washed with PBS for 10 min. For rISH-IF, samples were overnight incubated in 70% (*v/v*) ethanol at 4 °C. After rehydration in PBS for 30 min, samples were permeabilized with PBS 0.4% Triton X-100, 0.05% CHAPS for 10 min at room temperature, and pre-treated with hybridization buffer (10% formamide, 2X SSC, 0.2 mg/mL *E. coli* 522 tRNAs, 0.2 mg/mL sheared salmon sperm DNA and 2 mg/mL BSA) for 30 min at room temperature. Samples were then incubated overnight with 50 ng of an EBNA1-digoxigenin DNA probe (5′ CTTTCCAAACCACCCTCCTTTTTTGCGCCTGCCTCCATCAAAAA-digoxigenin 3′) in a humidified chamber at 37 °C. To avoid secondary structures, the probe was diluted in 5 µL of water, denaturated at 80 °C for 5 min, chilled on ice for 5 min, and resuspended in 35 µL of hybridization buffer. After hybridization, samples were serially washed for 20 min with 2X SSC 10% formamide, hybridization buffer (twice), 2X SSC, and PBS. Washes were carried out at room temperature, except with hybridization buffer (37 °C). Samples were saturated with PBS 3% BSA for 30 min and incubated with a mouse anti-digoxigenin (1/200, clone DI-22, Sigma) for 2 h at room temperature. A goat anti-mouse immunoglobulin G (IgG) secondary antibody conjugated to Alexa Fluor® 568 (Sigma) was used to detect immunocomplexes (1 h at 37 °C) and DAPI was used for nuclear counterstaining under standard conditions. For IF, fixed samples were saturated with PBS 3% BSA for 30 min, incubated with rabbit polyclonal antibody anti-NCL (1/1000, ab22758-Abcam) for 2 h and goat anti-rabbit Ig secondary antibody conjugated to Alexa Fluor® 488 (Sigma) for 1 h at 37 °C. DAPI was used for nuclear counterstaining.

2.3. Sequence of EBNA1 cDNA

The sequence of EBNA1 cDNA (GenBank: MG021311.1) is as follows (the GAr-encoding sequence which forms G4 is highlighted in cyan):

ATGTCTGACGAGGGACCAGGTACAGGACCTGGAAATGGCCTAGGACAGAAGGAAGACAC
ATCTGGACCAGACGGCTCCAGCGGCAGTGGACCTCAAAGAAGAGGGGGGGGATAACCATGGAC
GAGGACGGGGAAGAGGACGAGGACGAGGAGGCGGAAGACCAGGAGCTCCGGGCGGCTCAG
GATCAGGGCCAAGACATAGAGATGGTGTCCGGAGACCCCAAAAACGTCCAAGTTGCATTGGC
TGCAAAGGGGCCCACGGTGGAACAGGAGCAGGAGGAGGGGCAGGAGCAGGAGGGGCAGGA
GCAGGAGGAGGGGCAGGAGCAGGAGGAGGGGCAGGAGCAGGAGGAGCAGGAGGAGGGGC
AGGAGCAGGAGGAGGGGCAGGAGCAGGAGGAGGGGCAGGAGCAGGAGGAGGGGCAGGAG
CAGGAGGAGGGGCAGGAGCAGGAGGAGGGGCAGGAGGAGGAGGAGGGGCAGGAGCAGGA
GGAGGGGCAGGAGCAGGAGGAGGGGCAGGAGCAGGAGGAGGGGCAGGAGGGGCAGGAGC
AGGAGGAGGGGCAGGAGCAGGAGGAGGGGCAGGAGCAGGAGGAGGGGCAGGAGCAGGAG
GGGCAGGAGCAGGAGGAGGGGCAGGAGCAGGAGGGGCAGGAGCAGGAGGAGGGGCAGGA
GCAGGAGGAGGGGCAGGAGCAGGAGGGGCAGGAGCAGGAGGGGCAGGAGCAGGAGGGGC
AGGAGCAGGAGGGGCAGGAGGAGGAGGAGCAGGAGGGGCAGGAGGGGCAGGAGCAGGAG
GGGCAGGAGGGGCAGGAGCAGGAGGAGGGGCAGGAGGGGCAGGAGCAGGAGGAGGGGCA
GGAGGGGCAGGAGCAGGAGGGGCAGGAGGGGCAGGAGCAGGAGGGGCAGGAGGGGCAGG
AGCAGGAGGGGCAGGAGGGGCAGGAGCAGGAGGAGGGGCAGGAGCAGGAGGGGCAGGAG
CAGGAGGTGGAGGCCGGGGTCGAGGAGGCAGTGGAGGCCGGGGTCGAGGAGGTAGTGGA
GGCCGGGGTCGAGGAGGTAGTGGAGGCCGCCGGGGTAGAGGACGTGAAAGAGCCAGGGGG
GGAAGTCGTGAAAGAGCCAGGGGGGAGAGGTCGTGGACGTGGTGAAAAGAGGCCCAGGAGT
CCCAGTAGTCAGTCATCATCATCCGGGTCTCCACCGCGCAGGCCCCCTCCAGGTAGAAGGCC
ATTTTTCCACCCTGTAGGGGAAGCCGATTATTTTGAATACCACCAAGAAGGTGGCCCAGATGG
TGAGCCTGACATGCCCCCGGGAGCGATAGAGCAGGGCCCCGCAGATGACCCAGGAGAAGGC
CCAAGCACTGGACCCCGGGGTCAGGGTGATGGAGGCAGGCGCAAAAAAGGAGGGTGGTTT
GGAAAGCATCGTGGTCAAGGAGGTTCCAACCAGAAATTTGAGAACATTGCAGAAGGTTTAAG
AACTCTCCTGGCTAGGTGTCACGTAGAAAGGACTACCGATGAAGGAACTTGGGTCGCCGGTG
TGTTCGTATATGGAGGTAGTAAGACCTCCCTTTACAACCTCAGGCGAGGAATTGCCCTTGCTAT
TCCACAATGTCGTCTTACACCATTGAGTCGTCTCCCCTTTGGAATGGCCCCTGGACCCGGCCCA
CAACCTGGCCCACTAAGGGAGTCCATTGTCTGTTATTTCATTGTCTTTTTACAAACTCATATATTT
GCTGAGGGTTTGAAGGATGCGATTAAGGACCTTGTTATGCCAAAGCCCGCTCCTACCTGCAATA
TCAAGGCGACTGTGTGCAGCTTTGACGATGGAGTAGATTTGCCTCCCTGGTTTCCACCTATGGT
GGAAGGGGCTGCCGCGGAGGGTGATGACGGAGATGACGGAGATGAAGGAGGTGATGGAG
ATGAGGGTGAGGAAGGGCAGGAGTGA

2.4. Proximity Ligation Assay (PLA)

H1299 cells were plated and fixed as previously described. For experiments using B95-8, 12-mm-diameter coverslips were coated with poly-L-lysine 0.01% (Sigma) for 30 min and air-dried for 5 min in 24-well plates. B-cells were then resuspended in PBS, plated on pre-treated coverslips and incubated for 2 h at room temperature. After a wash with PBS for 5 min, cells were fixed with PBS 4% paraformaldehyde for 20 min and re-washed with PBS for 10 min. Following fixation, both cell lines were processed for in situ hybridization according to the rISH-IF protocol. Samples were then saturated with PBS 3% BSA for 30 min and incubated for 2 h at room temperature with a mix of primary antibody containing the mouse anti-digoxigenin and the rabbit anti-nucleolin previously described. Subsequently, PLA was carried out using the Duolink PLA in situ kit (Sigma), anti-rabbit plus and anti-mouse minus probes (Sigma) following the manufacturer's protocol.

2.5. Microscopy and Image Analysis

Samples were examined with an LSM 800 confocal laser microscope (Carl Zeiss MicroImaging, Jena, Germany). ImageJ [14] was used for analysis of images. PLA signals were quantified in 100 cells per sample according to the protocol provided as Supplementary materials. Data analysis was carried out by ANOVA with Tukey HSD test using GraphPad Prism 5 for Windows (GraphPad Software, San Diego, CA, USA). Data shown are mean $\pm$ SD of three independent experiments.

3. Results and Discussion

3.1. Detection of EBNA1 mRNA and NCL by rISH-IF and IF

EBNA1 is essential for EBV genome maintenance and, as such, is expressed in all EBV-carrying cells, including cancers. Because EBNA1 is highly antigenic, EBV has evolved a sophisticated strategy to evade the immune detection of latently infected cells by limiting *EBNA1* mRNA translation and, as a consequence, by minimizing the production of antigenic peptides for the major histocompatibility (MHC) class I pathway [13]. Nucleolin (NCL) directly binds G4 structures in the GAr (the glycine-alanine rich domain of EBNA1)-coding sequence of the *EBNA1* mRNA and this is essential for suppressing the translation of the *EBNA1* mRNA and the production of antigenic peptides (Figure 1A,B). A small G4 ligand, PhenDC3, can displace NCL from the *EBNA1* message and augment its translation, thereby increasing the production of antigenic peptides and triggering $CD8^+$ T cell response [11]. Interestingly, another study based on in vitro translation showed that pyridostatin (PDS), another G4-binding compound frequently used as benchmark, instead further suppressed *EBNA1* mRNA translation [15]. This observation is surprising, as it has previously not been appreciated that G4 ligands can have different effects on the function of the G4 or on their interaction with cellular factors. In this context, G4 structures might be targeted in a specific way by therapeutic intervention, opening a so far unknown field of drug target validation in cellulo. In order to shed light on the apparent discrepancy between how different G4 ligands act on the NCL-*EBNA1* mRNA interaction and thus their potential use as compounds that can trigger an immune reaction against EBV-carrying cancers, we developed a protocol based on proximity ligation (Figure 1C,D). This approach allows us to overcome difficulties with RNA folding in vitro to quantitatively study endogenous protein-mRNA interactions in cellulo and to avoid using large tags and overexpression system. By combining in-cellulo data with in vitro assays, this approach has the advantage of providing a straightforward and easy confirmation of the relevance of in vitro studies based on recombinant proteins and synthetic RNAs with in vivo data. In addition, we developed a method to quantify protein-mRNA interactions, which could allow structure-activity relationship (SAR) studies in cellulo to be carried out on a specific RNA-protein interaction.

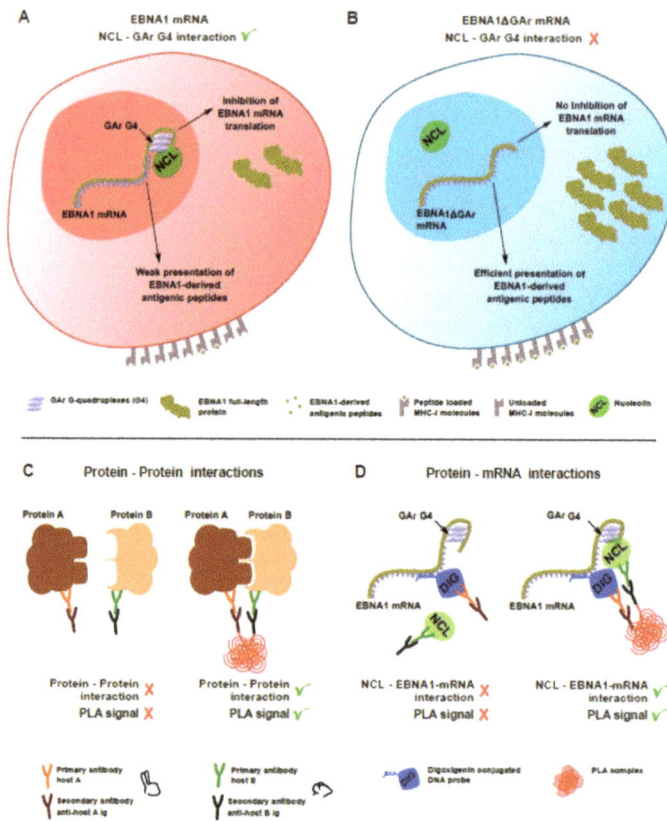

Figure 1. (**A**) cartoon depicting the interaction between nucleolin (NCL) and the G4 formed in the GAr-encoding sequence of *EBNA1* mRNA. This interaction is crucial for EBNA1/Epstein-Barr virus (EBV) immune evasion as it inhibits both *EBNA1* mRNA translation and the production of EBNA1-derived antigenic peptides, hence limiting the production of EBNA1 to the minimal level to fulfill its essential role in maintenance and replication of the viral genome and, at the same time, allowing EBNA1 to evade the immune system. (**B**) If the interaction between EBNA1 G4 and NCL is compromised or lost (e.g., when EBNA1ΔGAr, a form of EBNA1 deleted for its GAr domain, is expressed), then full length EBNA1ΔGAr protein as well as EBNA1-derived antigenic peptides are expressed at a higher level, leading to recognition of EBV-infected cells by the immune system of the host. (**C**) Schematic depicting the principle of the proximity ligation assay (PLA) between two proteins (or two epitopes of the same protein). (**D**) Schematic depicting the adaptation of the PLA to visualize protein/mRNA interactions in cellulo.

The proximity ligation assay (PLA) was originally conceived to detect proteins in close proximity. For this, one pair of primary antibodies raised in two different species is used to target the two proteins of interest (Figure 1C). Afterwards, DNA strand-conjugated secondary antibodies and enzymatic reactions are employed to generate fluorescent reporter molecules [16]. Since we aimed to explore a protein-mRNA interaction, a hybridization step was added in order to tag the mRNA of interest with a complex recognizable by antibodies (Figure 1D). A similar approach has been reported for DNA-protein interactions [17]. Therefore, as an initial step, EBV negative cells transfected, or not, with an EBNA1 construct were analyzed by RNA in situ hybridization coupled to immunofluorescence (rISH-IF). This enabled us to first validate the hybridization conditions using the digoxigenin-labelled EBNA1 probe and the mouse anti-digoxigenin primary antibody to be employed in the PLA (Figure 2A).

IF was also performed to determine the appropriate conditions for detecting endogenous NCL using a rabbit anti-NCL antibody (Figure 2B). Altogether, these assays demonstrated an accumulation of NCL and *EBNA1* mRNA in the nucleus.

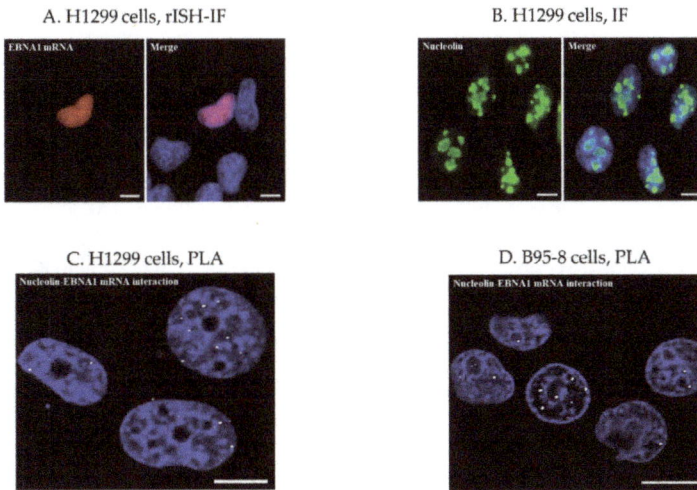

A. H1299 cells, rISH-IF

B. H1299 cells, IF

C. H1299 cells, PLA

D. B95-8 cells, PLA

Figure 2. Use of PLA for the study of a protein-mRNA interaction. (A) H1299 cells were transfected with *EBNA1* and analyzed by RNA in situ hybridization-immunofluorescence (rISH-IF) to verify the specificity of the *EBNA1*-digoxigenin probe and to validate the detection of probe-mRNA complexes using a mouse anti-digoxigenin antibody. Immunocomplexes were detected using an anti-mouse Alexa Fluor® 568-conjugated secondary antibody, revealing the accumulation of *EBNA1* mRNA in the nucleus. *EBNA1* mRNA is depicted in red. (**B**) Immunofluorescence (IF) was performed in H1299 cells using a rabbit anti-nucleolin antibody to set up the appropriate conditions for detection of endogenous NCL. The expected labelling of NCL in the nucleolus was confirmed. (**C**) PLA in *EBNA1*-transfected H1299 cells using mouse anti-digoxigenin and rabbit anti-nucleolin tested in (A) and (B). Anti-rabbit and anti-mouse Ig PLA probes were used following the manufacturer's protocol to generate PLA complexes depicted as white dots. Each dot represents an interaction between NCL and *EBNA1* mRNA. (**D**) The EBV-transformed B-cell line B95-8 was tested for endogenous NCL-*EBNA1* mRNA interaction under the same conditions used in (**C**). PLA uncovered this interaction in the nuclear compartment as in *EBNA1*-transfected H1299 cells shown in (**C**). Scale bars represent 10 μm.

3.2. Analysis of NCL-EBNA1 mRNA Interactions by Proximity Ligation

PLA was then carried out to detect the NCL-*EBNA1* mRNA interactions in situ using either transfected cells or EBV-infected cells. PLA complexes are depicted as white dots and each dot represents an interaction between NCL and *EBNA1* mRNA. In line with rISH-IF and IF results, interactions were uncovered in or at the close vicinity of the nuclear compartment of EBNA1-transfected cells (Figure 2C) and EBV-transformed lymphoblastic B95-8 cells (Figure 2D), confirming that NCL binds EBNA1 mRNA in the nucleus of virus-carrying cells. During and after transcription, mRNAs undergo a complex maturation process relying on a large repertoire of RBP and indeed, protein-mRNA interactions control pivotal steps of mRNA biogenesis and function [18]. In addition, evidence is accumulating that these interactions play a broader role in cellular processes, regulating multiple enzymatic and metabolic activities [19]. Hence, these results denote that EBV exploits host cell mRNA maturation process/es in order to hamper translation and thus immune responses.

3.3. Use of Quantitative PLA to Evaluate the Effect of RNA-Binding Drugs on NCL-EBNA1 mRNA Interactions

An estimated 2–3% of cancers are associated with EBV, making GAr-based EBNA1 immune evasion an important target for therapeutic approaches against EBV-related cancers [20,21]. Therefore, the binding of NCL to G4 in *EBNA1* mRNA represents a promising target for novel therapeutic strategies aimed at stimulating immune recognition of EBV-carrying cancers. This, and the fact that different compounds bind the G4 of the *EBNA1* mRNA, makes this an interesting model system for the identification of compounds that interfere with a specific RNA-protein interaction. Since NCL binds specifically G4 within EBNA mRNA [11], we treated, or not, B95.8 cells with the G4 ligands PDS or PhenDC3 (Figure 3) and evaluated the effect of treatments on this interaction using PLA. Of note, PhenDC3, but not PDS, reduced the NCL-*EBNA1* mRNA interaction (Figure 4A). This is surprising as both compounds bind strongly the *EBNA1* mRNA G4 structure in vitro [11,22]. In addition, a previous report has shown that PDS suppresses EBNA1 synthesis in vitro [15], while PhenDC3 increases the levels of EBNA1 in cellulo [11]. Altogether, these contrasting results indicate that different G4 ligands may induce distinct biological responses and complementary assays are required to determine the activity of these compounds in the cellular context. To refine this finding, we developed a protocol to quantify PLA results using the public domain image processing program ImageJ (Figure 4B and Supplementary materials). As advantages, quantitative PLA generates information suitable for statistical tests, avoids subjective data interpretation, and enables the estimation of differences less evident by the comparison of single images. This approach revealed a remarkable difference between the ability of PDS and PhenDC3 in preventing the NCL-*EBNA1* mRNA interaction (Figure 4C). It has been reported that by binding to an RNA fold, small molecules can alter RNA structure, inhibiting or enhancing protein-RNA associations [23]. Therefore, one could speculate that PDS and PhenDC3 may modify G4 structure in a different way, thereby preventing, or not, the binding of NCL, which can help to explain the discrepancy between these two G4 ligands. Alternatively, the difference between these two compounds in their ability to prevent NCL binding to G4 of *EBNA1* mRNA may be due to differential affinities for these G4. In line with this hypothesis, we have previously observed that PDS binding affinity for EBNA1 G4 is significantly weaker when compared to PhenDC3 as evaluated by G4-FID assay: DC_{50} (PDS) ≈ 0.47 μM; DC_{50} (PhenDC3) ≈ 0.26 μM. This was further confirmed by the thermal stabilization values (ΔTm) measured by the FRET-melting assay on EBNA1 G4 (ΔTm PDS = 14.3 °C; ΔTm PhenDC3 = 20.5 °C [11]. Although the two assays are calibrated for selecting high affinity binders, the difference is nonetheless significant. Thus, it is tempting to deduce that the higher affinity of PhenDC3 for the EBNA1 G4 might give it an advantage when placed in a complex cellular milieu, thereby allowing this compound, and not PDS, to prevent NCL binding by a competitive mechanism (Figure 4D). In support of this we have previously shown that PhenDC3 is able to inhibit the pulldown of NCL by EBNA1 G4-coated beads, whereas PDS has no effect in the same conditions [11]. However, one can consider this last possibility quite unlikely, as the affinity of PDS for the *EBNA1* mRNA G4 structure is quite high per se, at least in vitro. Hence, PDS should also prevent NCL binding, although less efficiently than PhenDC3. Finally, another possibility is that PDS and PhenDC3 may have different binding sites on *EBNA1* mRNA G4. In particular, a ternary interaction could exist between PDS/NCL/*EBNA1* mRNA G4 as has been observed in the case of TERRA G4, the G4 ligand carboxypyridostatin (cPDS, a chemical derivative of PDS), and anti-G4 antibodies [24], whereas PhenDC3 and NCL may share the same, or overlapping, binding site(s). The number of binding sites may also strongly differ from one G4 ligand to another, especially with long G4-forming domains like the GAr-encoding sequence of *EBNA1* mRNA [25]. All these possibilities highlight the importance of methods enabling the study of RNA-protein interactions and the control of these interactions by candidate molecules in presence of the multiple biological entities within the cell.

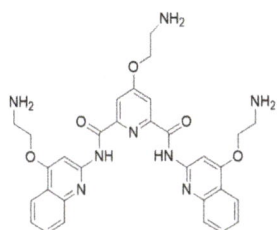

pyridostatin (PDS)

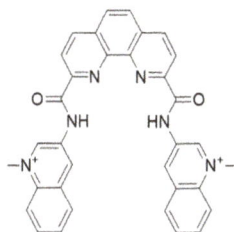

PhenDC3

Figure 3. Molecular structures of the G-quadruplex (G4) ligands pyridostatin (PDS) and PhenDC3.

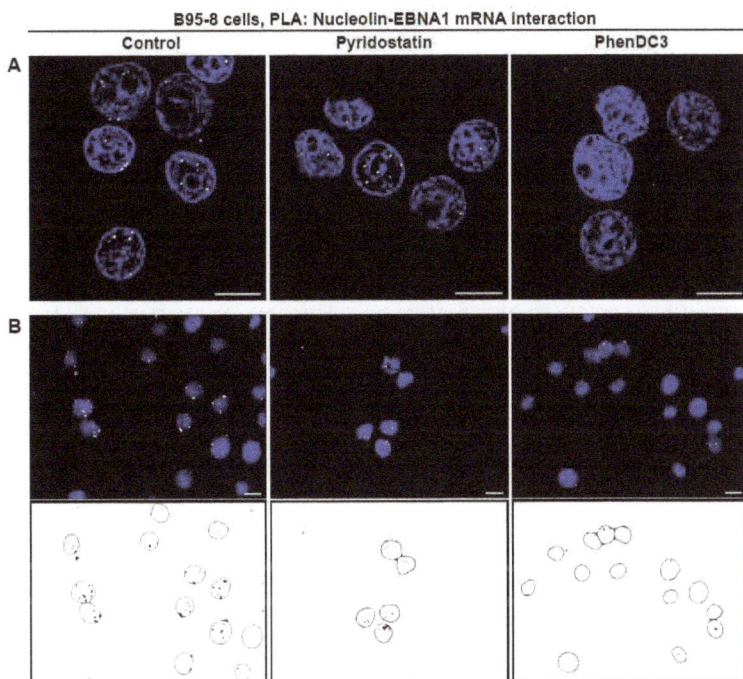

Figure 4. *Cont.*

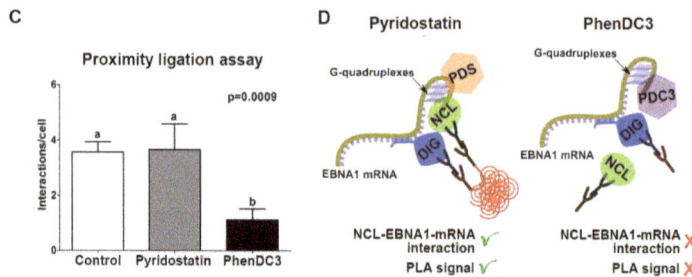

Figure 4. PLA as a tool for the characterization of RNA-binding drugs. (**A**) B95-8 cells treated with the G-quadruplex (G4) ligands pyridostatin (PDS) or PhenDC3 were tested for the NCL-*EBNA1* mRNA interaction using PLA. PhenDC3, but not PDS, was shown to prevent the interaction, denoting that PhenDC3 competes specifically with NCL for binding *EBNA1* mRNA G4. (**B**) Quantitative PLA was performed to quantify the effect of PDS and PhenDC3 on NCL-*EBNA1* mRNA interactions. One hundred cells from control (DMSO)-, PDS-, and PhenDC3-treated groups were imaged and the number of interactions per cell was estimated using a customized protocol in ImageJ. Upper and lower lanes depict images before and after analysis, respectively. Open circles represent the nucleus included in the analysis and red dots depict PLA complexes. Cells located in the border of images and dots found outside filtered nucleus were excluded from the analysis. (**C**) Histogram displaying the number of NCL-*EBNA1* mRNA interactions per cell from control (DMSO)-, PDS-, and PhenDC3-treated groups. Data shown are mean ± SD of three independent experiments performed as described in (**B**). (**D**) Schematic depicting the use of PLA to evaluate the effect of PDS and PhenDC3 on the NCL-*EBNA1* mRNA interactions in EBV-infected B95-8 cells. PhenDC3, but not PDS, competes with NCL for binding *EBNA1* mRNA G4. One possible explanation for this difference (differential binding sites for PhenDC3 and PDS, the latter forming a ternary complex EBNA1 mRNA/NCL/PDS, whereas PhenDC3 and NCL would share a common binding site) is shown. By preventing this interaction, PhenDC3 stimulates the translation of the *EBNA1* mRNA and the production of EBNA1-derived antigenic peptides for the MHC class I pathway. PDS and PDC3 mean pyridostatin and PhenDC3, respectively. Scale bars represent 10 µm.

4. Concluding Remarks

Protein-mRNA interactions influence multiple aspects of cellular function. However, in spite of progress experienced over the last decades, the study of these interactions has been restricted to assays technically demanding and unable to provide accurate information at subcellular levels. In this context, PLA represents an attractive alternative to overcome these limitations, opening new avenues for the study of protein-mRNA interactions in cellulo. We provided evidences that PLA can be coupled to quantitative analysis and be successfully employed to screen molecules interfering with target protein-mRNA interactions. Additionally, the approach described here can be adapted to other technologies, like flow cytometry, for medium to high throughput drug screening. This highlights the potential of mRNA-protein PLA as a tool for efforts focused not only on targeting specific G4 structures, but more generally for drug development based on disruption of specific protein-RNA structure complexes.

Supplementary Materials: The supplementary materials are available online.

Author Contributions: Conceptualization, R.P.M., M.B. and R.F.; Methodology, R.P.M., S.F. and C.D.; Software, R.P.M.; Validation, R.P.M., M.-P.T.-F., M.B. and R.F.; Formal Analysis, R.P.M., M.-P.T.-F., M.B. and R.F.; Resources, M.-P.T.-F. and R.F.; Writing-Original Draft Preparation, R.P.M., M.-P.T.-F., M.B. and R.F.; Writing-Review & Editing, R.P.M., M.-P.T.-F., M.B. and R.F.; Supervision, M.-P.T.-F., M.B. and R.F.; Funding Acquisition, R.F., M.B. and M.-P.T.-F.

Funding: This work was supported by the following grant agencies: La Ligue contre le cancer, La Ligue contre le cancer CSIRGO, Fondation ARC, Institut National du cancer (INCa), Cancerfonden (16059), Cancerforskningsfondedn Norr and Vetenskapsradet. This work was partially supported by the project MEYS-NPS

I-L01413. RF was partially supported by P206/12/G151. The International Centre for Cancer Vaccine Sciences is within the International Agendas program of the FNP co-financed by the European Union under the European Regional Development Fund.

Conflicts of Interest: The authors declare no commercial or financial conflict of interest.

References

1. Beckmann, B.M.; Castello, A.; Medenbach, J. The expanding universe of ribonucleoproteins: Of novel RNA-binding proteins and unconventional interactions. *Pflugers Arch.* **2016**, *468*, 1029–1040. [CrossRef] [PubMed]

2. Bao, H.L.; Ishizuka, T.; Sakamoto, T.; Fujimoto, K.; Uechi, T.; Kenmochi, N.; Xu, Y. Characterization of human telomere RNA G-quadruplex structures in vitro and in living cells using 19F NMR spectroscopy. *Nucleic Acids Res.* **2017**, *45*, 5501–5511. [CrossRef] [PubMed]

3. Bao, H.L.; Xu, Y. Investigation of higher-order RNA G-quadruplex structures in vitro and in living cells by (19)F NMR spectroscopy. *Nat. Protoc.* **2018**, *13*, 652–665. [CrossRef] [PubMed]

4. Haeusler, A.R.; Donnelly, C.J.; Periz, G.; Simko, E.A.; Shaw, P.G.; Kim, M.S.; Maragakis, N.J.; Troncoso, J.C.; Pandey, A.; Sattler, R.; et al. C9orf72 nucleotide repeat structures initiate molecular cascades of disease. *Nature* **2014**, *507*, 195–200. [CrossRef] [PubMed]

5. Taylor, J.P. Neurodegenerative diseases: G-quadruplex poses quadruple threat. *Nature* **2014**, *507*, 175–177. [CrossRef] [PubMed]

6. Wolfe, A.L.; Singh, K.; Zhong, Y.; Drewe, P.; Rajasekhar, V.K.; Sanghvi, V.R.; Mavrakis, K.J.; Jiang, M.; Roderick, J.E.; Van der Meulen, J.; et al. RNA G-quadruplexes cause eIF4a-dependent oncogene translation in cancer. *Nature* **2014**, *513*, 65–70. [CrossRef] [PubMed]

7. Largy, E.; Granzhan, A.; Hamon, F.; Verga, D.; Teulade-Fichou, M.P. Visualizing the quadruplex: From fluorescent ligands to light-up probes. *Top Curr. Chem.* **2013**, *330*, 111–177. [PubMed]

8. Mendoza, O.; Bourdoncle, A.; Boule, J.B.; Brosh, R.M., Jr.; Mergny, J.L. G-quadruplexes and helicases. *Nucleic Acids Res.* **2016**, *44*, 1989–2006. [CrossRef] [PubMed]

9. Song, J.; Perreault, J.P.; Topisirovic, I.; Richard, S. RNA G-quadruplexes and their potential regulatory roles in translation. *Translation (Austin)* **2016**, *4*. [CrossRef] [PubMed]

10. Lista, M.J.; Martins, R.P.; Angrand, G.; Quillevere, A.; Daskalogianni, C.; Voisset, C.; Teulade-Fichou, M.P.; Fahraeus, R.; Blondel, M. A yeast model for the mechanism of the Epstein-Barr virus immune evasion identifies a new therapeutic target to interfere with the virus stealthiness. *Microb. Cell.* **2017**, *4*, 305–307. [CrossRef] [PubMed]

11. Lista, M.J.; Martins, R.P.; Billant, O.; Contesse, M.A.; Findakly, S.; Pochard, P.; Daskalogianni, C.; Beauvineau, C.; Guetta, C.; Jamin, C.; et al. Nucleolin directly mediates Epstein-Barr virus immune evasion through binding to G-quadruplexes of EBNA1 mRNA. *Nat. Commun.* **2017**, *8*. [CrossRef] [PubMed]

12. De Cian, A.; Delemos, E.; Mergny, J.L.; Teulade-Fichou, M.P.; Monchaud, D. Highly efficient G-quadruplex recognition by bisquinolinium compounds. *J. Am. Chem. Soc.* **2007**, *129*, 1856–1857. [CrossRef] [PubMed]

13. Yin, Y.; Manoury, B.; Fahraeus, R. Self-inhibition of synthesis and antigen presentation by Epstein-Barr virus-encoded EBNA1. *Science* **2003**, *301*, 1371–1374. [CrossRef] [PubMed]

14. Schneider, C.A.; Rasband, W.S.; Eliceiri, K.W. NIH Image to ImageJ: 25 years of image analysis. *Nat. Methods* **2012**, *9*, 671–675. [CrossRef] [PubMed]

15. Murat, P.; Zhong, J.; Lekieffre, L.; Cowieson, N.P.; Clancy, J.L.; Preiss, T.; Balasubramanian, S.; Khanna, R.; Tellam, J. G-quadruplexes regulate Epstein-Barr virus-encoded Nuclear Antigen 1 mRNA translation. *Nat. Chem. Biol.* **2014**, *10*, 358–364. [CrossRef] [PubMed]

16. Soderberg, O.; Gullberg, M.; Jarvius, M.; Ridderstrale, K.; Leuchowius, K.J.; Jarvius, J.; Wester, K.; Hydbring, P.; Bahram, F.; Larsson, L.G.; et al. Direct observation of individual endogenous protein complexes in situ by proximity ligation. *Nat. Methods* **2006**, *3*, 995–1000. [CrossRef] [PubMed]

17. Gomez, D.; Shankman, L.S.; Nguyen, A.T.; Owens, G.K. Detection of histone modifications at specific gene loci in single cells in histological sections. *Nat. Methods* **2013**, *10*, 171–177. [CrossRef] [PubMed]

18. de Klerk, E.; t Hoen, P.A. Alternative mRNA transcription, processing, and translation: Insights from RNA sequencing. *Trends Genet.* **2015**, *31*, 128–139. [CrossRef] [PubMed]

Molecules **2018**, 23, 3124

19. Mitchell, S.F.; Parker, R. Principles and properties of eukaryotic mRNPs. *Mol. Cell.* **2014**, *54*, 547–558. [CrossRef] [PubMed]
20. Daskalogianni, C.; Pyndiah, S.; Apcher, S.; Mazars, A.; Manoury, B.; Ammari, N.; Nylander, K.; Voisset, C.; Blondel, M.; Fahraeus, R. Epstein-Barr virus-encoded EBNA1 and ZEBRA: Targets for therapeutic strategies against EBV-carrying cancers. *J. Pathol.* **2015**, *235*, 334–341. [CrossRef] [PubMed]
21. Wilson, J.B.; Manet, E.; Gruffat, H.; Busson, P.; Blondel, M.; Fahraeus, R. EBNA1: Oncogenic activity, immune evasion and biochemical functions provide targets for novel therapeutic strategies against Epstein-Barr virus-associated cancers. *Cancers (Basel)* **2018**, *10*, 109. [CrossRef] [PubMed]
22. Biffi, G.; Di Antonio, M.; Tannahill, D.; Balasubramanian, S. Visualization and selective chemical targeting of RNA G-quadruplex structures in the cytoplasm of human cells. *Nat Chem* **2014**, *6*, 75–80. [CrossRef] [PubMed]
23. Hermann, T. Strategies for the design of drugs targeting RNA and RNA-protein complexes. *Angew. Chem. Int. Ed. Engl.* **2000**, *39*, 1890–1904. [CrossRef]
24. Yangyuoru, P.M.; Di Antonio, M.; Ghimire, C.; Biffi, G.; Balasubramanian, S.; Mao, H. Dual binding of an antibody and a small molecule increases the stability of terra G-quadruplex. *Angew. Chem. Int. Ed. Engl.* **2015**, *54*, 910–913. [CrossRef] [PubMed]
25. Gabelica, V.; Maeda, R.; Fujimoto, T.; Yaku, H.; Murashima, T.; Sugimoto, N.; Miyoshi, D. Multiple and cooperative binding of fluorescence light-up probe thioflavin T with human telomere DNA G-quadruplex. *Biochemistry* **2013**, *52*, 5620–5628. [CrossRef] [PubMed]

Sample Availability: Samples of the compound PhenDC3 are available from the authors. PDS is commercially available (Sigma-Aldrich, now Merck).

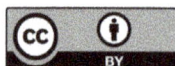

molecules

MDPI

Article

The Presence and Localization of G-Quadruplex Forming Sequences in the Domain of Bacteria

Martin Bartas [1,†], Michaela Čutová [2,†], Václav Brázda [2,3], Patrik Kaura [4], Jiří Šťastný [4,5], Jan Kolomazník [5], Jan Coufal [3], Pratik Goswami [3], Jiří Červeň [1] and Petr Pečinka [1,*]

[1]   Department of Biology and Ecology/Institute of Environmental Technologies, Faculty of Science, University of Ostrava, 710 00 Ostrava, Czech Republic; dutartas@gmail.com (M.B.); jiri.cerven@osu.cz (J.Č.)
[2]   Faculty of Chemistry, Brno University of Technology, Purkyňova 118, 612 00 Brno, Czech Republic; xcfricova@fch.vut.cz (M.Č.); vaclav@ibp.cz (V.B.)
[3]   Institute of Biophysics, Academy of Sciences of the Czech Republic v.v.i., Královopolská 135, 612 65 Brno, Czech Republic; jac@ibp.cz (J.C.); pratikgoswami@ibp.cz (P.G.)
[4]   Faculty of Mechanical Engineering, Brno University of Technology, Technicka 2896/2, 616 69 Brno, Czech Republic; 160702@vutbr.cz (P.K.); stastny@fme.vutbr.cz (J.Š.)
[5]   Department of Informatics, Mendel University in Brno, Zemedelska 1665/1, 61300 Brno, Czech Republic; jan.kolomaznik@gmail.com
*   Correspondence: petr.pecinka@osu.cz; Tel.: +420-553-46-2318
†   These authors contributed equally to this work.

Received: 16 April 2019; Accepted: 1 May 2019; Published: 2 May 2019

Abstract: The role of local DNA structures in the regulation of basic cellular processes is an emerging field of research. Amongst local non-B DNA structures, the significance of G-quadruplexes was demonstrated in the last decade, and their presence and functional relevance has been demonstrated in many genomes, including humans. In this study, we analyzed the presence and locations of G-quadruplex-forming sequences by G4Hunter in all complete bacterial genomes available in the NCBI database. G-quadruplex-forming sequences were identified in all species, however the frequency differed significantly across evolutionary groups. The highest frequency of G-quadruplex forming sequences was detected in the subgroup Deinococcus-Thermus, and the lowest frequency in Thermotogae. G-quadruplex forming sequences are non-randomly distributed and are favored in various evolutionary groups. G-quadruplex-forming sequences are enriched in ncRNA segments followed by mRNAs. Analyses of surrounding sequences showed G-quadruplex-forming sequences around tRNA and regulatory sequences. These data point to the unique and non-random localization of G-quadruplex-forming sequences in bacterial genomes.

Keywords: G-quadruplex; bacteria; bioinformatics; deinococcus; G4Hunter

---

1. Introduction

The discovery of the B-DNA structure by Crick and Watson started a rapid growth in genetic and molecular biology research [1]. However, it is now clear that, apart from this well-known double helical DNA structure, other forms of secondary structure participate in various basic processes [2]. The presence of various local DNA structures including cruciforms [3], quadruplexes [4] and triplexes [5] has been demonstrated by various methodological approaches. For example, G-quadruplexes (G4) were studied by crystallography as far back as 1962 [6]. G4s are secondary structures formed by guanine rich sequences which are widespread in DNA and RNA [4]. The building block for a G4 is a guanine quartet formed by G:G Hoogsteen base pairs (Figure 1). G4 formation requires the presence of monovalent cations such as Na^+ and K^+ [7]. Formation of this structure regulates various processes including gene expression [8], protein translation [9] and proteolysis pathways [10] in both prokaryotes and eukaryotes. In human, G4s are formed in various regions including sub-telomeres, gene bodies and gene regulatory regions [11] and in telomere regions to suppress degradation and maintain genomic stability [12]. Formation of G4s in this region decreases telomerase activity and decreases the chances of cancer development [13,14]. In addition, the proto-oncogene *MYC* is bound by nucleolin in its hypersensitive region III and enhances G4 folding and suppresses *MYC* transcription [15]. Therefore, it has been suggested that anticancer therapy will be possible by targeting G4s [16–18]. Moreover, it has been demonstrated that G4-stabilizing ligands modulate gene transcription [11]. It is already known that clusters of G4-forming sequences induce gene expression and that they are distributed near promoters and 5'UTRs. Replication-dependent DNA damage evidenced by G4 ligands have also been discovered in tumor suppressor genes and oncogenes [19]. Another potential therapeutic option is to target G4-binding proteins. Many proteins are known to bind to G4s, including some proteins important in cancer [20,21]. Moreover, novel G4 binding proteins have been suggested, sharing the NIQI amino acid motif (RGRGR GRGGG SGGSG GRGRG) [22].

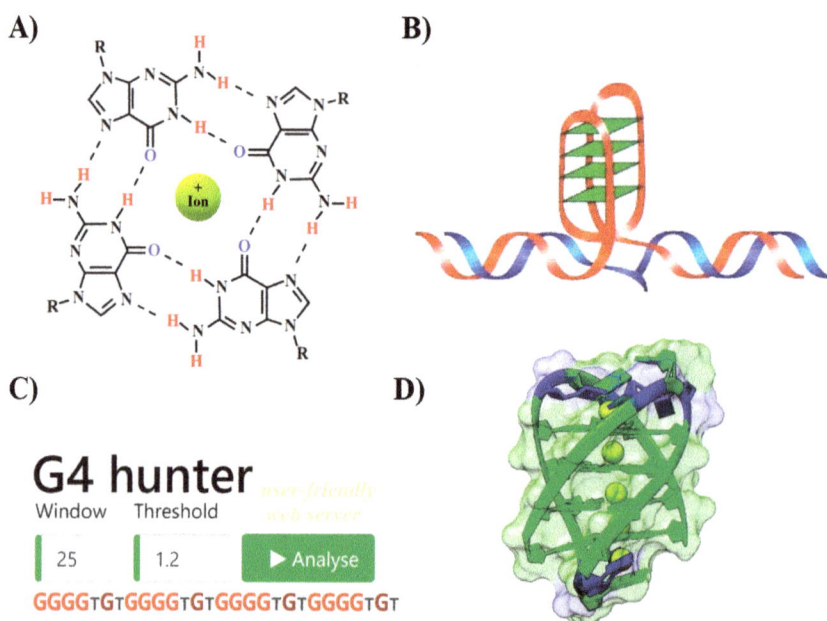

Figure 1. G-quadruplexes: (**A**) guanine tetrad stabilized by Hoogsten base pairing and positively charged central ion; (**B**) schematic drawing of intramolecular G4 structure arising from double stranded DNA; (**C**) G4Hunter, a new user-friendly web server for high throughput analyses of G4-forming sequences in DNA; and (**D**) 3D model of intramolecular antiparallel G4 formed from the sequence (5'-GGGGTGTGGGGTGT GGGGTGTGGGGTGT-3') found in *Microcystis aeruginosa* built using 3D-NuS webserver [23].

Due to the roles of G4s in regulating basic cellular processes, it is essential to identify the location of G4s in genomes. Several algorithms for detecting expected matching patterns for G4 formation are already described. The first algorithm [$G_n N_m G_n N_o G_n N_p G_n$] was created by Balasubramanian and colleagues [24] and the second algorithm considering occurrence of repeating unit G_n ($n \geq 2$) was created by the group of Maizels [25]. Nevertheless, these algorithms only produce binary (yes/no; match/no match) results, rather than the quantitative analyses that are mandatory for correlation with quadruplex strength metrics. G4Hunter was developed to overcome this limitation, in which G4 propensity is calculated depending on G richness and G skewness [26].

Bacterial genetic material is stored mostly in circular chromosomes and plasmids [27]. It was demonstrated that secondary structures in bacterial genomes are responsible for genomic stability [28]. In addition, G4 structures are more stable than double stranded DNA due to slower unfolding kinetics [29]. Nevertheless, fewer studies on role of G4 in bacterial survival and virulence have been carried out [30]. A comparative functional analysis by Pooja et al. revealed that open reading frame (ORF) formulated amino acids biosynthesis and signal transduction are restrained by/controlled by G4 DNA in prokaryotes [31]. There are have been many reports on the role of G4s in eukaryotes over many years [32], although advances in prokaryotic G4s are not fully elucidated [33].

The formation of an intramolecular G4 requires the presence of a loop sequence between the G-tracts [34] and the density of G4 therefore broadly correlates with GC content. The GC content in bacterial genomes varies remarkably, from 17% to 75% [35]. It was demonstrated that G4 forming sequences are enriched and biased around transcription start sites of genes in the order Deinococcales [36]. Another function of G-tracts is in sustaining and maintaining duplex stability at higher temperatures in thermophiles; for example, *Thermus aquaticus* has a GC content of 68% [37]. Interestingly, the soil bacterium *Paracoccus denitrificans* contains 494 G4-forming sequences, which play roles in digestion of NO_3- through G4 formation upstream of *NasT* [38]. The presence of G4-forming motifs in genes *hsdS*, *recD*, and *pmrA* of *Streptococcus pneumoniae* participate in host–pathogen interactions [30]. Such observations show the significance role of G4 in bacteria and also in eukaryotic cell organelles such as chloroplasts and mitochondria with circular DNAs that originated from prokaryotic organisms. Several papers show the importance of local DNA structures in mitochondrial DNA including G4 using G4Hunter [26] and inverted repeats [39] using palindrome analyzer [40]. Similarly, cruciforms exist in various regulatory regions in chloroplast DNA [41].

The presence of G4 in bacteria remains poorly understood. In our study, we comprehensively analyzed the presence and locations of G4 in 1627 bacterial genomes using G4Hunter. These data bring more information about evolutionary changes of G4 frequency between phyla and provide evidence for the importance of G4 in prokaryotes.

2. Results

2.1. Variation in Frequency for G4-forming Sequences in Bacteria

We analyzed the occurrence of putative G4 sequences (PQS) by G4Hunter in all 1627 known bacterial genomes. The length of bacterial genomes in the dataset varies from 298 kbp to 20.20 Mbp. The GC content average is 50.44%, with minimum 20.2% for *Buchnera aphidicola* (Gammaproteobacteria) and maximum 74.7% for *Corynebacterium sphenisci* (Actinobacteria). Using standard values for G4Hunter algorithm—window size 25 and G4Hunter score above 1.2—we found 9,202,364 PQS in all 1547 bacteria with 1627 genomes (some bacteria have two genomes). The most abundant PQS are those with G4Hunter scores of 1.2–1.4 (97.9% of all PQS), much less abundant are PQS with G4Hunter scores 1.4–1.6 (1.96% of all PQS), followed by 1.6–1.8 (0.128% of all PQS) and 1.8–2.0 (0.0056% of all PQS) and the lowest number of PQS is above G4Hunter score 2 (0.0009% of all PQS). In general, a higher G4Hunter score means a higher probability of G4s forming inside the PQS [26]. A summary of all PQS found in ranges of G4Hunter score intervals and precomputed PQS frequencies per 1000 bp is shown in Table 1.

According to NCBI taxonomy classification, the fully sequenced organisms of Bacteria domain are divided into 18 groups (6 with 10 or more sequenced genomes) and 39 subgroups (14 with 10 or more sequenced genomes), as shown in the phylogenetic tree (Figure 2). For statistical analyses, we used only groups with 10 or more sequenced genomes (highlighted by colors).

The number of all analyzed sequences in individual phylogenetic categories, together with median genome length, shortest genome, longest genome, mean, minimal and maximal observed frequency of PQS per 1000 bp and total PQS counts are shown in Table 2. Five subgroups (Actinobacteria, Chloroflexi, Deinococcus-Thermus, Alphaproteobacteria and Betaproteobacteria) show >60% GC content. On the other side, three subgroups (Spirochaetia, Thermotogae and Tenericutes) show < 40% GC content.

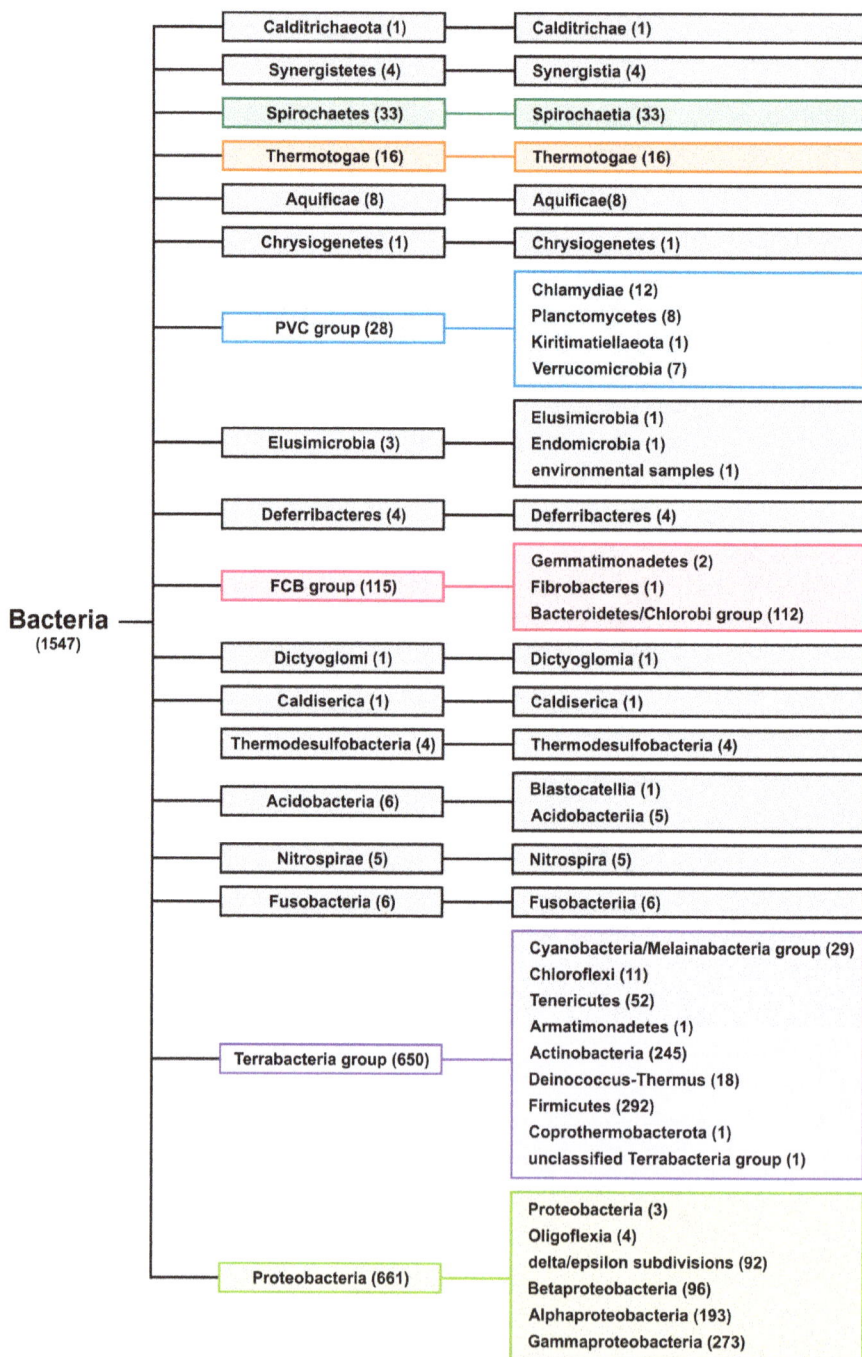

Figure 2. Phylogenetic tree of inspected Bacterial Groups and Subgroups.

Table 1. Total number of PQS and their resulting frequencies per 1000 bp in all 1547 representative bacteria, grouped by G4Hunter score. Frequency was computed by using total number of PQS in each category divided by total length of all analyzed sequences and multiplied by 1000.

Interval of G4Hunter Score	Number of PQS in Dataset	PQS Frequency per 1000 bp
1.2–1.4	9,009,593	1.315033
1.4–1.6	180,395	0.025058
1.6–1.8	11,779	0.00155
1.8–2.0	511	0.000055
2.0–more	86	0.000009

Table 2. Genomic sequences sizes, PQS frequencies and total counts. Seq (total number of sequences), Median (median length of sequences), Short (shortest sequence), Long (longest sequence), GC % (average GC content), PQS (total number of predicted PQS), Mean f (mean frequency of predicted PQS per 1000 bp), Min f (lowest frequency of predicted PQS per 1000 bp), Max f (highest frequency of predicted PQS per 1000 bp). Colors correspond to phylogenetic tree depiction.

Domain	Seq	Median	Short	Long	GC%	PQS	Mean f	Min f	Max f
Bacteria	1627	3,307,820	83,026	13,033,779	50.6	9,202,364	1.342	0.013	14.213
Group	**Seq**	**Median**	**Short**	**Long**	**GC%**	**PQS**	**Mean f**	**Min f**	**Max f**
Spirochaetes	38	2,646,038	277,655	4,653,970	39.7	87,109	0.809	0.079	6.668
Thermotogae	16	2,150,379	1,884,562	2,974,229	39.1	13,617	0.395	0.149	0.812
PVC group	28	2,917,407	1,041,170	9,629,675	50.7	198,358	1.646	0.388	4.802
FCB group	117	3,914,632	605,745	9,127,347	42.3	302,949	0.608	0.013	2.746
Terrabacteria	659	3,018,755	91,776	11,936,683	50.4	4,766,517	1.601	0.016	14.213
Proteobacteria	724	3,551,512	83,026	13,033,779	53.4	3,688,101	1.276	0.025	5.507
Other	45	2,157,835	1,012,010	6,237,577	44.3	145,713	1.103	0.062	5.855
Subgroup	**Seq**	**Median**	**Short**	**Long**	**GC%**	**PQS**	**Mean f**	**Min f**	**Max f**
Spirochaetia	38	2,646,038	277,655	4,653,970	39.7	87,109	0.809	0.079	6.668
Thermotogae	16	2,150,379	1,884,562	2,974,229	39.1	13617	0.395	0.149	0.812
Chlamydiae	12	1,168,953	1,041,170	3,072,383	40.3	12453	0.646	0.388	0.957
Bacteroidetes/Chlorobi	114	3,878,527	605,745	9,127,347	41.9	282,516	0.585	0.013	2.746
Cyanobacteria/Melaina	29	5,315,554	1,657,990	9,673,108	42.6	193,894	1.247	0.201	6.004
Chloroflexi	12	2,333,610	125,2731	5,723,298	60	62,688	1.89	1.223	3.222
Tenericutes	52	981,001	564,395	1,877,792	28	6460	0.136	0.016	0.834
Actinobacteria	246	3,960,961	775,354	11,936,683	66.2	3,590,884	2.821	0.143	8.556
Deinococcus-Thermus	18	2,895,913	2,035,182	3,881,839	66.8	311,949	6.626	1.885	14.213
Firmicutes	298	2,835,823	91,776	8,739,048	40.8	579,740	0.56	0.064	6.587
delta/epsilon subdiv.	92	3,136,746	1,457,670	13,033,779	50	807,251	1.681	0.034	5.282
Betaproteobacteria	110	3,763,620	820,037	6,987,670	60.6	585,984	1.306	0.195	4.007
Alphaproteobacteria	213	3,424,964	83,026	9,207,384	61.5	126,134	1.764	0.051	5.507
Gammaproteobacteria	302	3,777,066	298,471	7,783,862	48.8	31,686	0.799	0.025	4.264
other	75	2,406,157	1,012,010	9,629,675	48.4	432,683	1.406	0.0616	5.855

Mean frequency for all bacterial genomes was 1.342 PQS per 1000 bp. The lowest mean frequency is for Thermotogae (0.395) and the highest for the PVC group (1.646), followed by Terrabacteria (1.601). On the subgroup level, the lowest mean frequency was found in Tenericutes (0.136) and the highest in Deinococcus-Thermus (6.626), followed by Actinobacteria (2.821). The very highest PQS frequency of 14.213 PQS/kbp was found in *Thermus oshimai JL-2* (subgroup Deinococcus-Thermus) and the lowest frequency (0.013 PQS/kbp) in *Lacinutrix venerupis* (subgroup Bacteroidetes/Chlorobi) containing only 40 PQS in its 31,923,99 bp genome (0.0125 PQS/kbp). Detailed statistical inter group and inter subgroup comparisons are depicted in Supplementary Material S5 (SM_05).

Detailed statistical characteristics for PQS frequencies (including mean, variance, and outliers) are depicted in boxplots for all inspected subgroups (Figure 3).

Distribution of Quadruplex frequencies

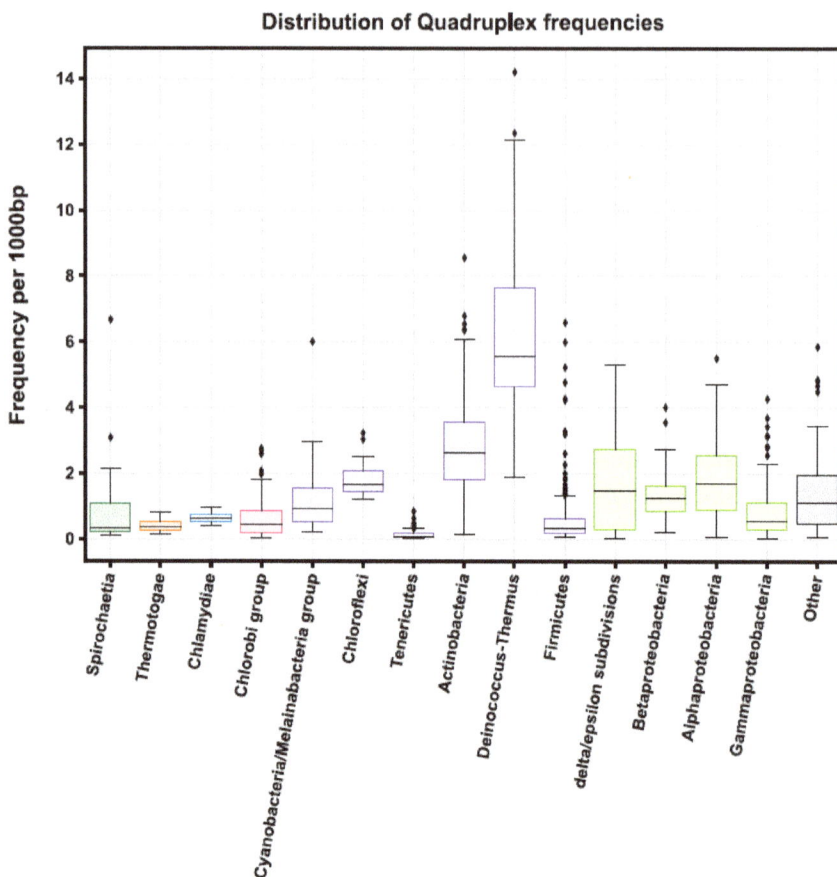

Figure 3. Frequencies of PQS in subgroups of the analyzed bacterial genomes. Data within boxes span the interquartile range and whiskers show the lowest and highest values within 1.5 interquartile range. Black diamonds denote outliers.

We visualized the relationship between %GC content in genomes with the frequency of PQS (Figure 4). In general, PQS frequencies usually correlate with GC content, however there are many exceptions to this rule. Organisms with high PQS frequencies relative to their GC content (over 50% of the maximal observed PQS frequency, Figure 4) are highlighted in color; the whole figure is separated into smaller segments according to inspected G4Hunter score intervals. Nearly all of the 10 outliers belong to the group Terrabacteria, except *Spirochaeta thermophila* DSM 6578 (group Spirochaetes). From the Terrabacteria group, six outliers belong to the small subgroup Deinococcus-Thermus (*Thermus oshimai* JL-2, *Thermus brockianus*, *Thermus aquaticus* Y51MC23, *Thermus scotoductus* SA-01, *Marinithermus hydrothermalis* DSM 14884, and *Deinococcus puniceus*), two outliers belong to the subgroup Actinobacteria (*Verrucosispora maris* AB-18-032 and *Rubrobacter xylanophilus* DSM 9941) and one outlier comes from the subgroup Cynobacteria/Melainabacteria (*Microcystis aeruginosa* NIES-843).

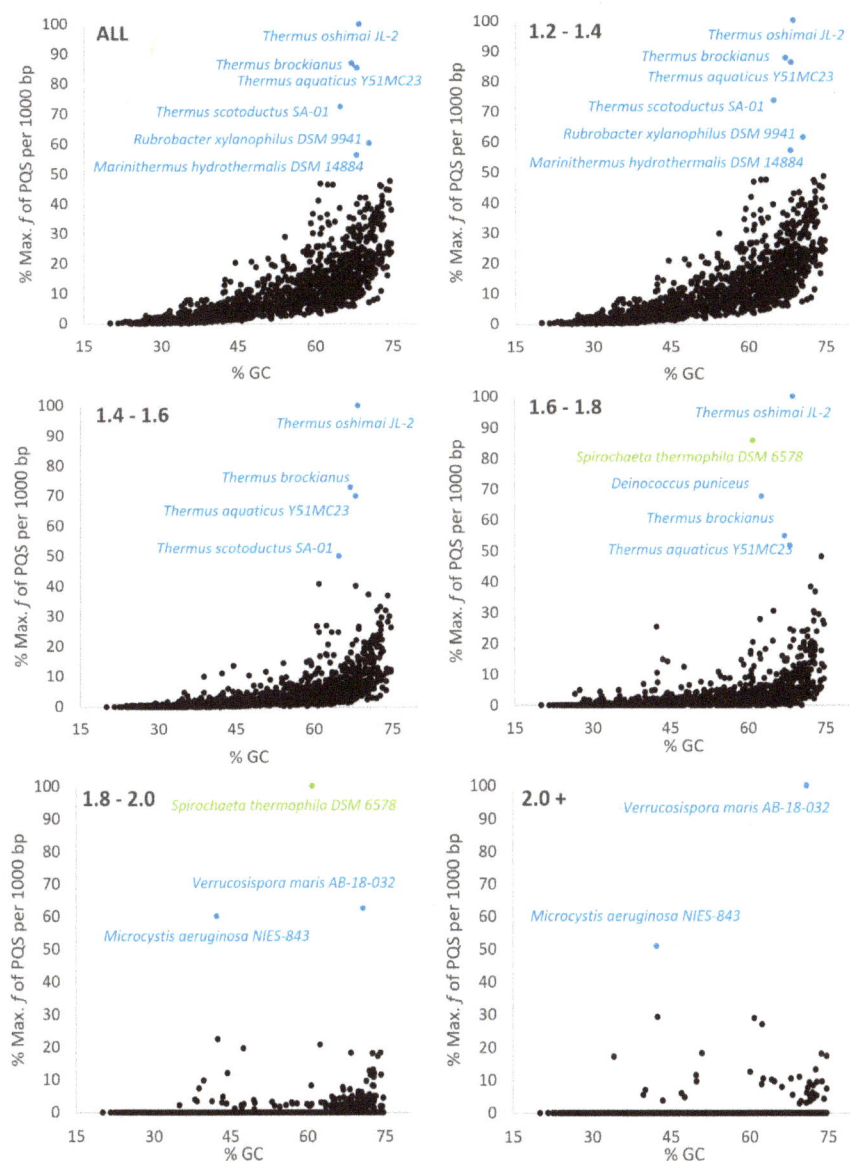

Figure 4. Relationship between observed frequency of PQS per 1000 bp and GC content in all analyzed prokaryotic sequences in various G4 Hunter score intervals. In each G4Hunter score interval miniplot, frequencies were normalized according to the highest observed frequency of PQS. Organisms with max. frequency per 1000 bp greater than 50% are described and highlighted in color.

2.2. Localization of PQS in Genomes

To evaluate the position of PQS in bacterial genomes, we downloaded the described "features" of all bacterial genomes and analyzed the presence of all PQS in each annotated sequences and its close proximity (100 bp before and after feature annotation). PQS frequencies around annotated genome sites are shown in Figure 5. The highest PQS frequencies are before and after transfer RNA (tRNA), then inside transfer-messenger RNA (tmRNA) and inside ribosomal (rRNA). The lowest PQS frequencies were noticed before and after sequence-tagged sites (STS), then after and before rRNA and after miscellaneous features. If we consider only "inside" regions of inspected features, the differences between features are much smaller than within "before" and "after" regions.

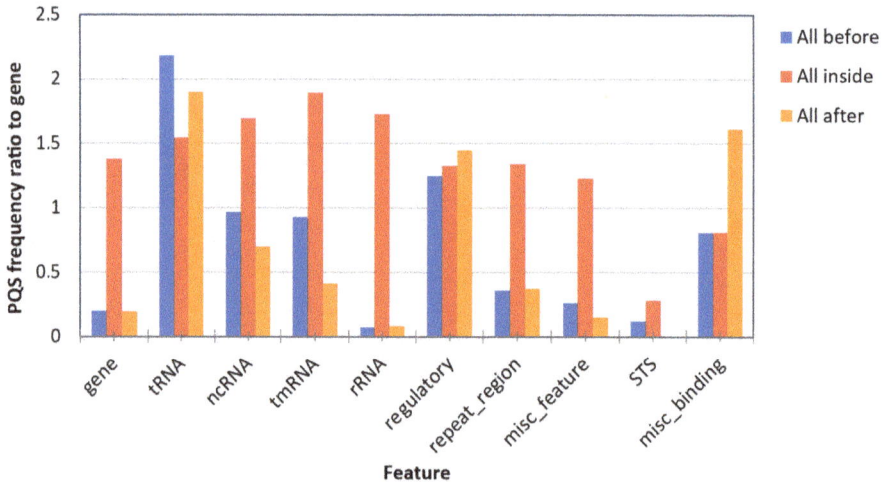

Figure 5. Differences in PQS frequency by DNA locus. The chart shows PQS frequencies according to "gene" annotation and other annotated locations from the NCBI database. We analyzed the frequencies of all PQS within (inside), before (100 bp) and after (100 bp) annotated locations.

As shown in Figure 5, there is no straight pattern in PQS occurrence in all annotated sequences but, in some groups, there are certain PQS distributions. For example, inside rRNA, tmRNA, ncRNA, misc_features, genes and repeat regions, there is higher amount of PQS in annotated sequences, but these PQS are not frequently present in DNA situated before and after these annotated sequences. In contrast, there is almost the same distribution of PQS before, inside and after annotated sequences in tRNA and regulatory groups.

3. Discussion

It has been demonstrated that G4s could be used as targets for therapy [42]. G4 ligands are suggested as a target in cancer [43] and show antiparasitic activity for *Trypanosoma brucei* binding to a G4 structure [44]. Therefore, it has been proposed that G4 sequences in bacterial genomes represent novel and promising targets for antimicrobial therapy [33], and dinuclear polypyridylruthenium(II) complexes are active against drug-resistant bacteria including Methicillin-resistant *Staphylococcus aureus* and Vancomycin-resistant *Enterococcus* [45,46]. Dinuclear ruthenium complexes are relatively well-characterized G4 DNA binding agents [47–49]. Interestingly, we found large numbers of PQS with G4Hunter scores greater than 1.8 in the cyanobacterium *Microcystis aeruginosa*. *Microcystis aeruginosa* is a ubiquitous cyanobacterium living in eutrophic fresh water, which produces harmful hepatotoxins and neurotoxins, and can cause economic loss and damage to the ecosystem [50]. Our analysis indicates that this organism contains unusual and perfectly repeated PQSs (for example, DNA repeat of $(GGGGTGT)_{58}$). Therefore, we hypothesize that this organism could be very sensitive to treatment with specific G4 binding compounds to inhibit its growth, as a possible alternative to commonly used algicides (the human genome does not contain these GGGGTGT repetitions). On the other hand, the lowest mean frequency of PQS was found in Terrabacteria subgroup Tenericutes (0.136 PQS/kbp) with the lowest average GC content (28%). The subgroup Tenericutes includes the genus *Mycoplasma* with many pathogens of clinical importance. On the other hand, a G4 was found in the promoter region of *Mycobacterium tuberculosis* and G4 ligands inhibited *M. tuberculosis* growth in the low micromolar range [51]. Therefore, the presence of a G4 could be important not only in antiviral [42,52] but also in antibacterial therapy. According to a recent study by Ding et al., eukaryotic organisms have similar PQS frequencies of 0.3 PQS per 1000 bp, whereas prokaryote frequencies are more diverse [36]. Based on our analysis, prokaryote PQS frequencies span a range of 0.013 (*Lacinutrix venerupis*) to 14.213 (*Thermus oshimai JL-2*) PQS per 1000 bp. A similar observation was shown by Quadparser algorithm and leads to the hypothesis that thermophilic organisms are enriched with PSQs due to their living at high temperatures [36]. However, similar enrichment has been demonstrated also for organisms with resistance to other stress factors such as radioresistance [53,54], thus the direct correlation between temperature and G4 presence is not supported by these finding. Validation of the G4Hunter score was made based on biophysical measurements at room temperature [26], therefore the number of G4 sequences in thermophiles could be overestimated, especially for those sequences with G4Hunter scores close to 1.2. Moreover, the mostly thermophilic and hyperthermophilic bacteria in phylum Thermotogae strains has one of the lowest PSQ frequencies. Thus, it seems that Gram-negative thermophilic bacteria evolved according to G4 structures in a completely different way than Gram-positive thermophilic bacteria, and that correlation among thermophiles and G4s depends on the phylum. Contrary to the enrichment of PQS near transcriptional start sites (TSS), 5′-3′UTR sequences and coding regions in eukaryotes [36], our analyses showed the highest PQS frequencies inside tmRNA, ncRNA and rRNA regions in prokaryotes (Figure 5). tmRNAs play a key role in the so-called ribosome rescue process, if ribosomes cannot finish translation, e.g. due to lost stop codon in translated mRNA. The physiological role of ncRNAs in prokaryotes is not fully elucidated, although they are considered to be important regulators of pathogenic processes by controlling virulence gene expression in *Staphylococcus aureus* and *Vibrio cholerae* [55]. The comparison of PQS frequencies between different studies could be complicated due to various PQS thresholds and algorithms. In our study, we used the state-of-the-art algorithm, G4Hunter, developed by Mergny and colleagues. This algorithm takes into account G-richness and G-skewness and has been experimentally validated [26]. Moreover, the current G4Hunter web version allows easy analyses of multiple genomes [56] and our comprehensive analysis showed the broad variations of PQS frequencies and their locations in bacterial genomes.

4. Methods

4.1. Selection of DNA Sequences

The set of all complete bacterial genomic DNA sequences was downloaded from the Genome database of the National Center for Biotechnology Information [57]. We used for our analyses only completely assembly level and we have selected one genome (representative) for each species (Supplementary Material S1 (SM_01)) to avoid non-complete sequences and duplications. In total, we analyzed the presence of G4 sequences in 1627 genomes from the domain Bacteria, representing 5886 Mbp.

4.2. Process of Analysis

We used the computational core of our DNA analyzer software written in Java [40]. For these analyses, we used the G4Hunter algorithm implementation [56]. Parameters for G4Hunter was set to "25" for window size and G4 score above 1.2. An example of a putative G4 sequence found using such search criteria is provided in Supplementary Material S2 (SM_02). The overall results for each species group contained a list of species with size of genomic DNA and number of putative G4 sequences found (Supplementary Material S3 (SM_03)). These data were processed by Python jupyter using Pandas (contains statistical tools). Graphs were generated from the Pandas tables using "seaborn" graphical library.

4.3. Analysis of Putative G4 Sequences Around Annotated NCBI Features

We downloaded the feature tables from the NCBI database along with the genomic DNA sequences. Feature tables contain annotations of known features found in the DNA sequence. We analyzed the occurrence of G4-forming sequences inside and around (before and after) recorded features. Features were grouped by the name stated in the feature table file. From this analysis, we obtained a file with feature names and numbers of putative G4 forming sequences found inside and around features for each group of species analyzed. Search for putative G4 forming sequences took place in a predefined feature neighborhood (we used ±100 bp—this figure is important for calculation of putative G4-forming sequence frequencies in feature neighborhoods) and inside feature boundaries. We calculated the amount of all predicted putative G4-forming sequences in regions before, inside and after features. An example of categorizing a putative G4-forming sequence according to its overlap with a feature or feature's neighborhood is shown in Supplementary Material S2 (SM_02). Further processing was performed in Microsoft Excel and the data are available as Supplementary Material S4 (SM_04).

4.4. Phylogenetic Tree Construction

Exact taxid IDs of all analyzed groups were obtained from Taxonomy Browser via NCBI Taxonomy Database [58], downloaded to phyloT: a tree generator (http://phylot.biobyte.de) and a phylogenetic tree was constructed using function "Visualize in iTOL" in Interactive Tree of Life environment [59]. The resulting tree is shown in Figure 2.

4.5. Statistical Analysis

Statistical evaluations of differences in G4-forming sequences in phylogenetic groups were made by Kruskal–Wallis test in STATISTICA, with *p*-value cut-off 0.05; data are available in Supplementary Material S5 (SM_05).

5. Conclusions

In this research, we analyzed the presence of PQS in bacterial genomes. PQS were identified in all species, but the number of PQS differ remarkably among individual subgroups, showing evolutionary adaptations connected with G4. While the highest frequency of PQS was detected in Gram-positive extremophiles Deinococcus-Thermus subgroup, the lowest PQS frequency was found in Gram-negative thermophilic bacteria in Bacteroidetes/Chlorobi subgroup. Thus, it seems that evolution of these subgroups was driven by different strategies. PQS are enriched in ncRNA segments followed by mRNAs; analyses of surrounding sequences showed PQS enrichment also around tRNA and regulatory sequences. These data point to the unique and non-random localization of PQS in bacterial genomes.

Supplementary Materials: The supplementary material are available online. Supplementary Material S1 (SM_01): The accession codes and phylogenetic classification of all 1627 representative prokaryotic complete genomic DNA sequences, Supplementary Material S2 (SM_02): Example putative G4 sequence and predefined feature neighborhood, Supplementary Material S3 (SM_03): Overall results of PQS frequencies found in each analyzed genomic sequence (group or subgroup) together with GC content, sequence length and other parameters, Supplementary Material S4 (SM_04): Detailed results of PQS occurrence around defined genomic features, Supplementary Material S5 (SM_05): Statistical evaluations of differences in G4-forming sequences in phylogenetic groups

Author Contributions: Conceptualization, M.B. and P.P.; Data curation, P.K.; Formal analysis, M.B. and P.K.; Funding acquisition, P.P.; Investigation, M.Č. and J.C.; Methodology, V.B.; Project administration, P.P.; Resources, M.Č., J.Š.; and J.K.; Software, P.K., J.Š.; and J.K.; Supervision, J.Č. and P.P.; Validation, V.B.; Visualization, M.B., P.K. and P.G.; Writing—original draft, M.B., M.Č., V.B., J.C. and P.G.; and Writing—review and editing, J.Č.

Funding: This work was supported by the Grant Agency of the Czech Republic (18-15548S); the Ministry of Education, Youth and Sports of the Czech Republic in the "National Feasibility Program I" (LO1208 TEWEP); EU structural funding Operational Programme Research and Development for innovation, project No. CZ.1.05/2.1.00/19.0388; and project SGS/09/PrF/2019 financed by University of Ostrava.

Acknowledgments: We thank Philip J. Coates for proofreading and editing the manuscript.

Molecules **2019**, *24*, 1711

Conflicts of Interest: The authors declare no conflict of interest.

References

1. Watson, J.D.; Crick, F.H. Molecular structure of nucleic acids. *Nature* **1953**, *171*, 737–738. [CrossRef]
2. Szlachta, K.; Thys, R.G.; Atkin, N.D.; Pierce, L.C.T.; Bekiranov, S.; Wang, Y.-H. Alternative DNA secondary structure formation affects RNA polymerase II promoter-proximal pausing in human. *Genome Biol.* **2018**, *19*, 89. [CrossRef] [PubMed]
3. Brázda, V.; Laister, R.C.; Jagelská, E.B.; Arrowsmith, C. Cruciform structures are a common DNA feature important for regulating biological processes. *BMC Mol. Biol.* **2011**, *12*, 33. [CrossRef]
4. Sun, Z.-Y.; Wang, X.-N.; Cheng, S.-Q.; Su, X.-X.; Ou, T.-M. Developing Novel G-Quadruplex Ligands: From Interaction with Nucleic Acids to Interfering with Nucleic Acid–Protein Interaction. *Molecules* **2019**, *24*, 396. [CrossRef]
5. Nelson, L.D.; Bender, C.; Mannsperger, H.; Buergy, D.; Kambakamba, P.; Mudduluru, G.; Korf, U.; Hughes, D.; Van Dyke, M.W.; Allgayer, H. Triplex DNA-binding proteins are associated with clinical outcomes revealed by proteomic measurements in patients with colorectal cancer. *Mol. Cancer* **2012**, *11*, 38. [CrossRef] [PubMed]
6. Gellert, M.; Lipsett, M.N.; Davies, D.R. Helix Formation by Guanylic acid. *Proc. Natl. Acad. Sci. USA* **1962**, *48*, 2013–2018. [CrossRef]
7. Harkness, R.W.; Mittermaier, A.K. G-quadruplex dynamics. *Biochim. Biophys. Acta Proteins Proteom.* **2017**, *1865*, 1544–1554. [CrossRef]
8. Siddiqui-Jain, A.; Grand, C.L.; Bearss, D.J.; Hurley, L.H. Direct evidence for a G-quadruplex in a promoter region and its targeting with a small molecule to repress c-MYC transcription. *Proc. Natl. Acad. Sci. USA* **2002**, *99*, 11593–11598. [CrossRef]
9. Lee, S.C.; Zhang, J.; Strom, J.; Yang, D.; Dinh, T.N.; Kappeler, K.; Chen, Q.M. G-Quadruplex in the NRF2 mRNA 5′ Untranslated Region Regulates De Novo NRF2 Protein Translation under Oxidative Stress. *Mol. Cell. Biol.* **2016**, *37*, e00122-16. [CrossRef] [PubMed]
10. Endoh, T.; Kawasaki, Y.; Sugimoto, N. Stability of RNA quadruplex in open reading frame determines proteolysis of human estrogen receptor α. *Nucleic Acids Res.* **2013**, *41*, 6222–6231. [CrossRef] [PubMed]
11. Lam, E.Y.N.; Beraldi, D.; Tannahill, D.; Balasubramanian, S. G-quadruplex structures are stable and detectable in human genomic DNA. *Nat. Commun.* **2013**, *4*, 1796. [CrossRef]
12. Long, X.; Stone, M.D. Kinetic Partitioning Modulates Human Telomere DNA G-Quadruplex StructuralPolymorphism. *PLoS ONE* **2013**, *8*, e83420. [CrossRef] [PubMed]
13. Sun, D.; Thompson, B.; Cathers, B.E.; Salazar, M.; Kerwin, S.M.; Trent, J.O.; Jenkins, T.C.; Neidle, S.; Hurley, L.H. Inhibition of human telomerase by a G-Quadruplex-Interactive compound. *J. Med. Chem.* **1997**, *40*, 2113–2116. [CrossRef] [PubMed]
14. Lee, H.-S.; Carmena, M.; Liskovykh, M.; Peat, E.; Kim, J.-H.; Oshimura, M.; Masumoto, H.; Teulade-Fichou, M.-P.; Pommier, Y.; Earnshaw, W.C.; et al. Systematic Analysis of Compounds Specifically Targeting Telomeres and Telomerase for Clinical Implications in Cancer Therapy. *Cancer Res.* **2018**, *78*, 6282–6296. [CrossRef]
15. Dickerhoff, J.; Onel, B.; Chen, L.; Chen, Y.; Yang, D. Solution Structure of a MYC Promoter G-Quadruplex with 1:6:1 Loop Length. *ACS Omega* **2019**, *4*, 2533–2539. [CrossRef]
16. Balasubramanian, S.; Hurley, L.H.; Neidle, S. Targeting G-quadruplexes in gene promoters: A novel anticancer strategy? *Nat. Rev. Drug Discov.* **2011**, *10*, 261–275. [CrossRef]
17. Cimino-Reale, G.; Zaffaroni, N.; Folini, M. Emerging Role of G-quadruplex DNA as Target in Anticancer Therapy. *Curr. Pharm. Design* **2016**, *22*, 6612–6624. [CrossRef]
18. Asamitsu, S.; Obata, S.; Yu, Z.; Bando, T.; Sugiyama, H. Recent Progress of Targeted G-Quadruplex-Preferred Ligands Toward Cancer Therapy. *Molecules* **2019**, *24*, 429. [CrossRef]
19. Yoshida, W.; Saikyo, H.; Nakabayashi, K.; Yoshioka, H.; Bay, D.H.; Iida, K.; Kawai, T.; Hata, K.; Ikebukuro, K.; Nagasawa, K.; et al. Identification of G-quadruplex clusters by high-throughput sequencing of whole-genome amplified products with a G-quadruplex ligand. *Sci. Rep.* **2018**, *8*, 1–8. [CrossRef] [PubMed]
20. Brázda, V.; Hároníková, L.; Liao, J.C.C.; Fojta, M. DNA and RNA Quadruplex-Binding Proteins. *Int. J. Mol. Sci.* **2014**, *15*, 17493–17517. [CrossRef]

21. Mishra, S.K.; Tawani, A.; Mishra, A.; Kumar, A. G4IPDB: A database for G-quadruplex structure forming nucleic acid interacting proteins. *Sci. Rep.* **2016**, *6*, 38144. [CrossRef] [PubMed]

22. Brázda, V.; Cerveň, J.; Bartas, M.; Mikysková, N.; Coufal, J.; Pečinka, P. The amino acid composition of quadruplex binding proteins reveals a shared motif and predicts new potential quadruplex interactors. *Molecules* **2018**, *23*, 2341. [CrossRef]

23. Patro, L.P.P.; Kumar, A.; Kolimi, N.; Rathinavelan, T. 3D-NuS: A web server for automated modeling and visualization of non-canonical 3-dimensional nucleic acid structures. *J. Mol. Biol.* **2017**, *429*, 2438–2448. [CrossRef]

24. Huppert, J.L.; Balasubramanian, S. Prevalence of quadruplexes in the human genome. *Nucleic Acids Res.* **2005**, *33*, 2908–2916. [CrossRef] [PubMed]

25. Eddy, J.; Maizels, N. Gene function correlates with potential for G4 DNA formation in the human genome. *Nucleic Acids Res.* **2006**, *34*, 3887–3896. [CrossRef]

26. Bedrat, A.; Lacroix, L.; Mergny, J.L. Re-evaluation of G-quadruplex propensity with G4Hunter. *Nucleic Acids Res.* **2016**, *44*, 1746–1759. [CrossRef]

27. diCenzo, G.C.; Finan, T.M. The Divided Bacterial Genome: Structure, Function, and Evolution. *Microbiol. Mol. Biol. Rev.* **2017**, *81*, e00019-17. [CrossRef]

28. Yadav, V.K.; Abraham, J.K.; Mani, P.; Kulshrestha, R.; Chowdhury, S. QuadBase: Genome-wide database of G4 DNA—Occurrence and conservation in human, chimpanzee, mouse and rat promoters and 146 microbes. *Nucleic Acids Res.* **2008**, *36*, D381–D385. [CrossRef]

29. König, S.L.B.; Huppert, J.L.; Sigel, R.K.O.; Evans, A.C. Distance-dependent duplex DNA destabilization proximal to G-quadruplex/i-motif sequences. *Nucleic Acids Res.* **2013**, *41*, 7453–7461. [CrossRef] [PubMed]

30. Mishra, S.K.; Jain, N.; Shankar, U.; Tawani, A.; Sharma, T.K.; Kumar, A. Characterization of highly conserved G-quadruplex motifs as potential drug targets in Streptococcus pneumoniae. *Sci. Rep.* **2019**, *9*, 1791. [CrossRef]

31. Rawal, P.; Kummarasetti, V.B.R.; Ravindran, J.; Kumar, N.; Halder, K.; Sharma, R.; Mukerji, M.; Das, S.K.; Chowdhury, S. Genome-wide prediction of G4 DNA as regulatory motifs: Role in Escherichia coli global regulation. *Genome Res.* **2006**, *16*, 644–655. [CrossRef]

32. Neidle, S. The structures of quadruplex nucleic acids and their drug complexes. *Curr. Opin. Struct. Biol.* **2009**, *19*, 239–250. [CrossRef] [PubMed]

33. Saranathan, N.; Vivekanandan, P. G-Quadruplexes: More than just a kink in microbial genomes. *Trends Microbiol.* **2018**, *27*, 148–163. [CrossRef]

34. Kaplan, O.I.; Berber, B.; Hekim, N.; Doluca, O. G-quadruplex prediction in E. coli genome reveals a conserved putative G-quadruplex-Hairpin-Duplex switch. *Nucleic Acids Res.* **2016**, *44*, 9083–9095. [PubMed]

35. Brocchieri, L. The GC Content of Bacterial Genomes. *J. Phylogenet. Evolut. Biol.* **2013**, *2*, 1–3. [CrossRef]

36. Ding, Y.; Fleming, A.M.; Burrows, C.J. Case studies on potential G-quadruplex-forming sequences from the bacterial orders Deinococcales and Thermales derived from a survey of published genomes. *Sci. Rep.* **2018**, *8*, 15679. [CrossRef]

37. Brumm, P.J.; Monsma, S.; Keough, B.; Jasinovica, S.; Ferguson, E.; Schoenfeld, T.; Lodes, M.; Mead, D.A. Complete Genome Sequence of Thermus aquaticus Y51MC23. *PLoS ONE* **2015**, *10*, e0138674. [CrossRef]

38. Waller, Z.A.E.; Pinchbeck, B.J.; Buguth, B.S.; Meadows, T.G.; Richardson, D.J.; Gates, A.J. Control of bacterial nitrate assimilation by stabilization of G-quadruplex DNA. *Chem. Commun.* **2016**, *52*, 13511–13514. [CrossRef] [PubMed]

39. Čechová, J.; Lýsek, J.; Bartas, M.; Brázda, V. Complex analyses of inverted repeats in mitochondrial genomes revealed their importance and variability. *Bioinformatics* **2018**, *34*, 1081–1085. [CrossRef]

40. Brázda, V.; Kolomazník, J.; Lýsek, J.; Hároníková, L.; Coufal, J.; Šťastný, J. Palindrome analyser—A new web-based server for predicting and evaluating inverted repeats in nucleotide sequences. *Biochem. Biophys. Res. Commun.* **2016**, *478*, 1739–1745. [CrossRef]

41. Brázda, V.; Lýsek, J.; Bartas, M.; Fojta, M. Complex Analyses of Short Inverted Repeats in All Sequenced Chloroplast DNAs. *BioMed Res. Int.* **2018**, *2018*, 1097018. [CrossRef]

42. Ruggiero, E.; Richter, S.N. G-quadruplexes and G-quadruplex ligands: Targets and tools in antiviral therapy. *Nucleic Acids Res.* **2018**, *46*, 3270–3283. [CrossRef]

43. Chen, B.-J.; Wu, Y.-L.; Tanaka, Y.; Zhang, W. Small Molecules Targeting c-Myc Oncogene: Promising Anti-Cancer Therapeutics. *Int. J. Biol. Sci.* **2014**, *10*, 1084–1096. [CrossRef] [PubMed]

44. Belmonte-Reche, E.; Martínez-García, M.; Guédin, A.; Zuffo, M.; Arévalo-Ruiz, M.; Doria, F.; Campos-Salinas, J.; Maynadier, M.; López-Rubio, J.J.; Freccero, M.; et al. G-Quadruplex Identification in the Genome of Protozoan Parasites Points to Naphthalene Diimide Ligands as New Antiparasitic Agents. *J. Med. Chem.* **2018**, *61*, 1231–1240. [CrossRef]

45. Li, F.; Mulyana, Y.; Feterl, M.; Warner, J.M.; Collins, J.G.; Keene, F.R. The antimicrobial activity of inert oligonuclear polypyridylruthenium(II) complexes against pathogenic bacteria, including MRSA. *Dalton Trans.* **2011**, *40*, 5032–5038. [CrossRef]

46. Li, F.; Grant Collins, J.; Richard Keene, F. Ruthenium complexes as antimicrobial agents. *Chem. Soc. Rev.* **2015**, *44*, 2529–2542. [CrossRef] [PubMed]

47. Xu, L.; Chen, X.; Wu, J.; Wang, J.; Ji, L.; Chao, H. Dinuclear Ruthenium(II) Complexes That Induce and Stabilise G-Quadruplex DNA. *Chem. Eur. J.* **2015**, *21*, 4008–4020. [CrossRef]

48. Xu, L.; Zhang, D.; Huang, J.; Deng, M.; Zhang, M.; Zhou, X. High fluorescence selectivity and visual detection of G-quadruplex structures by a novel dinuclear ruthenium complex. *Chem. Commun.* **2010**, *46*, 743–745. [CrossRef] [PubMed]

49. Wilson, T.; Williamson, M.P.; Thomas, J.A. Differentiating quadruplexes: Binding preferences of a luminescent dinuclear ruthenium (II) complex with four-stranded DNA structures. *Org. Biomol. Chem.* **2010**, *8*, 2617–2621. [CrossRef] [PubMed]

50. Codd, G.A.; Lindsay, J.; Young, F.M.; Morrison, L.F.; Metcalf, J.S. Harmful cyanobacteria. In *Harmful Cyanobacteria*; Springer: Dordrecht, The Netherlands, 2005; pp. 1–23.

51. Perrone, R.; Lavezzo, E.; Riello, E.; Manganelli, R.; Palù, G.; Toppo, S.; Provvedi, R.; Richter, S.N. Mapping and characterization of G-quadruplexes in Mycobacterium tuberculosis gene promoter regions. *Sci. Rep.* **2017**, *7*, 5743. [CrossRef] [PubMed]

52. Lavezzo, E.; Berselli, M.; Frasson, I.; Perrone, R.; Palù, G.; Brazzale, A.R.; Richter, S.N.; Toppo, S. G-quadruplex forming sequences in the genome of all known human viruses: A comprehensive guide. *PLOS Comput. Biol.* **2018**, *14*, e1006675. [CrossRef]

53. Beaume, N.; Pathak, R.; Yadav, V.K.; Kota, S.; Misra, H.S.; Gautam, H.K.; Chowdhury, S. Genome-wide study predicts promoter-G4 DNA motifs regulate selective functions in bacteria: Radioresistance of D. radiodurans involves G4 DNA-mediated regulation. *Nucleic Acids Res.* **2013**, *41*, 76–89. [CrossRef]

54. Kota, S.; Dhamodharan, V.; Pradeepkumar, P.I.; Misra, H.S. G-quadruplex forming structural motifs in the genome of Deinococcus radiodurans and their regulatory roles in promoter functions. *Appl. Microbiol. Biotechnol.* **2015**, *99*, 9761–9769. [CrossRef]

55. Repoila, F.; Darfeuille, F. Small regulatory non-coding RNAs in bacteria: Physiology and mechanistic aspects. *Biol. Cell* **2009**, *101*, 117–131. [CrossRef] [PubMed]

56. Brázda, V.; Kolomazník, J.; Lýsek, J.; Bartas, M.; Fojta, M.; Šťastný, J.; Mergny, J.-L. G4Hunter web application: A web server for G-quadruplex prediction. *Bioinformatics* **2019**, btz087. [CrossRef]

57. Sayers, E.W.; Agarwala, R.; Bolton, E.E.; Brister, J.R.; Canese, K.; Clark, K.; Connor, R.; Fiorini, N.; Funk, K.; Hefferon, T.; et al. Database resources of the National Center for Biotechnology Information. *Nucleic Acids Res.* **2019**, *47*, D23–D28. [CrossRef]

58. Federhen, S. The NCBI taxonomy database. *Nucleic Acids Res.* **2011**, *40*, D136–D143. [CrossRef]

59. Letunic, I.; Bork, P. Interactive tree of life (iTOL) v3: An online tool for the display and annotation of phylogenetic and other trees. *Nucleic Acids Res.* **2016**, *44*, W242–W245. [CrossRef]

Sample Availability: Not available.

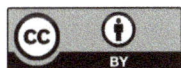

molecules

MDPI

Article

Conformational Dynamics of the RNA G-Quadruplex and its Effect on Translation Efficiency

Tamaki Endoh [1] and Naoki Sugimoto [1,2,*]

[1] Frontier Institute for Biomolecular Engineering Research (FIBER), Konan University,
7-1-20 Minatojima-Minamimachi, Chuo-ku, Kobe 650-0047, Japan; t-endoh@konan-u.ac.jp

[2] Graduate School of Frontiers of Innovative Research in Science and Technology (FIRST), Konan University,
7-1-20 Minatojima-Minamimachi, Chuo-ku, Kobe 650-0047, Japan

* Correspondence: sugimoto@konan-u.ac.jp; Tel.: +81-78-303-1147; Fax: +81-78-303-1495

Academic Editor: Sara Richter
Received: 12 April 2019; Accepted: 22 April 2019; Published: 24 April 2019

Abstract: During translation, intracellular mRNA folds co-transcriptionally and must refold following the passage of ribosome. The mRNAs can be entrapped in metastable structures during these folding events. In the present study, we evaluated the conformational dynamics of the kinetically favored, metastable, and hairpin-like structure, which disturbs the thermodynamically favored G-quadruplex structure, and its effect on co-transcriptional translation in prokaryotic cells. We found that nascent mRNA forms a metastable hairpin-like structure during co-transcriptional folding instead of the G-quadruplex structure. When the translation progressed co-transcriptionally before the metastable hairpin-like structure transition to the G-quadruplex, function of the G-quadruplex as a roadblock of the ribosome was sequestered. This suggested that kinetically formed RNA structures had a dominant effect on gene expression in prokaryotes. The results of this study indicate that it is critical to consider the conformational dynamics of RNA-folding to understand the contributions of the mRNA structures in controlling gene expression.

Keywords: conformational dynamics; co-transcriptional folding; co-translational refolding; metastable structure; G-quadruplex; translation suppression

1. Introduction

An mRNA sequence not only determines the sequence of amino acids in protein but also controls gene expression by the formation of secondary and tertiary structures [1–4]. Thus, RNA structures present in the transcriptome of an organism are of interest since the structural elements formed by the RNA directly impact gene expression [5–8].

Owing to the directional nature of the transcription reaction, RNA structure elements are folded from 5′ to 3′ direction, a process referred to as co-transcriptional folding [9,10]. Co-transcriptional RNA folding restricts the landscape of its structure formation, which also engages the formation of metastable RNA structures [11]. These metastable structures are transient and show conformational transition to thermodynamically stable ones during the directional folding or post-transcriptional organization of the RNAs. The structures of coding regions of mRNAs are also reorganized co-translationally following passage of the ribosome, which incorporates and discharges single-stranded mRNA as the template strand. Thus, the intracellular RNA structures are transient and fluctuate dynamically over time as the processes involved in gene expressions occur.

G-quadruplexes are non-canonical structure elements formed by guanine-rich (G-rich) sequences in the DNA and RNA [12,13]. Since G-quadruplexes are stabilized under molecular crowding conditions, which mimics intracellular molecular environment [14–16], it is speculated that these structures have biological functions [17,18]. Previous studies have indicated that G-quadruplexes formed on the template strands of DNAs and RNAs become a roadblock of proteins that moves progressively on the template strands such as DNA polymerase, RNA polymerase and ribosome [19–23]. G-quadruplexes formed by mRNAs suppress progression of the ribosome along both non-coding (5′-untranslated) and coding (open reading frame, ORF) regions, and reduce their levels of protein expression [23–27]. G-quadruplex-mediated suppression of elongation during translation in the coding region also affects the ribosomal frameshift and nascent protein folding [28–30]. While multiple studies have implicated various functions of the G-quadruplex [17,31–34], a recent study suggested that the G-quadruplexes in eukaryotic cells are found in a globally unfolded state [35]. Additionally, an impairment in the translation and growth of bacteria caused by the G-quadruplex suggested an evolutionary depletion of G-quadruplex–forming sequences in prokaryotes [35]. However, we previously found five G-quadruplex–forming sequences in the ORF of the *E. coli* genes, including *glyQ*, which encodes the glycyl-tRNA synthetases and is fundamental for gene expression [23]. Since these findings are contradictory, to ascertain their accuracy, it would be necessary to discuss the dynamic behavior of RNA G-quadruplexes in cells [36]. The kinetics of formation and dissociation of the G-quadruplex are significantly slower than those of the canonical secondary structures [37–40]. The slow folding rate of the G-quadruplex is disadvantageous for its co-transcriptional folding and increases the possibility to form alternative metastable structures such as hairpins. When the translation reaction progresses before the metastable mRNA structure transitions to the stable G-quadruplex, its effect as a roadblock of the ribosome would be sequestered. Particularly, in prokaryotic systems, translation begins during transcription immediately after the ribosomal binding site is synthesized on the mRNA and discharged from the RNA polymerase. If metastable RNA structures are formed prior to formation of the G-quadruplex, a balance between the rates of transition from the metastable to the G-quadruplex structures and progress of the translation reaction may have a significant effect on gene expression. Thus, effects of the folding dynamics of G-quadruplexes on translation reactions should be elucidated to understand the characteristic processes involved in gene expression by co-transcriptional translation.

In the current study, we demonstrated that the metastable hairpin-like structure formed co-transcriptionally or co-translationally and the time lag between transcription and translation are the key factors that affect formation of the G-quadruplex, and thereby, suppression of translation both in vitro and in *E. coli* cells. The rate of transition from metastable to stable structures enables dynamic control of gene expression suggesting that a code for temporal gene expression is present in many mRNA structures.

2. Results

2.1. Design of RNAs that Potentially Form Metastable Hairpin-Like and Stable G-Quadruplex Structures

It has been demonstrated that the G-rich sequence derived from the ORF of the *E. coli EutE* gene forms a stable G-quadruplex and suppresses the process of elongation during translation in mammalian cells [23]. The wild-type G-rich sequence contains two cytosine nucleobases at the 5′ end that flanking of the G-rich region and several cytosines in regions of the loops, which connect the guanine tracts involved in G-quartets formation. The sequence forms a metastable hairpin-like structure with several G-C base pairs, in which the thermodynamic stability ($\Delta G°$) predicted by the Mfold program [41] is −11.3 kcal mol^{-1} (Figure 1b). The metastable hairpin-like structure transitions to the thermodynamically stable G-quadruplex in response to the potassium ion [42]. Thus, we expected a dynamic behavior of the G-rich sequence during its involvement in the processes of gene expression in the cells. Here, we designed RNA derivatives based on the wild-type G-rich sequence. Mutant A was designed to disrupt formation of the G-quadruplex. It has five mutations from guanine to adenine at positions involved in the formation of G-quartets. Mutant B and mutant C were designed to destabilize the metastable hairpin-like structure, while they maintained the numbers of the guanine tracts. Predicted hairpin-like structures in mutant B (with two mutations compared to the wild-type sequence) and mutant C (with four mutations) are significantly less stable than those of the wild-type sequence (Figure 1b). All sequences encode the same amino acids to enable evaluation of gene expression levels by analyzing the luminescence signal of the reporter protein, *Renilla* luciferase (Figure 1a).

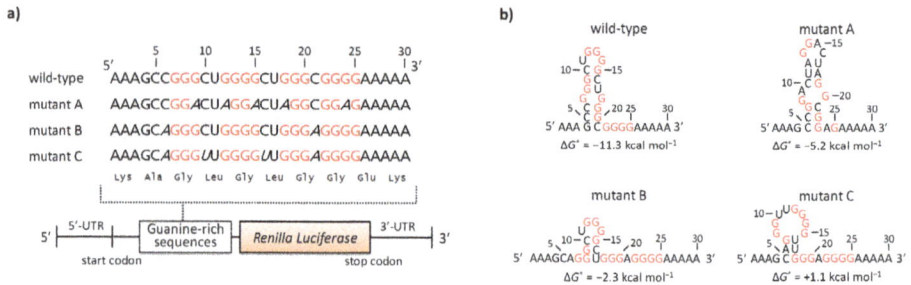

Figure 1. G-rich sequence variants designed to form metastable hairpin-like structures with different stabilities. (**a**) G-rich sequence elements and reporter mRNA constructs. Guanine nucleobases expected to be involved in the formation of the G-quadruplex structure are given in red. Nucleotides mutated from the wild-type sequence are indicated in italics. The amino acid sequence is indicated below the sequence of the nucleic acids and the reporter construct is shown schematically. (**b**) Secondary structures of the G-rich sequence variants predicted using the Mfold program. Thermodynamic stabilities ($\Delta G°$) of the secondary structures predicted by the Mfold program are given.

Formation of G-quadruplexes by the RNA oligonucleotides (shown in Figure 1b) was evaluated by circular dichroism (CD) spectroscopy and RNase T1 digestion after refolding in buffers containing potassium at physiological concentrations (100 mM KCl). The CD spectra of the wild-type, mutant B and mutant C oligonucleotides were characterized by positive and negative peaks at 265 nm and 240 nm, respectively (Supporting Figure S1a). These peaks are characteristics of parallel G-quadruplex structures. While the CD spectrum of mutant A had peaks at around 265 nm and 240 nm, a large negative peak at 210 nm suggested the formation of a hairpin-like structure partially forming an A-form RNA duplex (Figure 1b) [43]. Formation of G-quadruplexes by wild-type, mutant B, and mutant C, and hairpin-like structure by mutant A was also suggested by RNase T1 cleavage of the oligonucleotides (Supporting Figure S1b). RNase T1 cleaved the wild-type, mutant B, and mutant C oligonucleotides at guanines G_{15} and G_{25}, which are located at 3′ positions of the tracts of four guanines. Other guanines in the tracts were protected from the nuclease probably due to their involvement in the G-quartets. These results suggested that wild-type, mutant B, and mutant C oligonucleotides predominantly form parallel G-quadruplex structures containing three G-quartets in a buffer containing physiological concentrations of potassium (Supporting Figure S1c). In contrast, significant RNase T1 cleavage was observed at G_{13}, G_{14}, and G_{25}, which are locating loop and 3′ tail regions of the hairpin-like structure of mutant A (Figure 1b).

2.2. Formation of Metastable Hairpin-Like Structure during Transcription

Wild-type and mutant sequences were inserted into the 5′ region of the ORF encoding *Renilla* luciferase as the reporter gene (Figure 1a). DNA templates prepared using PCR were transcribed in vitro by T7 RNA polymerase in a buffer containing 100 mM potassium. After a transcription reaction at 37 °C for 30 min, TURBO DNase was added to the reaction mixture to degrade the DNA templates. Using agarose gel electrophoresis, it was confirmed that similar amounts of mRNA transcripts were obtained from all the templates (Figure 2a). N-methyl mesoporphyrin (NMM), a fluorescence indicator of the G-quadruplex structure [23,25,30], was added to the intact transcripts to evaluate formation of the G-quadruplex during transcription (Figure 2b). The fluorescence signals of NMM mixed with the mRNAs of mutant B and mutant C were significantly higher than those mixed with the control sample, which consisted of a solution for performing the transcription reaction without the DNA template, and with mutant A mRNA, which does not form a G-quadruplex. In contrast, the fluorescence signal of NMM mixed with the wild-type mRNA was almost equivalent to that of the mutant A mRNA. These results indicated that the wild-type mRNA does not form a G-quadruplex, whereas the mRNAs of mutant B and mutant C, which have the same guanine tracts as well as the wild-type mRNA but contain mutations, formed G-quadruplexes during transcription.

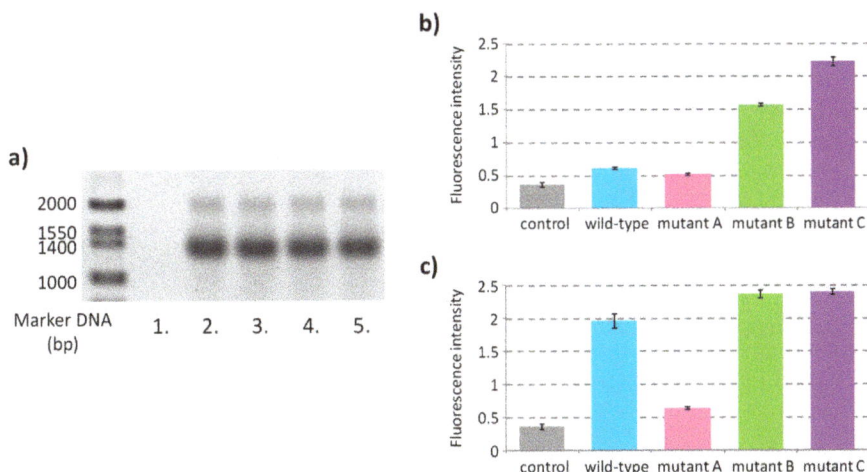

Figure 2. Co-transcriptional formation of the G-quadruplex depending on the stability of metastable hairpin-like structures. (**a**) mRNA transcripts of the reaction without DNA template (lane 1), with DNA template for wild-type (lane 2), mutant A (lane 3), mutant B (lane 4), and mutant C (lane 5) were electrophoresed on an agarose gel. mRNAs were stained with ethidium bromide and imaged at 532 nm excitation and 575 nm emission wavelengths. (**b,c**) Fluorescence intensities of NMM mixed with mRNA transcripts immediately after transcription (**b**) or after refolding by heating to 70 °C and then cooling to 25 °C (**c**). mRNA transcripts were diluted in a buffer containing 50 mM HEPES-KOH (pH 7.6), 5 mM magnesium acetate, 100 mM potassium glutamate, 2 mM spermidine, 0.01% Tween 20, 0.01% DMSO, and 500 nM NMM. NMM fluorescence was measured at 37 °C at 400 nm excitation and 615 nm emission wavelengths. Values are expressed as means ± S.D. of experiments performed in triplicates.

The NMM fluorescence signals were also evaluated with mRNAs that were denatured at 70 °C and refolded by cooling to 25 °C (Figure 2c); this treatment favors the formation of the structure that has maximum thermodynamic stability. Fluorescence of NMM mixed with the wild-type mRNA had increased significantly after refolding compared to that mixed with the intact wild-type mRNA without refolding (Figure 2b,c). This indicated that the G-quadruplex was more stable than the kinetically favored structure formed during transcription as an oligonucleotide of the wild-type G-rich sequence formed a G-quadruplex in a buffer containing 100 mM potassium (Supporting Figure S1). It is considered that the hairpin-like structure of wild type mRNA (as shown in Figure 1b) was formed as a kinetically favored metastable structure during transcription and had suppressed formation of the G-quadruplex. The fluorescence of NMM mixed with mutant B also increased after refolding of the mRNA. The small hairpin structure of mutant B is predicted to have a $\Delta G°$ of −2.3 kcal mol^{-1} (Figure 1b). The small increase of NMM fluorescence after refolding of mutant B mRNA suggests that some population of this mRNA formed the small hairpin structure co-transcriptionally. The fluorescence signals of NMM mixed with mRNAs of mutant A and mutant C were similar before and after the refolding, suggesting that the mRNA of mutant A does not adopt a G-quadruplex structure, whereas that of mutant C forms one irrespective of the folding conditions.

Time-course analyses of NMM fluorescence during in vitro transcription [44] were found to support co-transcriptional folding of metastable hairpin-like structures in the wild-type and mutant B mRNAs (Supporting Figure S2). Although the fluorescence signal of NMM increased with the reaction time of transcription for both mutant C and mutant B mRNAs, the rate of increase in signal in the mRNA of mutant B was slower. This indicated that the mRNA of mutant B first formed the metastable small hairpin structure co-transcriptionally and then transitioned to the more stable G-quadruplex. The $\Delta G°$ of the predicted hairpin-like secondary structure of the mutant C oligonucleotide was positive (Figure 1b); therefore, the mutant C mRNA had probably adopted the G-quadruplex structure during transcription without competition from any other metastable structure. In the case of wild-type mRNA, an increase of NMM fluorescence with the reaction time, which is slightly faster than that of mutant A mRNA, suggested that a small population of mRNAs formed the G-quadruplex during or after transcription. An increase in fluorescence with the mRNA of mutant A is possibly due to a non-specific interaction of NMM with the long mRNA [30].

2.3. Effects of G-Quadruplex Sequestering on In Vitro Translation

Translation of mRNAs with and without refolding was carried out in vitro. After reactions at 37 °C for 30 min, the translation was terminated by addition of RNase A and puromycin; the nuclease degrades the transcript and the antibiotic immediately terminates the elongation process [45]. Protein expression levels in the *E. coli* S30 extract were determined based on the luminescence signal obtained after addition of the substrate for *Renilla* luciferase (Figure 3a). The relative intensities of luminescence were inversely correlated to those of the fluorescence observed when transcripts were incubated with NMM (Figure 2b,c). There was a large difference between the levels of protein expression observed in mRNA of the wild-type with and without refolding. When mRNAs were not refolded, the *Renilla* luciferase signal obtained from the wild-type was similar to that of the mutant A. When the mRNAs were refolded prior to translation, the level of signal from the wild-type was similar to those from mutant B and mutant C. These results indicate that translation was suppressed by the G-quadruplex, which is consistent with our previous reports [23,25]. Contrarily, even though the G-quadruplex is a thermodynamically stable structure, the translation reaction was found to progress smoothly and the level of protein expression had increased when the kinetically favored, metastable, secondary structure was sequestering the G-quadruplex (Figure 3b).

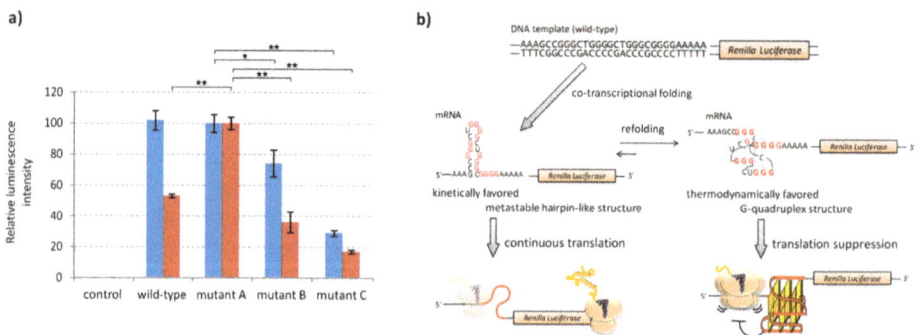

Figure 3. Protein expression levels from intact mRNA and after its refolding using the in vitro translation system of *E. coli* S30 extract. (**a**) Relative luminescence intensities from *Renilla* luciferase translated from mRNA transcripts with (red) and without (blue) refolding. Luminescence signals were measured after addition of coelenterazine (5 μM) to the translated products and were normalized to the signal obtained from mutant A mRNA. Values are expressed as mean ± S.D. of triplicate experiments. Asterisks indicate two-tailed *P*-values for Student's *t*-test: * $P < 0.05$ and ** $P < 0.01$. (**b**) Effect of the mRNA structure elements formed during co-transcriptional folding or refolding of wild-type G-rich sequence on translation reaction.

2.4. Effects of Co-Transcriptional Translation and Co-Translational mRNA Refolding on Gene Expression

To evaluate the effects of continuous co- and post-transcriptional translation systems on the reporter gene expression, the time courses of the protein expressions were evaluated in multiple turn-over translation reactions. Here, in vitro protein synthesis using recombinant elements (PURE) system (PUREfrex®; GeneFrontier) [46,47] was used to circumvent the obscurant effect of degradation of the DNA templates and mRNAs during the reaction. To mimic the co-transcriptional translation system in prokaryotes, DNA templates were mixed with T7 RNA polymerase and a translation solution of the PURE system. Protein expression levels in the coupled reaction were evaluated over a time course of 120 min (Figure 4a). At 15 min, the levels of protein expression were comparable among the sequence variants. These results suggested that translation began immediately after the mRNA was discharged from the RNA polymerase before formation of the G-quadruplex, which suppresses the translation. In contrast, after the 60 min reaction time point, the protein expression levels from the mRNA of mutant C were significantly reduced compared to those of the other sequence variants. It is expected that the mRNA of mutant C formed the G-quadruplex without the formation of any metastable secondary structure after the ribosome had passed through the G-rich sequence region as it efficiently formed the G-quadruplex during transcription (Figure S2). Thus, the numbers of mutant C mRNA, which formed the G-quadruplex, possibly accumulated with the reaction time and progressively suppressed post-transcriptional translation in the multiple turn-over system (Figure 4b).

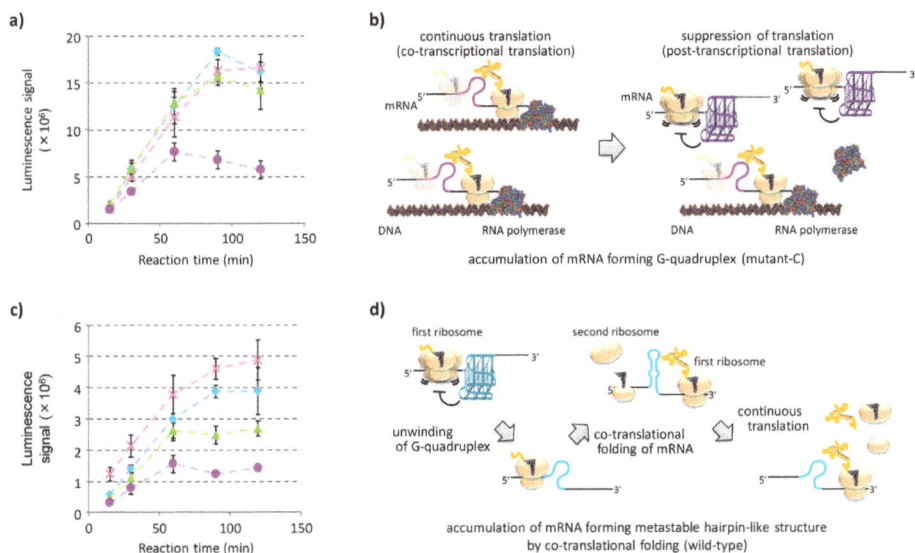

Figure 4. Time course of the levels of protein expression affected by co-transcriptional and co-translational RNA conformational dynamics within the hairpin-like and G-quadruplex structures. (**a**) Time course of co-transcriptional translation of reporter genes encoding wild-type (blue), mutant A (pink), mutant B (green), and mutant C (purple) sequences. DNA templates were mixed with the PURE system solution in the presence of T7 RNA polymerase and incubated at 37 °C. (**b**) Predicted suppression of translation caused by accumulation of the mutant C mRNA, which formed the G-quadruplex, with increasing reaction time. (**c**) Time course of translation of the refolded mRNAs with G-rich sequence of the wild-type (blue), mutant A (pink), mutant B (green), and mutant C (purple). Transcribed mRNAs refolded at 70 °C were mixed with PURE system solution and incubated at 37 °C. (**d**) Schematic of co-translational folding of metastable hairpin-like structure in wild-type mRNA that allows uninhibited translation by a subsequent ribosome. In (**a**) and (**c**), luminescence intensities of *Renilla* luciferase are expressed as mean ± S.D. of triplicate experiments.

Time course of protein expression levels after addition of refolded mRNAs were also evaluated (Figure 4c). After translation for 15 min, the levels of protein expression of wild-type, mutant B, and mutant C mRNAs were found to be significantly lesser than those of the mRNA of mutant A. We had expected these results because all mRNAs except the mutant A adopted a G-quadruplex structure after refolding and suppressed translation (Figure 3a). Signals of relative luminescence in mRNAs of the wild-type, mutant B, and mutant C at the 15-min time point were 46%, 37%, and 24%, respectively, compared to that of the mutant A mRNA. Despite significant differences in the levels of protein expression at 15 min, an increase in the rate of protein expression after 15-min time point for the wild-type mRNA was very similar to that of the mutant A mRNA. This result suggests that wild-type mRNA co-translationally refolded the metastable hairpin-like structure after the ribosome passed through the G-rich sequence region and was no longer able to suppress the translation (Figure 4d). The levels of relative protein expressions of the wild-type, mutant B, and mutant C mRNAs at the 120-min time point were 80%, 55%, and 29% compared to that of mutant A mRNA, respectively. The metastable small hairpin structure formed during co-translational folding of the mutant B mRNA transitioned to the G-quadruplex significantly faster than that formed by the wild-type mRNA. Thus, in the experimental condition without additional transcription from the DNA template, it was observed that the mRNA of mutant B caused moderate repression of translation.

2.5. Protein Expression in E. coli Influenced by the Metastable mRNA Structure

Plasmid vectors which code the reporter gene constructs were transformed into the *E. coli* strain BL21(DE3). Expression of reporter proteins was induced by the addition of 100 μM isopropyl β-D-1-thiogalactopyranoside either in the absence or presence of 0.5 μM tetracycline. Tetracycline prevents binding of the aminoacyl-tRNA to its ribosomal acceptor site by interaction with the 30S ribosomal subunit [48]. After incubation for 60 min, the protein expression levels in *E. coli* were evaluated based on the luminescence signals from the cell lysates. The luminescence signals were normalized based on the optical density at 600 nm when the *E. coli* were lysed. In the absence of tetracycline, the levels of protein expression were very similar among all the mRNA variants (Figure 5a). Based on the results of the in vitro translation coupled with transcription at the 15-min time point, it was conjectured that the levels of protein expression were similar among the variants, because the mRNAs were translated before they formed the G-quadruplex (Figure 4a). Contrary to the normal translation conditions, in the presence of tetracycline, the level of protein expression from the mRNA of mutant C was significantly reduced compared to that of the other sequence variants (Figure 5b). Reduction in the activity of the ribosome would provide a time lag between the transcription of mRNA and initiation of the translation. Under these conditions, mutant C mRNA was expected to form the G-quadruplex structure without formation of the metastable secondary structure and suppressed the translation reaction in *E. coli*. Similar results were also observed in the presence of 2 μM chloramphenicol, which inhibits the elongation reaction during translation by binding to the 50S ribosomal subunit (Supporting Figure S3).

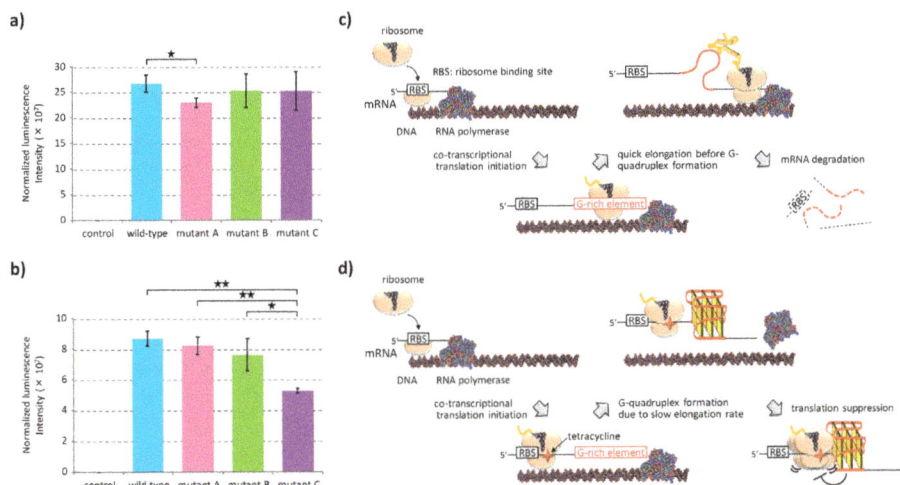

Figure 5. Gene expression in *E. coli* dominated by kinetically favored metastable mRNA structure. (**a,b**) Normalized luminescence intensities of the *E. coli* lysate cultured in the absence (**a**) or presence (**b**) of 0.5 μM tetracycline. Protein expression was induced by 100 μM β-D-1-thiogalactopyranoside in 2× YT medium containing 100 mM potassium glutamate for 1 h. Luminescence signals were normalized by adjusting to an optical density of 600 nm of *E. coli* cells. Values are expressed as mean ± S.D. of triplicated *E. coli* culturing wells. Asterisks indicate two-tailed *P*-values for the Student's *t*-test: * $P < 0.05$ and ** $P < 0.01$. (**c**) Illustration of the co-transcriptional translation in usual culturing conditions of *E. coli*, in which the ribosome translates a region of G-rich elements before forming the G-quadruplex. (**d**) Illustration of co-transcriptional translation in the presence of tetracycline, in which the level of protein expression is dominated by kinetically favored mRNA structures. Only mRNA of mutant C, which forms the G-quadruplex by bypassing any metastable structure, reduces the level of protein expression due to the roadblock function of the G-quadruplex.

3. Discussion

The rate of folding of RNA G-quadruplexes is generally slower than other simple secondary structures and, thus, would be influenced by their entrapment into kinetically favored metastable structures. Here, we designed mRNA derivatives based on G-rich sequences located in the ORF of the *E. coli* EutE mRNA to evaluate the effect of metastable hairpin-like structures with different stabilities (Figure 1b) that compete with the formation of thermodynamically stable G-quadruplexes during protein expression. To facilitate a direct comparison between the levels of protein expressions using luminescence signals, mutations were designed without changing the sequence of their amino acids (Figure 1a). The CD spectra and RNase T1 digestion revealed that all the designed sequences except mutant A adopted the thermodynamically favored G-quadruplex structure after refolding (Figure S1). In contrast, when NMM fluorescence was used as a probe for G-quadruplex formation, it was indicated that, if the G-rich sequence has a potential to form alternative secondary structures, kinetically favored metastable secondary structures are formed during transcription instead of the thermodynamically stable G-quadruplex; this suppressed its function as a roadblock of ribosomes (Figures 2 and 3). In vitro multi turnover translation also indicated that the metastable secondary structures were co-translationally formed and consequently sequestered the G-quadruplex (Figure 4).

In *E. coli*, mRNAs are quickly degraded by endogenous nucleases with an average half-life of several minutes [49,50]. It was considered that the protein expression in all the sequence variants were similar levels in *E. coli* (Figure 5a) because the mRNAs were translated and degraded before the sequences transitioned to the G-quadruplex (Figure 5c). Additionally, inhibition of ribosomal activity by antibiotics in *E. coli* facilitated the suppression of translation from mutant C mRNA (Figure 5b and Figure S4). It is considered that a decrease in the ribosome activity provided a window time to the mutant C mRNA to form the G-quadruplex structure that resulted in the translation suppression. These results suggested that in prokaryotic gene expression with a co-transcriptional translation system, the effect of RNA structure elements on the translation reaction was dominated by kinetically formed RNA structures.

While G-quadruplex is a thermodynamically stable structure, the wild-type sequence derived from the ORF of the *E. coli EutE* gene did not reduce the level of protein expression due to formation of the kinetically favored metastable structure. Our data suggested that formation of a metastable hairpin-like structure enables *E. coli* to express the *EutE* gene, which encodes acetaldehyde dehydrogenase, to utilize ethanolamine as a carbon source [51]. All five G-quadruplex-forming sequences found previously in the ORF of the *E. coli* genes efficiently suppressed the ribosome progression under conditions in which the thermodynamically favored G-quadruplex was formed after refolding [23]. In each of these natural sequences, the mRNAs are predicted to form relatively stable hairpin-like structures that potentially sequester the G-quadruplex structure. These hairpin-like structures have $\Delta G°$ values ranging from -5.1 to -11.9 kcal mol^{-1} which are more stable than those of the mutant B mRNA (Supporting Figure S4). These metastable hairpin-like structures should form co-transcriptionally to enable efficient expression of the genes by disrupting formation of the thermodynamically stable G-quadruplex. This may be one of the reasons for these secondary structures to be evolutionarily conserved within the coding regions [52,53].

Co-transcriptional folding of RNA is one of the general mechanisms to functionalize both noncoding and coding transcripts in vivo [9]. The translation reaction in which a ribosome incorporates and discharges the mRNA as single strand also forces directional folding of the mRNA co-translationally. The directionality of RNA folding may lead to the formation of kinetically entrapped metastable structures that would, in turn, influence the resulting function of the RNA [54–58]. The dynamic features of intracellular RNAs are probably a reason why predictions of RNA structures based on thermodynamics have a less than perfect correlation with those characterized in vivo [6]. Evidences suggest that metastable RNA structures formed during directional folding transition rapidly to thermodynamically stable ones in vivo [59,60]. However, as demonstrated in the present study, if the metastable structures are sufficiently stable over a considerable timeframe from a biological standpoint, the metastable structures existing transiently will impact the biological reactions [11]. Particularly, in microorganisms, which have a relatively short lifecycle, the influence of metastable RNA structures would be relatively significant [54,57]. Even in eukaryotes, recent computational studies of RNA structures have suggested that the metastable RNA structures have an impact on gene modulations [61–63]. The impacts of the metastable RNA structure elements will vary depending on various kinetic factors such as the rates of transcription and translation, transition of the metastable structures, and translocation and degradation of the RNAs, respectively. Therefore, when the influence of metastable RNA structures on gene expressions is compared between eukaryotes and prokaryotes with different kinetic factors involved in the processes of gene expression, we will be able to provide important findings on the role of metastable RNA structures in biological systems.

4. Materials and Methods

4.1. CD Spectrum Acquisition

RNA oligonucleotides purchased from Japan Bio Services Co., Ltd. (Saitama, Japan). were incubated in a buffer containing 50 mM Tris-HCl (pH 7.6), 5 mM magnesium acetate, 100 mM KCl, 2 mM spermidine, and 0.01% (*v/v*) Tween 20 at 70 °C for 5 min and cooled to 4 °C at a rate of 1 °C min^{-1}. The CD spectra were collected on a JASCO (Tokyo, Japan) J-820 spectropolarimeter at 37 °C in cuvettes of 1.0 mm path length. The CD spectra shown are averages of three scans. The temperature of the cell holder was regulated by a JASCO PTC-348 temperature controller.

4.2. Partial Digestion of RNA Oligonucleotide by RNase T1

RNA oligonucleotides were labelled with Alexa Fluor 546 C5-maleimide (Thermo Fisher Scientific, Waltham, MA, USA) using the 5′ EndTag Nucleic Acid Labelling System (Vector Laboratories, Burlingame, CA, USA). Labelled RNAs were purified using a denaturing polyacrylamide gel and precipitated with ethanol in the presence of 20 µg glycogen. Five pmol labelled RNAs in a transcription-buffer (T-buffer) containing 50 mM HEPES-KOH (pH 7.6), 5 mM magnesium acetate, 100 mM potassium glutamate, 2 mM spermidine and 0.01% (v/v) Tween 20 were incubated at 70 °C for 5 min and cooled to 37 °C at a rate of 1 °C min^{-1}. The samples were incubated with 0.02 U of RNase T1 (Roche, Basel, Switzerland) at 37 °C for 10 min and electrophoresed on a 20% denaturing polyacrylamide gel at 70 °C. The fluorescence signal in the gel was imaged using a FLA-5100 fluorescence image scanner (Fuji Film, Tokyo, Japan) with 532 nm excitation and 575 nm emission.

4.3. Construction of Reporter Plasmids

Plasmid vectors encoding wild-type or mutant A sequences in the ORF of *Renilla* luciferase (pCMV-TnT-G-rich-RL) were previously constructed based on pCMV-TnT vector (Promega, Madison, WI, USA) [19]. The reporter gene constructs on the pCMV-TnT-G-rich-RL plasmids were digested by *EcoRI* and *NotI*, and appropriate DNA fragments were inserted into same restriction enzyme sites of pET21a (+) (Novagen, Madison, WI, USA). DNA fragments encoding G-rich sequences of mutant B and mutant C (Table S1) were purchased from Hokkaido System Science Co., Ltd. (Hokkaido, Japan) and inserted into the *EcoR* I and *Sal* I sites to yield variants of the pET21-G-rich-RL plasmids.

4.4. Preparation of the DNA Template

DNA templates encoding the G-rich sequences followed by the *Renilla* luciferase ORF were amplified from the pET21-G-rich-RL plasmids by PCR using the T7 promoter and terminator primers. Amplified DNA fragments were purified using the QIAquick PCR Purification Kit (Qiagen, Hilden, Germany).

4.5. In Vitro Transcription

DNA templates (20 ng/µL) were mixed with T7 RNA polymerase (2 U/µL) in T-buffer containing 1 mM rNTPs and incubated at 37 °C for 30 min. TURBO DNase (Thermo Fisher Scientific) was subsequently added to the reaction mixture at a concentration of 0.048 U/µL and incubated at 37 °C for 30 min. In order to refold the mRNA, transcripts were incubated at 70 °C for 3 min followed by cooling from 50 °C to 25 °C at a rate of 1 °C min^{-1}.

4.6. Fluorescence Analysis of NMM

Aliquots (5 µL) of mRNA transcripts with or without refolding were diluted into 50 µL of T-buffer containing 500 nM NMM and 0.01% (v/v) dimethyl sulfoxide. Fluorescence signal of NMM was measured using a microwell plate reader (Varioskan Flash, Thermo Fisher Scientific) at 400 nm excitation and 615 nm emission wavelengths after incubation at 37 °C for 30 min.

4.7. In Vitro Translation

Aliquots (1 µL) of mRNA transcripts with or without refolding were diluted into 4 µL reaction solutions of the *E. coli* S30 Extract System (Promega) and incubated at 37 °C for 30 min. For in vitro translation using PUREfrex (Gene Frontier, Chiba, Japan), aliquots (0.5 µL) of intact or refolded mRNA were diluted into reaction solutions of 2 µL and incubated at 37 °C. The translation reaction was terminated by a 10-fold dilution of the translated product in phosphate buffered saline (PBS) containing RNase A (20 µg/mL) and puromycin (20 µM) followed by incubation at 37 °C for 10 min. Levels of *Renilla* luciferase were determined by measuring the luminescence signal after addition of 5 µM coelenterazine (Promega) on the Varioskan Flash.

4.8. Evaluation of Protein Expression Levels in E. coli

Cells of the *E. coli* strain BL21(DE3) were transformed with the pET21-G-rich-RL plasmids. The cells were cultured over night at 37 °C in 2 × YT media containing 50 µg/mL ampicillin. The cultured cells were diluted 200 times into fresh 2 × YT media and incubated at 37 °C. When they reached an optical density of 0.5–1.0, the cells were transferred to the wells of a 96-well plate and diluted 2-fold with fresh 2× YT media containing final concentrations of 100 µM β-D-1-thiogalactopyranoside and indicated antibiotics. After incubation for 60 min at 37 °C, the optical density of *E. coli* was measured at 600 nm using a microwell plate reader (Infinite M200 Pro, Tecan, Mannedorf, Switzerland). Cells were lysed in 10 µL media using 50 µL of Passive Lysis Buffer (Promega) and the luminescence signal of 2 µL aliquot of the lysate was measured after addition of coelenterazine (5 µM) using Varioskan Flash.

Supplementary Materials: The following are available online at http://www.mdpi.com/1420-3049/24/8/1613/s1, Figure S1: CD spectra and partial digestion of RNA oligonucleotides, Figure S2: Real time monitoring of co-transcriptional G-quadruplex formation, Figure S3: Protein expression levels in *E. coli* in the presence of chloramphenicol, Figure S4: Sequences and secondary structures of G-rich elements found in open reading frames of *E. coli* mRNAs, Table S1: DNA oligonucleotides for synthesis of G-rich sequence variants.

Author Contributions: T.E. and N.S. conceived the study; T.E. designed the constructs and performed experiments; and T.E. and N.S. wrote the paper.

Funding: This work was supported by Grants-in-Aid for Scientific Research from the Ministry of Education, Culture, Sports, Science and Technology (MEXT) and Japan Society for the Promotion of Science (JSPS), especially a Grant-in-Aid for Scientific Research on Innovative Areas "Chemistry for Multimolecular Crowding Biosystems" (JSPS KAKENHI Grant No. JP17H06351), the MEXT-Supported Program for the Strategic Research Foundation at Private Universities (2014–2019), Japan, and The Hirao Taro Foundation of KONAN GAKUEN for Academic Research.

Acknowledgments: The authors thank Misa Kinoshita, Nobuaki Hattori, Akihiro Isumi, and Kenichi Hase for their help with experiments. We would like to thank Editage (www.editage.jp) for English language editing.

Conflicts of Interest: The authors declare no conflict of interest.

References

1. Jin, Y.; Yang, Y.; Zhang, P. New insights into RNA secondary structure in the alternative splicing of pre-mRNAs. *RNA Biol.* **2011**, *8*, 450–457. [CrossRef] [PubMed]
2. Kozak, M. Regulation of translation via mRNA structure in prokaryotes and eukaryotes. *Gene* **2005**, *361*, 13–37. [CrossRef] [PubMed]
3. Smith, A.M.; Fuchs, R.T.; Grundy, F.J.; Henkin, T.M. Riboswitch RNAs: Regulation of gene expression by direct monitoring of a physiological signal. *RNA Biol.* **2008**, *7*, 104–110. [CrossRef]
4. Mauger, D.M.; Siegfried, N.A.; Weeks, K.M. The genetic code as expressed through relationships between mRNA structure and protein function. *FEBS Lett.* **2013**, *587*, 1180–1188. [CrossRef]
5. Ding, Y.; Tang, Y.; Kwok, C.K.; Zhang, Y.; Bevilacqua, P.C.; Assmann, S.M. In vivo genome-wide profiling of RNA secondary structure reveals novel regulatory features. *Nature* **2014**, *505*, 696–700. [CrossRef]
6. Rouskin, S.; Zubradt, M.; Washietl, S.; Kellis, M.; Weissman, J.S. Genome-wide probing of RNA structure reveals active unfolding of mRNA structures in vivo. *Nature* **2014**, *505*, 701–705. [CrossRef] [PubMed]
7. Wan, Y.; Qu, K.; Zhang, Q.C.; Flynn, R.A.; Manor, O.; Ouyang, Z.; Zhang, J.; Spitale, R.C.; Snyder, M.P.; Segal, E.; et al. Landscape and variation of RNA secondary structure across the human transcriptome. *Nature* **2014**, *505*, 706–709. [CrossRef] [PubMed]
8. Mortimer, S.A.; Kidwell, M.A.; Doudna, J.A. Insights into RNA structure and function from genome-wide studies. *Nat. Rev. Genet.* **2014**, *15*, 469–479. [CrossRef]
9. Lai, D.; Proctor, J.R.; Meyer, I.M. On the importance of cotranscriptional RNA structure formation. *RNA* **2013**, *19*, 1461–1473. [CrossRef]
10. Zemora, G.; Waldsich, C. RNA folding in living cells. *RNA Biol.* **2010**, *7*, 634–641. [CrossRef]
11. Endoh, T.; Sugimoto, N. Conformational Dynamics of mRNA in Gene Expression as New Pharmaceutical Target. *Chem. Rec.* **2017**, *17*, 817–832. [CrossRef]
12. Collie, G.W.; Parkinson, G.N. The application of DNA and RNA G-quadruplexes to therapeutic medicines. *Chem. Soc. Rev.* **2011**, *40*, 5867–5892. [CrossRef]

13. Williamson, J.R. G-quartet structures in telomeric DNA. *Annu. Rev. Biophys. Biomol. Struct.* **1994**, *23*, 703–730. [CrossRef] [PubMed]
14. Miyoshi, D.; Fujimoto, T.; Sugimoto, N. Molecular crowding and hydration regulating of G-quadruplex formation. *Top. Curr. Chem.* **2013**, *330*, 87–110.
15. Miyoshi, D.; Karimata, H.; Sugimoto, N. Hydration regulates thermodynamics of G-quadruplex formation under molecular crowding conditions. *J. Am. Chem. Soc.* **2006**, *128*, 7957–7963. [CrossRef] [PubMed]
16. Trajkovski, M.; Endoh, T.; Tateishi-Karimata, H.; Ohyama, T.; Tanaka, S.; Plavec, J.; Sugimoto, N. Pursuing origins of (poly)ethylene glycol-induced G-quadruplex structural modulations. *Nucleic Acids Res.* **2018**, *46*, 4301–4315. [CrossRef]
17. Bugaut, A.; Balasubramanian, S. 5′-UTR RNA G-quadruplexes: Translation regulation and targeting. *Nucleic Acids Res.* **2012**, *40*, 4727–4741. [CrossRef] [PubMed]
18. Millevoi, S.; Moine, H.; Vagner, S. G-quadruplexes in RNA biology. *Wiley Interdiscip. Rev. RNA* **2012**, *3*, 495–507. [CrossRef] [PubMed]
19. Takahashi, S.; Brazier, J.A.; Sugimoto, N. Topological impact of noncanonical DNA structures on Klenow fragment of DNA polymerase. *Proc. Natl. Acad. Sci. USA* **2017**, *114*, 9605–9610. [CrossRef] [PubMed]
20. Tateishi-Karimata, H.; Kawauchi, K.; Sugimoto, N. Destabilization of DNA G-Quadruplexes by Chemical Environment Changes during Tumor Progression Facilitates Transcription. *J. Am. Chem. Soc.* **2018**, *140*, 642–651. [CrossRef]
21. Tateishi-Karimata, H.; Isono, N.; Sugimoto, N. New insights into transcription fidelity: Thermal stability of non-canonical structures in template DNA regulates transcriptional arrest, pause, and slippage. *PLoS ONE* **2014**, *9*, e90580. [CrossRef] [PubMed]
22. Takahashi, S.; Kim, K.T.; Podbevsek, P.; Plavec, J.; Kim, B.H.; Sugimoto, N. Recovery of the Formation and Function of Oxidized G-Quadruplexes by a Pyrene-Modified Guanine Tract. *J. Am. Chem. Soc.* **2018**, *140*, 5774–5783. [CrossRef] [PubMed]
23. Endoh, T.; Kawasaki, Y.; Sugimoto, N. Suppression of gene expression by G-quadruplexes in open reading frames depends on G-quadruplex stability. *Angew. Chem. Int. Ed.* **2013**, *52*, 5522–5526. [CrossRef] [PubMed]
24. Halder, K.; Wieland, M.; Hartig, J.S. Predictable suppression of gene expression by 5′-UTR-based RNA quadruplexes. *Nucleic Acids Res.* **2009**, *37*, 6811–6817. [CrossRef] [PubMed]
25. Endoh, T.; Kawasaki, Y.; Sugimoto, N. Translational halt during elongation caused by G-quadruplex formed by mRNA. *Methods* **2013**, *64*, 73–78. [CrossRef]
26. Kumari, S.; Bugaut, A.; Huppert, J.L.; Balasubramanian, S. An RNA G-quadruplex in the 5′ UTR of the NRAS proto-oncogene modulates translation. *Nat. Chem. Biol.* **2007**, *3*, 218–221. [CrossRef]
27. Gomez, D.; Guedin, A.; Mergny, J.L.; Salles, B.; Riou, J.F.; Teulade-Fichou, M.P.; Calsou, P. A G-quadruplex structure within the 5′-UTR of TRF2 mRNA represses translation in human cells. *Nucleic Acids Res.* **2010**, *38*, 7187–7198. [CrossRef] [PubMed]
28. Yu, C.H.; Teulade-Fichou, M.P.; Olsthoorn, R.C. Stimulation of ribosomal frameshifting by RNA G-quadruplex structures. *Nucleic Acids Res.* **2013**, *42*, 1887–1892. [CrossRef]
29. Endoh, T.; Sugimoto, N. Unusual-1 ribosomal frameshift caused by stable RNA G-quadruplex in open reading frame. *Anal. Chem.* **2013**, *85*, 11435–11439. [CrossRef]
30. Endoh, T.; Kawasaki, Y.; Sugimoto, N. Stability of RNA quadruplex in open reading frame determines proteolysis of human estrogen receptor alpha. *Nucleic Acids Res.* **2013**, *41*, 6222–6231. [CrossRef]
31. Marcel, V.; Tran, P.L.; Sagne, C.; Martel-Planche, G.; Vaslin, L.; Teulade-Fichou, M.P.; Hall, J.; Mergny, J.L.; Hainaut, P.; Van Dyck, E. G-quadruplex structures in TP53 intron 3: Role in alternative splicing and in production of p53 mRNA isoforms. *Carcinogenesis* **2011**, *32*, 271–278. [CrossRef] [PubMed]
32. Hershman, S.G.; Chen, Q.; Lee, J.Y.; Kozak, M.L.; Yue, P.; Wang, L.S.; Johnson, F.B. Genomic distribution and functional analyses of potential G-quadruplex-forming sequences in Saccharomyces cerevisiae. *Nucleic Acids Res.* **2008**, *36*, 144–156. [CrossRef] [PubMed]
33. Morris, M.J.; Negishi, Y.; Pazsint, C.; Schonhoft, J.D.; Basu, S. An RNA G-quadruplex is essential for cap-independent translation initiation in human VEGF IRES. *J. Am. Chem. Soc.* **2010**, *132*, 17831–17839. [CrossRef] [PubMed]
34. Sundquist, W.I.; Heaphy, S. Evidence for interstrand quadruplex formation in the dimerization of human immunodeficiency virus 1 genomic RNA. *Proc. Natl. Acad. Sci. USA* **1993**, *90*, 3393–3397. [CrossRef] [PubMed]

35. Guo, J.U.; Bartel, D.P. RNA G-quadruplexes are globally unfolded in eukaryotic cells and depleted in bacteria. *Science* **2016**, *353*, aaf5371. [CrossRef]
36. Yang, S.Y.; Lejault, P.; Chevrier, S.; Boidot, R.; Robertson, A.G.; Wong, J.M.Y.; Monchaud, D. Transcriptome-wide identification of transient RNA G-quadruplexes in human cells. *Nat. Commun.* **2018**, *9*, 4730. [CrossRef]
37. Zhang, A.Y.; Balasubramanian, S. The kinetics and folding pathways of intramolecular G-quadruplex nucleic acids. *J. Am. Chem. Soc.* **2012**, *134*, 19297–19308. [CrossRef]
38. Ansari, A.; Kuznetsov, S.V. Is hairpin formation in single-stranded polynucleotide diffusion-controlled? *J. Phys. Chem. B* **2005**, *109*, 12982–12989. [CrossRef]
39. Kuznetsov, S.V.; Ansari, A. A kinetic zipper model with intrachain interactions applied to nucleic acid hairpin folding kinetics. *Biophys. J.* **2012**, *102*, 101–111. [CrossRef]
40. Gray, R.D.; Trent, J.O.; Chaires, J.B. Folding and unfolding pathways of the human telomeric G-quadruplex. *J. Mol. Biol.* **2014**, *426*, 1629–1650. [CrossRef]
41. Zuker, M. Mfold web server for nucleic acid folding and hybridization prediction. *Nucleic Acids Res.* **2003**, *31*, 3406–3415. [CrossRef]
42. Rode, A.B.; Endoh, T.; Sugimoto, N. tRNA Shifts the G-quadruplex-Hairpin Conformational Equilibrium in RNA towards the Hairpin Conformer. *Angew. Chem. Int. Ed.* **2016**, *55*, 14315–14319. [CrossRef]
43. Gray, D.M.; Ratliff, R.L. Circular dichroism spectra of poly[d(AC):d(GT)], poly[r(AC):r(GU)], and hybrids poly[d(AC):r(GU)] and poly[r(AC):d(GT)] in the presence of ethanol. *Biopolymers* **1975**, *14*, 487–498. [CrossRef]
44. Endoh, T.; Rode, A.B.; Takahashi, S.; Kataoka, Y.; Kuwahara, M.; Sugimoto, N. Real-Time Monitoring of G-Quadruplex Formation during Transcription. *Anal. Chem.* **2016**, *88*, 1984–1989. [CrossRef]
45. Takahashi, S.; Iida, M.; Furusawa, H.; Shimizu, Y.; Ueda, T.; Okahata, Y. Real-time monitoring of cell-free translation on a quartz-crystal microbalance. *J. Am. Chem. Soc.* **2009**, *131*, 9326–9332. [CrossRef]
46. Shimizu, Y.; Inoue, A.; Tomari, Y.; Suzuki, T.; Yokogawa, T.; Nishikawa, K.; Ueda, T. Cell-free translation reconstituted with purified components. *Nat. Biotechnol.* **2001**, *19*, 751–755. [CrossRef]
47. Shimizu, Y.; Kanamori, T.; Ueda, T. Protein synthesis by pure translation systems. *Methods* **2005**, *36*, 299–304. [CrossRef]
48. Chopra, I.; Roberts, M. Tetracycline antibiotics: Mode of action, applications, molecular biology, and epidemiology of bacterial resistance. *Microbiol. Mol. Biol. Rev.* **2001**, *65*, 232–260. [CrossRef]
49. Rauhut, R.; Klug, G. mRNA degradation in bacteria. *FEMS Microbiol. Rev.* **1999**, *23*, 353–370. [CrossRef]
50. Bernstein, J.A.; Khodursky, A.B.; Lin, P.H.; Lin-Chao, S.; Cohen, S.N. Global analysis of mRNA decay and abundance in Escherichia coli at single-gene resolution using two-color fluorescent DNA microarrays. *Proc. Natl. Acad. Sci. USA* **2002**, *99*, 9697–9702. [CrossRef]
51. Bertin, Y.; Girardeau, J.P.; Chaucheyras-Durand, F.; Lyan, B.; Pujos-Guillot, E.; Harel, J.; Martin, C. Enterohaemorrhagic Escherichia coli gains a competitive advantage by using ethanolamine as a nitrogen source in the bovine intestinal content. *Environ. Microbiol.* **2011**, *13*, 365–377. [CrossRef] [PubMed]
52. Gu, W.; Li, M.; Xu, Y.; Wang, T.; Ko, J.H.; Zhou, T. The impact of RNA structure on coding sequence evolution in both bacteria and eukaryotes. *BMC Evol. Biol.* **2014**, *14*, 87. [CrossRef] [PubMed]
53. Chursov, A.; Frishman, D.; Shneider, A. Conservation of mRNA secondary structures may filter out mutations in Escherichia coli evolution. *Nucleic Acids Res.* **2013**, *41*, 7854–7860. [CrossRef] [PubMed]
54. Nagel, J.H.; Gultyaev, A.P.; Gerdes, K.; Pleij, C.W. Metastable structures and refolding kinetics in hok mRNA of plasmid R1. *RNA* **1999**, *5*, 1408–1418. [CrossRef] [PubMed]
55. Linnstaedt, S.D.; Kasprzak, W.K.; Shapiro, B.A.; Casey, J.L. The role of a metastable RNA secondary structure in hepatitis delta virus genotype III RNA editing. *RNA* **2006**, *12*, 1521–1533. [CrossRef] [PubMed]
56. Repsilber, D.; Wiese, S.; Rachen, M.; Schroder, A.W.; Riesner, D.; Steger, G. Formation of metastable RNA structures by sequential folding during transcription: Time-resolved structural analysis of potato spindle tuber viroid (-)-stranded RNA by temperature-gradient gel electrophoresis. *RNA* **1999**, *5*, 574–584. [CrossRef]
57. Poot, R.A.; Tsareva, N.V.; Boni, I.V.; van Duin, J. RNA folding kinetics regulates translation of phage MS2 maturation gene. *Proc. Natl. Acad. Sci. USA* **1997**, *94*, 10110–10115. [CrossRef]
58. Simon, A.E.; Gehrke, L. RNA conformational changes in the life cycles of RNA viruses, viroids, and virus-associated RNAs. *Biochim. Biophys. Acta* **2009**, *1789*, 571–583. [CrossRef]
59. Mahen, E.M.; Watson, P.Y.; Cottrell, J.W.; Fedor, M.J. mRNA secondary structures fold sequentially but exchange rapidly in vivo. *PLoS Biol.* **2010**, *8*, e1000307. [CrossRef]

60. Mahen, E.M.; Harger, J.W.; Calderon, E.M.; Fedor, M.J. Kinetics and thermodynamics make different contributions to RNA folding in vitro and in yeast. *Mol. Cell* **2005**, *19*, 27–37. [CrossRef]

61. Meyer, I.M.; Miklos, I. Statistical evidence for conserved, local secondary structure in the coding regions of eukaryotic mRNAs and pre-mRNAs. *Nucleic Acids Res.* **2005**, *33*, 6338–6348. [CrossRef]

62. Haas, U.; Sczakiel, G.; Laufer, S.D. MicroRNA-mediated regulation of gene expression is affected by disease-associated SNPs within the 3′-UTR via altered RNA structure. *RNA Biol.* **2012**, *9*, 924–937. [CrossRef]

63. Day, L.; Abdelhadi Ep Souki, O.; Albrecht, A.A.; Steinhofel, K. Accessibility of microRNA binding sites in metastable RNA secondary structures in the presence of SNPs. *Bioinformatics* **2014**, *30*, 343–352. [CrossRef]

Sample Availability: Samples of the compounds are available from the authors.

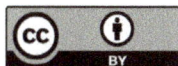

molecules

MDPI

Article

A Novel G-Quadruplex Binding Protein in Yeast—Slx9

Silvia Götz [1,2,†], Satyaprakash Pandey [1,4,†], Sabrina Bartsch [2], Stefan Juranek [3] and Katrin Paeschke [1,2,3,*]

1   University of Groningen, University Medical Center Groningen, European Research Institute for the Biology of Ageing, 9713 AV Groningen, The Netherlands
2   University of Würzburg, Department of Biochemistry, Biocentre, 97074 Würzburg, Germany
3   University Hospital Bonn, Department of Oncology, Hematology and Rheumatology, 53127 Bonn, Germany
4   Current address: Indian Institute of Technology, Department of Biosciences and Bioengineering, Powai, Mumbai 400076, India
*   Correspondence: katrin.paeschke@ukbonn.de; Tel.: +49-228-2875-1706
†   These authors contributed equally to this paper.

Academic Editor: Sara N. Richter
Received: 26 March 2019; Accepted: 3 May 2019; Published: 7 May 2019

Abstract: G-quadruplex (G4) structures are highly stable four-stranded DNA and RNA secondary structures held together by non-canonical guanine base pairs. G4 sequence motifs are enriched at specific sites in eukaryotic genomes, suggesting regulatory functions of G4 structures during different biological processes. Considering the high thermodynamic stability of G4 structures, various proteins are necessary for G4 structure formation and unwinding. In a yeast one-hybrid screen, we identified Slx9 as a novel G4-binding protein. We confirmed that Slx9 binds to G4 DNA structures in vitro. Despite these findings, Slx9 binds only insignificantly to G-rich/G4 regions in *Saccharomyces cerevisiae* as demonstrated by genome-wide ChIP-seq analysis. However, Slx9 binding to G4s is significantly increased in the absence of Sgs1, a RecQ helicase that regulates G4 structures. Different genetic and molecular analyses allowed us to propose a model in which Slx9 recognizes and protects stabilized G4 structures in vivo.

Keywords: protein–DNA interaction; *S. cerevisiae*; G-quadruplex formation; genome stability; RecQ helicase

---

1. Introduction

The observation that secondary structures within DNA or RNA can influence biological processes had a great impact on modern biology (reviewed in [1–4]). One prominent example of such a nucleic acid structure is a G-quadruplex (G4). G4 structures are polymorphic and thermodynamic stable structures that can form within DNA and RNA harboring a specific guanine-rich motif (G4 motif) (reviewed in [2,5]).

Although the in vivo existence of G4 structures was controversially discussed in the past, recent results from computational, biochemical, molecular, and genetic studies provided essential data that G4 structures exist in various organisms and can act as a regulatory tool [2,5–10].

G4 structures are discussed as being a regulatory tool in the cell for telomere maintenance, transcription, translation, and even origin activation [7,10–13]. This assumption is further supported by computational and in vitro and in vivo experiments. These data demonstrated that G4 structures form at specific sites (e.g., promoters) and regulate a specific pathway (e.g., transcription) [6,10,14–18] and can thereby become potential therapeutic targets. In contrast to their regulatory role, stable G4 structures can also block biological processes (e.g., replication, transcription) and, in doing so, increase genome instability (reviewed in [2,19]). G4 structures challenge genome stability by interfering with the normal regulatory machinery and/or stalling of cellular processes (e.g., replication). This can result in genomic mutations and deletions [8,20–22]. To ensure genome stability, controlled formation and unfolding of G4 structures is essential. Cellular machinery is necessary to regulate the kinetics of formation and unfolding of G4 structures in response to specific stimuli. To this date, multiple helicases, like members of the RecQ (e.g., Sgs1 in yeast or WRN or BLM in human) or Pif1 family and a few other proteins (e.g., CNBP) have been identified to support G4 unfolding [23,24]. Mutation or dysregulation of G4-binding proteins, especially helicases, are implicated in many human diseases [25]. Most helicases exhibit the ability to unwind G4 structures in vitro [26]. Some helicases recognize specific G4 motifs, in vivo, during certain biological processes [23,27]. How these helicases gain specificity is still unclear. A few examples are known where an additional protein supports the function of a given helicase. For example, in yeast, Mms1 supports the binding of Pif1 to a specific subset of G4 targets—those which are located on the lagging strand [28]. Identification of G4-recognizing proteins supports the detection of in vivo-relevant G4 structures. Additionally, the characterization of these proteins indirectly helps to gain insights into G4 function in vivo.

In this study, we used a yeast one-hybrid approach to identify *Saccharomyces cerevisiae* Slx9 as a novel G4-interacting protein. In vitro experiments confirmed the specific binding of Slx9 to G4 structures. Slx9 is a non-essential yeast protein that genetically interacts with the yeast RecQ helicase Sgs1 [29]. Sgs1 is involved in various processes that are linked to genome stability, such as DNA repair and G4 unwinding [27,30,31]. However, the functional relationship between Slx9 and Sgs1 is unclear. To further address Slx9 function at G4 structures in vivo, we mapped Slx9-binding sites, genome-wide, by chromatin immunoprecipitation (ChIP) followed by deep sequencing (ChIP-seq). These analyses revealed that Slx9 does not significantly bind, genome-wide, to G4 motifs. However, in the absence of Sgs1, Slx9 binds robustly to G4 motifs. Similarly, in the presence of hydroxyurea (HU), when more G4 structures are detectable [32], Slx9 binding to G4 motifs is increased. Additional genetic analyses allowed us to propose a mechanistic model addressing how Slx9 recognizes stabilized G4 structures.

2. Results

2.1. Identification of Slx9 as a Novel G4-Binding Protein in Vivo

G4 structures are evolutionary conserved, dynamic structures involved in various biological processes [2,5,14,17]. To understand the interaction of G4 structures with various proteins in vivo, an unbiased yeast one-hybrid (Y1H) screen was performed. A G4 motif from chromosome IX ($G4_{IX}$) and a mutated version of the same G4 motif (mut-$G4_{IX}$) were cloned upstream of the aureobasidin A resistance gene (*AUR-1C*) (Figure 1A). Mut-$G4_{IX}$ served as a control to remove any non-specific DNA-binding proteins and select for specific G4-binding proteins. A cDNA library comprising of yeast proteins tagged with the galactose activation domain (GAL4-AD) (Dualsystems Biotech) was transformed in the bait strain. An interaction of a protein with the $G4_{IX}$ motif resulted in the expression of the *AUR-1C* gene and, consequently, growth on aureobasidin A medium. In two independent screens, 156 different proteins were identified (SG, KP unpublished data). One of these proteins was Slx9. Slx9 binding to only the $G4_{IX}$ motif, and not to mut-$G4_{IX}$, was observed. Slx9 is a yeast-specific protein that was demonstrated to genetically interact with the yeast RecQ helicase Sgs1 [29]. Most RecQ helicases, including Sgs1, are potent G4 unwinders [26,31], and their function is linked to DNA repair, telomere maintenance, and transcriptional regulation [27–34].

A

B

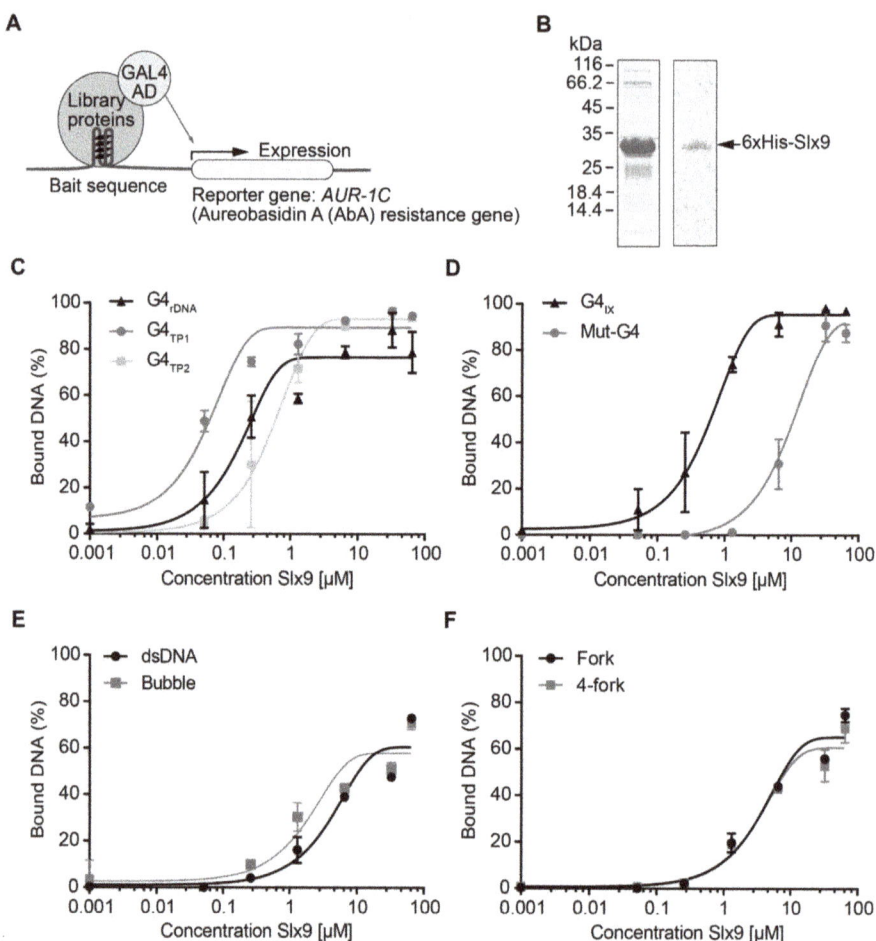

Figure 1. Slx9 is a novel in vitro G4-binding protein. (**A**) Illustration of the yeast one-hybrid screen experimental setup. (**B**) Coomassie staining and Western blot analysis of purified Slx9 protein. The Western blot was performed using an anti-His antibody. 6×His-Slx9 (30 kDa) was detectable between the 25 and 35 kDa marker (arrow). (**C**) Quantification of Slx9 binding to different G4 structures by filter-binding assay, plotted in log scale. Slx9 shows binding to all tested G4 structures with K_d values of 0.55 ± 0.08 μM (G4$_{IX}$), 0.21 ± 0.04 μM (G4$_{rDNA}$), 0.04 ± 0.01 μM (G4$_{TP1}$), and 0.53 ± 0.10 μM (G4$_{TP2}$). (**D**) Slx9 binding to a G4 structure from a selected region of chromosome IX (black) and a mutated version of this G4 motif which cannot fold G4 structures but is 95% identical (grey). (**E,F**) Slx9 binding to other DNA structures such as dsDNA, bubble, forked, and 4-fork substrates. Slx9 showed less affinity to the tested control DNA structures: K_d 15.69 ± 3.57 μM (G4$_{mut}$), 5.27 ± 1.18 μM (dsDNA), 1.73 ± 0.42 μM (bubble), 4.21 ± 0.64 μM (fork), 3.72 ± 0.62 μM (4-fork). Plotted results were based on the average of three independent experiments (n = 3).

To confirm the interaction between Slx9 and G4 structures, we cloned, expressed, and purified Slx9 from *Escherichia coli* (Figure 1B). Purified protein was subjected to standard filter-binding assays to determine the affinity of Slx9 to G4 structures [35] (Supplemental Materials S5A). Binding of Slx9 to different G4 motifs (G4$_{IX}$, G4$_{TP}$, and G4$_{rDNA}$) and other DNA controls (mut-G4$_{IX}$, dsDNA, forked DNA, and 4-way junctions) was tested. Slx9 showed preferential binding to all tested G4 structures with binding affinity for G4 structures ranging between 210 to 550 nM. Slx9 exhibited binding to the control sequences, but this binding was weaker and never reached 100% (Figure 1C–F, see figure legend for K_d values). The selective binding of Slx9 to G4 structures was confirmed using microscale thermophoresis (MST) analysis (Supplementary Materials S5B–C). MST is a powerful tool to analyze ligand–molecule interactions [36]. Fluorescently labelled G4$_{IX}$ and mut-G4$_{IX}$ were incubated with Slx9 in increasing concentrations and subjected to MST to quantify the binding affinities. MST analysis confirmed that Slx9 binds G4$_{IX}$ with a better binding affinity than linear G-rich DNA (mut-G4$_{IX}$) (Supplementary Materials S5B–C). These binding studies further strengthened the Y1H data that Slx9 binds G4 structures.

So far, there are three classes of G4-interacting proteins described in the literature: proteins that support or stabilize G4 formation, proteins that assist their unfolding, and those which recognize formed G4 structures [23,24]. As we detected no unfolding of G4 structures in both binding analyses, we tested whether G4 structures were stabilized by Slx9 binding. G4 structures have a characteristic CD spectrum owing to the π–π interactions between Hoogsteen hydrogen bonds. We assessed the effect of Slx9 on CD spectra of G4$_{IX}$ and mut-G4$_{IX}$. If the G4 structure is stabilized due to Slx9 binding, changes of the characteristic maxima or minima peaks should be detected after addition of the protein. However, Slx9 titration did not result in any observable changes in the signals of G4$_{IX}$ and mut-G4$_{IX}$ spectra, suggesting that the interaction between Slx9 and the G4 motif does not significantly alter the structure and stability of G4 structures (Supplementary Materials S5D–E).

2.2. Slx9 Binds to G-Rich Regions Genome-Wide

To test if in vitro Slx9 binding to G4 structures could be confirmed in vivo, we performed chromatin immunoprecipitation (ChIP) followed by genome-wide sequencing analysis (ChIP-seq) in asynchronous yeast cultures expressing C-terminal Myc-tagged Slx9. Using MACS 2.0, we identified 205 chromosomal binding sites for Slx9 (n = 3) (see Supplementary Materials S3 for peak locations). Peaks were compared to annotated genomic features (centromeres, ARS, promoters), previously identified protein-binding regions (Pif1, γ-H2AX, DNA Pol2), and regions that harbor annotated G4 motifs [14,17,37,38]. Slx9 did not bind significantly to ARS, centromeres, promoters, yH2AX, and Pif1-binding sites. However, we observed a strong correlation of Slx9 peaks to regions with high DNA Pol2 occupancy ($p = 0.0001$) that indicated that the replication fork slows or stalls near Slx9-binding sites. Surprisingly, we did not detect any overlap between annotated G4 motifs and Slx9 peaks. Despite this data, a MEME search resulted in identification of a specific binding motif in 32 of 205 sites (~15.5%) with high G-richness (>60%), greater than the average GC content of the *S. cerevisiae* genome (38%) (Figure 2A). In the past, G4 motifs have been described with a consensus motif $G_3N_{1-7}G_3N_{1-7}G_3N_{1-7}G_3$. However, in recent years, alternative, more flexible G4 motifs that can form metastable G4 structures have been described [39–42]. Slx9-bound regions contained potentially metastable G4 structures with two guanines next to each other (Figure 2A). This indicated that Slx9 did not bind to G4 motifs harboring a consensus sequence in vivo, but can recognize G4 motifs that form flexible, less stable G4 structures. To note, most Slx9-binding sites were detected in non-G-rich regions.

A

B

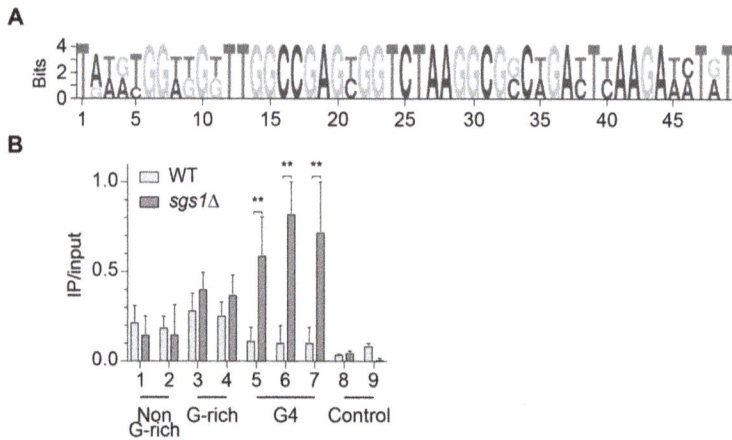

Figure 2. Slx9 binds, genome-wide, to G-rich regions. (**A**) Using Slx9-Myc, two independent ChIP-seq analyses were obtained. Peaks were called using MACS 2.0. A G-rich binding motif was obtained by MEME using the mean of two independent Slx9-Myc ChIP-seq experiments. The binding motif was identified in ~16% of the peaks. (**B**) Slx9 binding was determined to nine endogenous regions (see Supplementary Materials S4 for primer information) by ChIP and qPCR analysis. Selected regions have been identified as binding and non-binding regions in ChIP-seq. Different sequence compositions were chosen for analysis: non-G-rich (binding) and G-rich (binding) sequences, G4 motifs (no binding), and control regions (no binding). G4 motifs contained G-tracts of 3 guanines, resulting in stable G4 structure formation under G4-forming conditions. G-rich sequences could adopt less stable G4 structures, if at all. Binding of Slx9-Myc was monitored in wild type (light) and *sgs1Δ* (dark) cells. Significance was calculated based on Student's *t*-test (** *p*-value < 0.001). All depicted experiments were performed with at least n ≥ 3 biological replicates.

2.3. Slx9 Binds in a Sgs1-Dependent Manner to G4 Motifs

It has been discussed, in recent years, that it is unlikely that all G4 structures form simultaneously in a cell. There would be a selective set of G4s that form during specific biological processes, e.g., replication control, under specific conditions (differentiation, stress, starvation) or in the absence of regulatory proteins (e.g., helicases). The RecQ helicase Sgs1 can efficiently unwind G4 structures in vitro [26,30]. Among other non-G4 related defects, G4-dependent transcriptional changes were detected in Sgs1-deficient cells [14,27]. Due to the published genetic interaction between Sgs1 and Slx9, we speculated that without Sgs1, more G4 structures persist in the cell and, consequently, more Slx9 binds to G4 structures. Thus, we monitored Slx9 binding at G4 motifs in the absence of Sgs1. We performed ChIP–qPCR experiments in two different strains. In the first strain, Slx9 was endogenously Myc-tagged in a wild type background (light), and in the second strain, Slx9 was tagged in a *sgs1Δ* (dark) background (Figure 2B). For qPCR analysis, nine different primer pairs were selected to test Slx9 binding: two non-G-rich regions identified as Slx9-binding sites, two G-rich regions (relaxed G4, identified as Slx9-binding sites), three regions harboring a G4 motif (no detectable Slx9 binding by ChIP-seq), and two control regions (no peaks detected by ChIP-seq). Here, and in all subsequent ChIP and qPCR analyses, binding enrichment was plotted as IP values normalized to input values. In concordance with our ChIP-seq results, Slx9 is significantly associated with the four putative Slx9-binding sites (selected from ChIP-seq: non-G-rich, G-rich) in the wild type background, but did not show significant binding to G4 regions or control regions (Figure 2B). On the contrary, in the absence of Sgs1, Slx9 binding was enhanced at regions that could form G4 structures (Figure 2B), whereas binding to the controls and non-G-rich targets was unaffected by the absence of Sgs1. These results indicate that Slx9 binding to G4 structures is enhanced if they are not unfolded by the helicase Sgs1.

2.4. Slx9 Recognizes G4 Structures That Are Stabilized In Vivo

To further investigate the connection of Slx9 and Sgs1, we analyzed the doubling time of *slx9Δ*, *sgs1Δ*, and the double mutant (Figure 3A). Wild type yeast cells have a doubling time of 90 min, as expected. Cells lacking Sgs1 (*sgs1Δ*) or Slx9 (*slx9Δ*) showed minor growth changes in comparison to wild type (94.5 and 97.5 min, respectively). The double mutant (*sgs1Δ slx9Δ*) has a doubling time of 110.9 min, which is slower than any of the single mutants alone (Figure 3A). Although the differences are not huge, they support previously published data indicating that *SLX9* and *SGS1* genetically interact [29]. To test if G4 formation is the cause of these growth defects, we measured the growth of wild type and *slx9Δ* in the presence of G4-stabilizing ligands. *N*-methyl mesoporphyrin IX (NMM) and Phen-DC$_3$ are two G4-specific ligands that have been shown to stabilize G4 structures in yeast [14,43]. Yeast cells were incubated with the G4-specific ligand, and the doubling time was calculated. Incubation with either G4 ligand resulted in faster growth in *slx9Δ* in comparison to untreated. The doubling time of *slx9Δ* cells treated with Phen-DC$_3$ was 84.8 min, and with NMM 79.2 min, indicating that the deletion of *SLX9* imparts resistance to G4 stabilization (Figure 3B). Notably, the growth of wild type cells did not change upon treatment (Figure 3B). These data are in accordance with previously published screening results using NMM, in which Slx9 was identified as supporting G4 resistance [14].

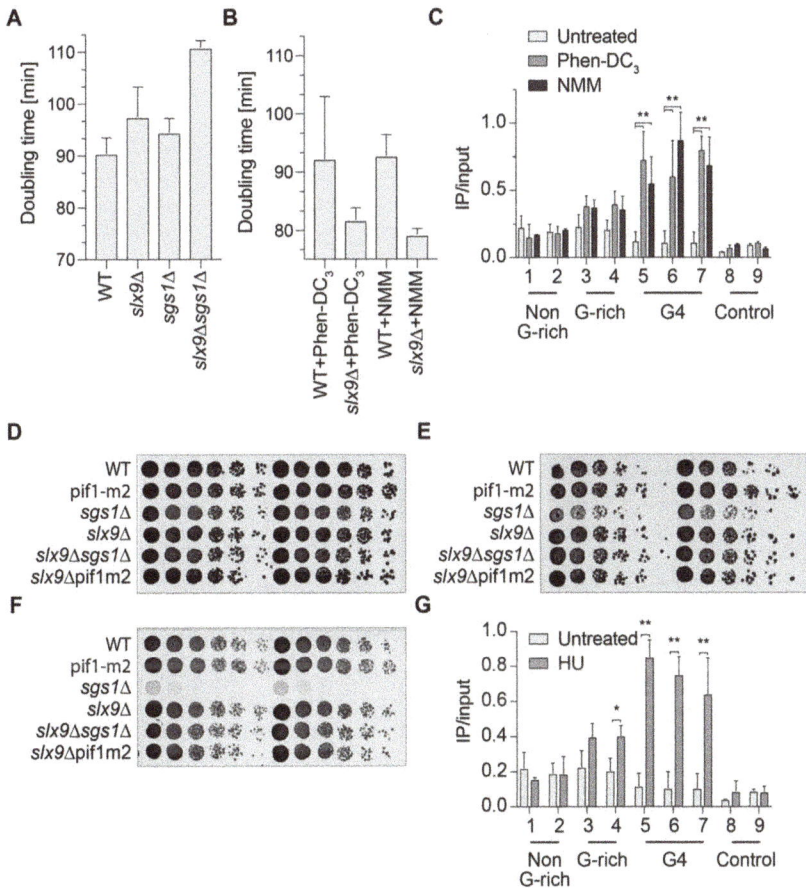

Figure 3. Slx9 supports the recognition of G4 structures in vivo.

(**A**) Growth curves were performed and doubling times (minutes) were calculated using the indicated yeast strains. (**B**) Doubling times in the presence of 10 μM Phen-DC$_3$ and 8 μM NMM. (**C**) ChIP analysis and qPCR of Slx9 binding in untreated (light) and in the presence of either Phen-DC$_3$ (grey) or NMM (dark). (**D–F**) Different concentrations of yeast cells were spotted on rich media in a serial dilution to determine growth changes and sensitivity. (**D**) Yeast growth on untreated YPD plates. (**E**) Yeast cells spotted on rich media containing 100 mM hydroxyurea (HU). (**F**) Yeast cells spotted on rich media and incubated with 25 J/m^2 UV light (254 nm). (**G**) ChIP analysis and qPCR of Slx9 binding in the presence (dark) and absence (light—see also Figure 2B) of 50 mM HU. Significance was calculated based on the Student's *t*-test (** *p*-value < 0.001, * *p*-value < 0.01). All depicted experiments were performed with at least n ≥ 3 biological replicates.

Slx9 binding to G4 motifs is not detectable in wild type cells, but increased in the absence of Sgs1 (Figure 2B). To test if this enhanced binding is due to G4 structures, we measured Slx9 binding in the presence of Phen-DC$_3$ and NMM when the formation of G4 structures is enhanced. For these analyses, the same Slx9-Myc-tagged strains as in the previous experiment were grown in the presence of either 10 μM Phen-DC$_3$ or 8 μM NMM. ChIP analysis was performed in an attempt to understand Slx9 binding to G4 and control regions. Both G4-stabilizing ligands caused a 2- to 8-fold increase of Slx9 binding at all tested G4 motifs (Figure 3C). This elevated binding is similar to the binding of Slx9 in the absence of the Sgs1 helicase (Figure 2B). The stronger binding of Slx9 to ligand-stabilized G4 structures supports the claim that Slx9 binds to folded G4 structures.

2.5. Slx9 Binding to G4 Structures Affects the "Repair" of These Structures

As a next step, we aimed to identify the process/pathway in which Slx9 acts at folded G4 structures. Due to the link to Sgs1, we hypothesized that Slx9 functions similarly to Sgs1 at G4s. Sgs1 is a multifunctional enzyme with proposed functions during transcription, telomere maintenance, and DNA repair [14,27,30,31]. Cells lacking Sgs1 are HU-sensitive and have transcriptional changes in genes with G4 motifs in their promoters [14,44–46]. We analyzed the impact of Slx9 on G4-mediated changes during transcription. We analyzed if *slx9Δ* cells, similar to *sgs1Δ*, show a selective downregulation of mRNAs with G4 motifs in their promoters. To assess this, we monitored changes in mRNA levels of 11 different endogenous loci that harbor G4 motifs and one control region (actin) using qPCR. Five out of 11 regions showed elevated mRNA levels in *slx9Δ* cells compared to wild type (Supplementary Materials S6A). These transcriptional changes indicated that Slx9 affected mRNA levels of a few genes, but these changes did not directly correlate to the presence of G4 motifs in their promoter.

Sgs1 has a role in homologous recombination and *sgs1Δ* cells are sensitive to HU and UV [44,47]. We tested if *slx9Δ* cells are also sensitive to DNA damage agents. Different cell numbers were spotted in a serial dilution on plates with 100 mM HU or were irradiated with 25 J/cm^2 UV light (254 nm). We found that *slx9Δ* cells did not show any growth defect under any of the tested conditions (Figure 3D–F). As expected, cells lacking Sgs1 (*sgs1Δ*) were sensitive to UV irradiation and HU treatment. Strikingly, the double deletion *slx9Δ sgs1Δ* showed no growth defects in either of the DNA damaging conditions, indicating that deletions of Slx9 rescued the HU and UV sensitivity of *sgs1Δ* cells (Figure 3E,F).

Treatment of yeast cells with HU is tightly correlated with increased genome instability. To test if our experimental observations can be explained by increased genome instability, we measured the direct correlation between G4 motifs and genome stability in *slx9Δ* cells. We performed a previously published gross chromosomal rearrangement assay (GCR), which measures telomere addition, recombination, deletions, and mutations as a result of a specific insert [48,49]. The GCR assay can quantitatively detect complex genome rearrangements by the loss of two counter-selectable markers (*URA3*, *CAN1*). The two markers are located downstream of the *PRB1* locus. If the inserted sequence increases genome instability, the markers are lost, and the cells can grow on selective media. The growth of colonies can be directly used as a quantitative readout for genome instability, and GCR rates can be determined via fluctuation analysis [50]. Wild type cells have a GCR rate of 0.1×10^{-9} events per generation [8].

We monitored genome instability using either a non-G-rich, a G-rich or a G4 insert in either wild type, *sgs1Δ*, or *slx9Δ* cells. Depicted GCR rates were normalized to wild type. No changes in GCR rates were detected in any of the experimental conditions, suggesting Slx9 does not have a direct influence on genome stability (Supplementary Materials S6B).

HU increases genome instability by depleting the dNTP pool of the cell, resulting in replication fork progression changes and, consequently, genome instability [51,52]. It has been observed that HU treatment results in elevated G4 structure formation [32]. We speculated that G4 stabilization by HU was the reason why *sgs1Δ* cells were HU-sensitive, and Slx9 recognized these stabilized G4s. We performed ChIP and qPCR experiments using strains with tagged Slx9 in the presence of HU. qPCR analyses using the same primers as used above revealed that Slx9 binding to G4 targets was stimulated in the presence of HU (Figure 3G). These observations further strengthened our previous results and establish a link between Slx9 and Sgs1 under stress conditions.

3. Discussion

Different in vitro and in vivo experiments in various organisms demonstrated the regulatory potential of G4 structures, but also highlight the challenges that such a structure poses for the cell [2,8,20,21,26]. Spatiotemporal regulation of the formation and unwinding of G4 structures is necessary for maintaining genome stability. However, it is not fully understood which proteins support G4 structure formation or recognize folded G4 structures in the cell.

In this study, we performed an unbiased Y1H screen to identify G4-interacting proteins. Among the identified putative G4-binding proteins, Slx9 was chosen for further analysis of its role in G4-mediated processes. Slx9 is a yeast-specific protein and has been reported to function during ribosome biogenesis [53]. Filter-binding assays and MST was used to analyze the binding affinity of Slx9 to G4 structures in vitro. Both techniques showed a preferential binding of Slx9 to G4 structures compared to other DNA structures (Figure 1C–F, Supplementary Materials S5B–C). The specific binding to G4 structures in vitro is interesting, and points towards a similar binding preference in vivo. However, ChIP-seq experiments did not show a significant correlation of Slx9 binding to previously identified G4 motifs (Figure 2) [17]. Recent findings demonstrated that G4 structures could also form within more flexible G4 motifs [39–42]. These metastable G4 motifs have two guanines in the G-tract and longer loop regions. Although 15.5% of all Slx9-binding sites (Figure 2A) harbor such flexible G4 motifs, the in vivo G4-specific interaction of Slx9 is rather poor. This indicated to us that Slx9 has no or only a minor function at G4 structures in wild type yeast cells. We went on to determine the specific conditions of G4-binding by Slx9. Due to the published connection of Slx9 and Sgs1 [29] and the link of Sgs1 to G4 motifs [27,31], we checked if G4 structures which remain folded in *sgs1Δ* cells are bound by Slx9. Indeed, we observed a 2- to 6-fold enrichment of Slx9 binding to these G4 structures if Sgs1 was not present in the cell (Figure 2B). No significant changes of Slx9 binding to relaxed G4s was determined by this method, indicating that Sgs1 did not target these regions. These data led to the speculation that either Slx9 at G4s is displaced by Sgs1 and, therefore, little or no binding can be observed in wild type, or that Slx9 cannot bind to G4 region because these structures are too efficiently regulated by the cellular machinery and not stably folded enough in wild type conditions.

Since Slx9 did not alter genome stability (as measured by GCR) or cause transcriptional changes in a G4-specific manner (Supplementary Materials S6B) we speculated that Slx9 binds to folded G4 structures. To test this hypothesis, we stabilized G4 structures by adding the G4-stabilization ligand NMM, or Phen-DC$_3$, to yeast cells [14,43]. ChIP analysis showed a 2- to 8-fold enrichment in Slx9 binding to G4s, similar to *sgs1Δ* cells (Figure 3C). In addition to helicase depletion and addition of G4-stabilizing ligand, it has been observed that HU favors G4 structure formation [32]. We speculated that Slx9 binding will be enhanced at G4 structures after HU treatment. ChIP analyses of Slx9 binding confirmed that Slx9 binding is enhanced at G4 motifs in the presence of HU (Figure 3G). Interestingly, the binding of Slx9 only increased mildly at relaxed G4 motifs, which might indicate that these relaxed

G4s are not affected by NMM or PhenDC3, and that their formation is only mildly stimulated under HU conditions.

In the past, it has been demonstrated that folded G4 structures stimulate genome instability [8,19,25, 26,54–57]. A reference for genome stability is cellular fitness or doubling time. We observed that the doubling time of wild type cells was not affected by the addition of a G4-stabilization ligand. However, in the absence of Slx9, cells displayed a faster growth rate than wild type cells if G4s were stabilized by G4-stabilization ligands (Figure 3B). This result was in agreement with previously published screening result using NMM, in which Slx9 was identified to support G4 resistance [14]. In line with our model, we speculated that Slx9 protects folded G4 structures, meaning that Slx9 blocks access to G4. This can be further expanded to HU conditions: in the absence of Sgs1, cells are HU-sensitive. Whether this is due to folded G4 structures or other features is not known [44]. We observed that cells lacking Slx9 and Sgs1 were not HU-sensitive (Figure 3E,F). Taking these results together, we propose that under HU conditions, more G4 structures form, and more Slx9 proteins recognize and bind these folded structures. In the absence of Sgs1, cells are sensitive to HU because Slx9 still binds and recognizes folded G4 structures and prevents other proteins unfolding them. In the double deletion mutant (*slx9Δ sgs1Δ*), similar to the NMM or Phen-DC3 conditions, G4 structures are accessible by other proteins and can be regulated.

From this yeast study, we gained two important insights. First, we revealed that Slx9 recognizes and protects folded G4 structures (Figure 4). Second, although a protein is a strong G4 binder in vitro, the in vivo binding might be different. The identification and characterization of the correct binding condition is essential not only for understanding the correct function of the protein, but also to understand the impact and function on G4 structures in the cell, in the case of Slx9. We speculate that more proteins will be identified that recognize and control G4 formation only under specific conditions, because G4 structures are highly dynamic structures that are altered during the cell cycle, different cellular conditions, and during cellular differentiation.

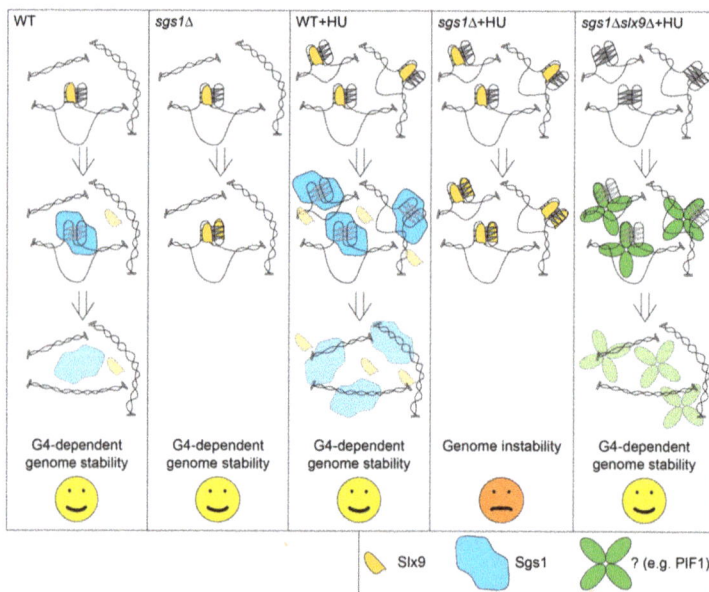

Figure 4. Model detailing how Slx9 recognizes folded G4 structures.

4. Materials and Methods

4.1. Yeast One-Hybrid Screen

The yeast one-hybrid screen was performed using the Matchmaker^{TM} Gold Yeast One-Hybrid Library Screening (Clontech, Kyoto, Japan). All yeast strains used in this assay are listed in the Supplementary Materials (Supplementary Materials S1). To construct the screening strain, a *S. cerevisiae* G4 motif from chromosome IX (G4$_{IX}$) with short flanking regions was cloned into the *S. cerevisiae* Y1HGold genome as described in the manual. The control bait, mut-G4$_{IX}$, was cloned using the same strategy. After determination of the minimal inhibitory concentration of aureobasidin A (AbA), screens were performed using an *S. cerevisiae* DUALhybrid cDNA library (Supplementary Materials) and 5 and 10 mM hydroxyurea (HU) in the plates. cDNA library plasmid (7 µg) was transformed into the screening strain bait G4 according to the manufacturer's protocol.

After streaking out each yeast colony twice on selective plates, the library plasmids were isolated from overnight cultures. Lysis was performed using DNA lysis buffer (2% Triton X-100, 1% SDS, 100 mM NaCl, 10 mM Tris/HCl pH 8.0, 1 mM EDTA) and glass beads in a FastPrep instrument (MP Biomedicals, Santa Ana, CA, USA) for 1 min at 4 °C, followed by phenol/chloroform extraction and ethanol precipitation. Plasmids were transformed in *E. coli* (XL-1 Blue), and overnight cultures were used to isolate plasmids by alkaline lysis. The obtained library plasmid was sent for sequencing using the primer GAL4ADseq (sequence from Dualsystems Biotech): 5′-ACCACTACAATGGATGATG-3′.

4.2. Cloning, Expression, and Purification of Slx9

SLX9 was amplified by PCR from *S. cerevisiae* genomic DNA and PCR primers SG304 (5′-AAAAAA*gaattc*ATGGTTGCTAAGAAGAGAAACA-3′) and SG305 (5′-AAAAAA*gcggccgc*TCATTGTTTTTGCAGCTTGATAA-3′). *SLX9* was cloned into the *Eco*RI and *Not*I sites of a pET28a vector (Novagen, Darmstadt, Germany). The resulting construct was confirmed by sequencing. 6×His-tagged Slx9 was expressed in Rosetta pLysS cells grown in LB medium supplemented with 25 µg/mL kanamycin and 30 µg/mL chloramphenicol. Expression was induced by 1 mM isopropyl β-ᴅ-thiogalactoside (IPTG) at 18 °C overnight, following the manufacturer's protocol and established protocols [58].

All purification steps were carried out at 4 °C. Cell lysis was performed in lysis buffer (300 mM NaCl, 20 mM HEPES pH 7.5, 10% (*v/v*) glycerol, 1 mM DTT, 5 mM imidazole) by sonication (6 × 45 s, 50% pulse intensity) using a Branson sonifier W250-D (Brandson, Danbury, CT, USA). After centrifugation of the lysate (10,000 g, 30 min) the supernatant was applied onto a Ni-NTA agarose column (equilibrated with two column volume lysis buffer) by gravity. After three washing steps with one column volume wash buffer (300 mM NaCl, 20 mM HEPES pH 7.5, 10% (v/v) glycerol, 1 mM DTT, 15 mM imidazole), the bound protein was eluted with one column volume elution buffer (300 mM NaCl, 20 mM HEPES, pH 7.5, 10% (v/v) glycerol, 1 mM DTT, 300 mM imidazole). The eluate was separated by SDS-PAGE. Fractions containing Slx9 were identified by Coomassie staining and Western blot analysis using an anti-His antibody (Santa Cruz, Dallas, TX, USA). Positive fractions were combined, and the buffer was exchanged, by dialysis, to elution buffer without imidazole. The protein was concentrated using a Vivaspin 6 Centrifugal Concentrator (10 kDa cutoff, Sartorius, Goettingen, Germany). The protein concentration was measured by Bradford and by SDS-PAGE using known amounts of bovine serum albumin (BSA) as a standard.

4.3. In Vitro Folding and Analysis of G4 Structures and Annealing of Control DNA Structures

The folding of DNA oligodeoxynucleotides into G4 structures was performed as previously described [33]. G4 structure formation was confirmed by 7% SDS-PAGE and circular dichroism (CD) measurements. Oligodeoxynucleotides for control DNA structures were also used as previously published [34] (Supplementary Materials S2). Annealing was performed in annealing buffer (50 mM HEPES, 2 mM magnesium acetate, 100 mM potassium acetate) for 1 min at 98 °C, 60 min at 37 °C, and 30 min at 22 °C. G4 structures and annealed control DNA structures for binding studies were desalted using illustra MicroSpin G-25 columns (GE Healthcare, Boston, MA, USA).

4.4. Binding Studies

DNA (20 pmol) was 5′-labelled with 25 µCi [γ-^{32}P] ATP by T4 polynucleotide kinase (NEB, Ipswich, UK). G4 and G4$_{mut}$ structures were purified by 7 % SDS-PAGE. Control DNA (ds, bubble, fork, 4 fork) was purified using illustra MicroSpin G-25 columns (GE Healthcare).

DNA–protein binding was analyzed by double-filter-binding assays [35] using a 96-well Bio-Dot SF apparatus (Bio-Rad, Hercules, CA, USA) and 10 nM DNA in binding buffer (50 mM Tris/HCl pH 8.0, 125 mM KCl, 5 mM DTT, 10% (v/v) glycerol [13]). Protein concentrations increased from 0 to 65 µM Slx9. After incubation on ice for 30 min, the reactions were filtered through a nitrocellulose and a positively charged nylon membrane, followed by three washing steps with binding buffer with no glycerol. The membranes were dried and analyzed by phosphorimaging on a Typhoon FLA 7000 (GE Healthcare). Percentage values of bound Slx9 were determined using ImageQuant, and were used to obtain dissociation equilibrium constants (K_d) by curve fitting using nonlinear regression (GraphPad Prism, San Diego, CA, USA).

4.5. ChIP-Seq -and ChIP Plus qPCR Analysis

ChIP experiments were performed as previously described [8,59]. For ChIP-Seq, chromatin was sheared to an average length of 200 bp using a S220 focused ultrasonicator (Covaris, Brighton, UK). For conventional ChIP, the DNA was sheared to an average length of 250 bp using a Branson sonifier W250-D (50% amplitude, 50% duty cycle, 5 × 5 pulses). The applied parameters for Covaris were 140 W, 5% duty, and 200 cycles/burst for 20 min at 4 °C. The pulldown was performed using a c-Myc antibody (Clontech, Kyoto, Japan). For genome-wide sequencing, DNA was treated according to manufacturer's instructions (NEBNext ChIP-seq Library Prep Master Mix Set for Illumina, NEB) and submitted to deep sequencing (Illumina Nextseq500 sequencer, San Diego, CA, USA). Obtained sequence reads were aligned to the yeast reference genome (sacCer3) with bowtie [60]. After the alignment, the number of reads was normalized to the sample with the lowest number of reads. Binding regions were identified by using the program 'Model-based Analysis for ChIP-Seq' (MACS 2.0) with default settings for narrow peaks [61]. Supplementary Materials S3 contains all Slx9 peaks. The ChIP input sample was used as a control. MEME-based motif elicitation was used to identify a consensus motif within the FASTA file from the binding regions identified by MACS 2.0 (Liu lab, Boston, MA, USA) [62]. Overlap of binding sites with other genomic features and binding regions was determined using in house PERL scripts based on a permutation analysis between query and subject features.

For ChIP-qPCR analyses, Slx9 was endogenously Myc-tagged at the C-terminal [63]. Asynchronous cultures were grown to OD (660 nm) of 0.4–0.6 and crosslinked with 1% formaldehyde for 5 min followed by quenching of the crosslinking by the addition of 125 mM glycine. ChIP experiments were carried out as described above, and the immunoprecipitated sample (IP) was subjected to real-time PCR using a SYBR green mix (Roche, Basel, Swiss). Details of the primers used in this study are in Supplementary Materials S4. Binding was calculated as ratio of IP/Input for the specific regions. Student's *t*-test was used to calculate the statistical significance.

4.6. Growth Assay

The strains used for growth assays are listed in Supplementary Materials S1. Overnight cultures of *S. cerevisiae* strains were used to inoculate YPD to a starting OD (660 nm) of 0.1. Cultures were grown at 30 °C until OD (660 nm) ≥ 1 was reached. Measurements were taken in 60 min intervals, and doubling times were calculated from log-phase OD (660 nm) values. Phen-DC$_3$ (10 µM) or 8 µM N-methyl mesoporphyrin IX (NMM) was added to the medium to perform growth assays under G4-stabilizing conditions. Growth curves were performed in triplicates.

4.7. Spot Assay

Yeast cultures were inoculated at an OD (660 nm) of 0.15 using a stationary *S. cerevisiae* culture, and grown at 30 °C until OD (660 nm) ≥ 0.8 was reached. All yeast cultures were diluted to OD (660 nm) = 0.8 and a dilution series with six 1:5 dilutions were prepared in a sterile 96-well plate. From each dilution, 3 µL were spotted on a plate, and after drying, incubated at 30 °C. After 2 days, the plates were scanned and growth of strains on different media was compared to estimate the growth defects.

Supplementary Materials: The following are available online at http://www.mdpi.com/1420-3049/24/9/1774/s1: Supplemental File S1: Yeast and bacteria strains used in this study, Supplemental File S2: List of G4 folding oligodeoxynucleotides, Supplemental File S3: List of peaks of ChIP-seq, Supplemental File S4: List of primers used in this study, Supplemental File S5: Supporting information for binding analysis, Supplemental File S6: Slx9 has no G4-mediated effect on genome stability or transcriptional changes.

Author Contributions: Conceptualization, K.P., S.G., S.P.: Methodology K.P., S.G., S.P., S.J., S.B.: Data analysis, K.P., S.G., S.P., S.J.: Writing—original Draft, K.P., S.G., Writing—Review & Editing, K.P., S.P., S.G., S.J. Funding Acquisition, K.P., Resources K.P., Supervision K.P.

Funding: The work in the Paeschke laboratory is supported by an European Research Council Starting grant (638988—G4DSB) as well as an DFG Emmy Noether fellowship.

Acknowledgments: We thank Wesley Browne (University of Groningen) for his help with circular dichroic measurements and Arnold Driessen and Inge Kazemier for help with MST analysis. We thank Diana Spierings and Nancy Halsema for support with ChIP-seq analysis. We thank Markus Sauer for careful reading of the manuscript and Alessio De Magis for experimental support during review process.

Conflicts of Interest: The authors declare no competing financial interests.

References

1. Bikard, D.; Loot, C.; Baharoglu, Z.; Mazel, D. Folded DNA in Action: Hairpin Formation and Biological Functions in Prokaryotes. *Microbiol. Mol. Biol. Rev.* **2010**, *74*, 570–588. [CrossRef]

2. Bochman, M.L.; Paeschke, K.; Zakian, V.A. DNA Secondary Structures: Stability and Function of G-Quadruplex Structures. *Nat. Rev. Genet.* **2012**, *13*, 770–780. [CrossRef] [PubMed]

3. Doherty, E.A.; Doudna, J.A. Ribozyme Structures and Mechanisms. *Annu. Rev. Biochem.* **2000**, *69*, 597–615. [CrossRef]

4. Mirkin, S.M. Discovery of Alternative DNA Structures: A Heroic Decade (1979–1989). *Front. Biosci.* **2008**, *13*, 1064–1071. [CrossRef]

5. Rhodes, D.; Lipps, H.J. G-Quadruplexes and Their Regulatory Roles in Biology. *Nucleic Acids Res.* **2015**, *43*, 8627–8837. [CrossRef]

6. Chambers, V.S.; Marsico, G.; Boutell, J.M.; di Antonio, M.; Smith, G.P.; Balasubramanian, S. High-Throughput Sequencing of DNA G-Quadruplex Structures in the Human Genome. *Nat. Biotechnol.* **2015**, *33*, 877–881. [CrossRef] [PubMed]

7. Biffi, G.; Tannahill, D.; McCafferty, J.; Balasubramanian, S. Quantitative Visualization of DNA G-Quadruplex Structures in Human Cells. *Nat. Chem.* **2013**, *5*, 182–186. [CrossRef]

8. Paeschke, K.; Capra, J.A.; Zakian, V.A. DNA Replication through G-Quadruplex Motifs Is Promoted by the Saccharomyces Cerevisiae Pif1 DNA Helicase. *Cell* **2011**, *145*, 678–691. [CrossRef] [PubMed]

9. Juranek, S.A.; Paeschke, K. Cell Cycle Regulation of G-Quadruplex DNA Structures at Telomeres. *Curr. Pharm. Des.* **2012**, *18*, 1867–1872. [CrossRef] [PubMed]

10. Siddiqui-Jain, A.; Grand, C.L.; Bearss, D.J.; Hurley, L.H. Direct Evidence for a G-Quadruplex in a Promoter Region and Its Targeting with a Small Molecule to Repress C-Myc Transcription. *Proc. Natl. Acad. Sci. USA* **2002**, *99*, 11593–11598. [CrossRef]

11. Wolfe, A.L.; Singh, K.; Zhong, Y.; Drewe, P.; Rajasekhar, V.K.; Sanghvi, V.R.; Mavrakis, K.J.; Jiang, M.; Roderick, J.E.; Van der Meulen, J.; et al. Rna G-Quadruplexes Cause Eif4a-Dependent Oncogene Translation in Cancer. *Nature* **2014**, *513*, 65–70. [CrossRef] [PubMed]

12. Besnard, E.; Babled, A.; Lapasset, L.; Milhavet, O.; Parrinello, H.; Dantec, C.; Marin, J.M.; Lemaitre, J.M. Unraveling Cell Type-Specific and Reprogrammable Human Replication Origin Signatures Associated with G-Quadruplex Consensus Motifs. *Nat Struct. Mol. Biol.* **2012**, *19*, 837–844. [CrossRef] [PubMed]

13. Paeschke, K.; Simonsson, T.; Postberg, J.; Rhodes, D.; Lipps, H.J. Telomere End-Binding Proteins Control the Formation of G-Quadruplex DNA Structures in Vivo. *Nat. Struct. Mol. Biol.* **2005**, *12*, 847–854. [CrossRef]
14. Hershman, S.G.; Chen, Q.; Lee, J.Y.; Kozak, M.L.; Yue, P.; Wang, L.S.; Johnson, F.B. Genomic Distribution and Functional Analyses of Potential G-Quadruplex-Forming Sequences in Saccharomyces Cerevisiae. *Nucleic Acids Res.* **2008**, *36*, 144–156. [CrossRef]
15. Balasubramanian, S.; Hurley, L.H.; Neidle, S. Targeting G-Quadruplexes in Gene Promoters: A Novel Anticancer Strategy? *Nat. Rev. Drug Discov.* **2011**, *10*, 261–275. [CrossRef] [PubMed]
16. Huppert, J.L.; Balasubramanian, S. G-Quadruplexes in Promoters Throughout the Human Genome. *Nucleic Acids Res.* **2007**, *35*, 406–413. [CrossRef]
17. Capra, J.A.; Paeschke, K.; Singh, M.; Zakian, V.A. G-Quadruplex DNA Sequences Are Evolutionarily Conserved and Associated with Distinct Genomic Features in Saccharomyces Cerevisiae. *PLoS Comput. Biol.* **2010**, *6*. [CrossRef] [PubMed]
18. Simonsson, T.; Pecinka, P.; Kubista, M. DNA Tetraplex Formation in the Control Region of C-Myc. *Nucleic Acids Res.* **1998**, *26*, 1167–1172. [CrossRef] [PubMed]
19. Mendoza, O.; Bourdoncle, A.; Boule, J.B.; Brosh, R.M., Jr.; Mergny, J.L. G-Quadruplexes and Helicases. *Nucleic Acids Res.* **2016**, *44*, 1989–2006. [CrossRef]
20. Bharti, S.K.; Sommers, J.A.; Zhou, J.; Kaplan, D.L.; Spelbrink, J.N.; Mergny, J.L.; Brosh, R.M., Jr. DNA Sequences Proximal to Human Mitochondrial DNA Deletion Breakpoints Prevalent in Human Disease Form G-Quadruplexes, a Class of DNA Structures Inefficiently Unwound by the Mitochondrial Replicative Twinkle Helicase. *J. Biol. Chem.* **2014**, *289*, 29975–29993. [CrossRef]
21. Cheung, I.; Schertzer, M.; Rose, A.; Lansdorp, P.M. Disruption of Dog-1 in Caenorhabditis Elegans Triggers Deletions Upstream of Guanine-Rich DNA. *Nat. Genet.* **2002**, *31*, 405–409. [CrossRef]
22. Tarsounas, M.; Tijsterman, M. Genomes and G-Quadruplexes: For Better or for Worse. *J. Mol. Biol.* **2013**, *425*, 4782–4789. [CrossRef]
23. Sauer, M.; Paeschke, K. G-Quadruplex Unwinding Helicases and Their Function in Vivo. *Biochem. Soc. Trans.* **2017**, *45*, 1173–1182. [CrossRef]
24. Brazda, V.; Haronikova, L.; Liao, J.C.; Fojta, M. DNA and Rna Quadruplex-Binding Proteins. *Int. J. Mol. Sci.* **2014**, *15*, 17493–17517. [CrossRef]
25. Maizels, N. G4-Associated Human Diseases. *EMBO Rep.* **2015**, *16*, 910–922. [CrossRef]
26. Paeschke, K.; Bochman, M.L.; Garcia, P.D.; Cejka, P.; Friedman, K.L.; Kowalczykowski, S.C.; Zakian, V.A. Pif1 Family Helicases Suppress Genome Instability at G-Quadruplex Motifs. *Nature* **2013**, *497*, 458–462. [CrossRef]
27. Smith, J.S.; Chen, Q.; Yatsunyk, L.A.; Nicoludis, J.M.; Garcia, M.S.; Kranaster, R.; Balasubramanian, S.; Monchaud, D.; Teulade-Fichou, M.P.; Abramowitz, L.; et al. Rudimentary G-Quadruplex-Based Telomere Capping in Saccharomyces Cerevisiae. *Nat. Struct. Mol. Biol.* **2011**, *18*, 478–485. [CrossRef]
28. Wanzek, K.; Schwindt, E.; Capra, J.; Paeschke, K. Mms1 Binds to G-Rich Regions in Saccharomyces Cerevisiae and Influences Replication and Genome Stability. *Nucleic Acids Res.* **2017**, *45*, 7796–7806. [CrossRef]
29. Ooi, S.L.; Shoemaker, D.D.; Boeke, J.D. DNA Helicase Gene Interaction Network Defined Using Synthetic Lethality Analyzed by Microarray. *Nat. Genet.* **2003**, *35*, 277–286. [CrossRef] [PubMed]
30. Zhu, Z.; Chung, W.H.; Shim, E.Y.; Lee, S.E.; Ira, G. Sgs1 Helicase and Two Nucleases Dna2 and Exo1 Resect DNA Double-Strand Break Ends. *Cell* **2008**, *134*, 981–994. [CrossRef]
31. Sun, H.; Bennett, R.J.; Maizels, N. The Saccharomyces Cerevisiae Sgs1 Helicase Efficiently Unwinds G-G Paired Dnas. *Nucleic Acids Res.* **1999**, *27*, 1978–1984. [CrossRef]
32. Papadopoulou, C.; Guilbaud, G.; Schiavone, D.; Sale, J.E. Nucleotide Pool Depletion Induces G-Quadruplex-Dependent Perturbation of Gene Expression. *Cell Rep.* **2015**, *13*, 2491–2503. [CrossRef]
33. Bachrati, C.Z.; Hickson, I.D. Analysis of the DNA Unwinding Activity of Recq Family Helicases. *Methods Enzymol.* **2006**, *409*, 86–100.
34. Mohaghegh, P.; Karow, J.K.; Brosh, R.M., Jr.; Bohr, V.A.; Hickson, I.D. The Bloom's and Werner's Syndrome Proteins Are DNA Structure-Specific Helicases. *Nucleic Acids Res.* **2001**, *29*, 2843–2849. [CrossRef]
35. Wong, I.; Lohman, T.M. A Double-Filter Method for Nitrocellulose-Filter Binding: Application to Protein-Nucleic Acid Interactions. *Proc. Natl. Acad. Sci. USA* **1993**, *90*, 5428–5432. [CrossRef]
36. Zhang, W.; Duhr, S.; Baaske, P.; Laue, E. Microscale Thermophoresis for the Assessment of Nuclear Protein-Binding Affinities. *Methods Mol. Biol.* **2014**, *1094*, 269–276.

37. Steinmetz, E.J.; Warren, C.L.; Kuehner, J.N.; Panbehi, B.; Ansari, A.Z.; Brow, D.A. Genome-Wide Distribution of Yeast Rna Polymerase Ii and Its Control by Sen1 Helicase. *Mol. Cell* **2006**, *24*, 735–746. [CrossRef]

38. Szilard, R.K.; Jacques, P.E.; Laramee, L.; Cheng, B.; Galicia, S.; Bataille, A.R.; Yeung, M.; Mendez, M.; Bergeron, M.; Robert, F.; et al. Systematic Identification of Fragile Sites Via Genome-Wide Location Analysis of Gamma-H2ax. *Nat. Struct. Mol. Biol.* **2010**, *17*, 299–305. [CrossRef]

39. Guedin, A.; Gros, J.; Alberti, P.; Mergny, J.L. How Long Is Too Long? Effects of Loop Size on G-Quadruplex Stability. *Nucleic Acids Res.* **2010**, *38*, 7858–7868. [CrossRef]

40. Mukundan, V.T.; Phan, A.T. Bulges in G-Quadruplexes: Broadening the Definition of G-Quadruplex-Forming Sequences. *J. Am. Chem. Soc.* **2013**, *135*, 5017–5028. [CrossRef]

41. Tippana, R.; Xiao, W.; Myong, S. G-Quadruplex Conformation and Dynamics Are Determined by Loop Length and Sequence. *Nucleic Acids Res.* **2014**, *42*, 8106–8114. [CrossRef]

42. Agrawal, P.; Lin, C.; Mathad, R.I.; Carver, M.; Yang, D. The Major G-Quadruplex Formed in the Human Bcl-2 Proximal Promoter Adopts a Parallel Structure with a 13-Nt Loop in K+ Solution. *J. Am. Chem. Soc.* **2014**, *136*, 1750–1753. [CrossRef]

43. Piazza, A.; Boule, J.B.; Lopes, J.; Mingo, K.; Largy, E.; Teulade-Fichou, M.P.; Nicolas, A. Genetic Instability Triggered by G-Quadruplex Interacting Phen-Dc Compounds in Saccharomyces Cerevisiae. *Nucleic Acids Res.* **2010**, *38*, 4337–4348. [CrossRef]

44. Saffi, J.; Pereira, V.R.; Henriques, J.A. Importance of the Sgs1 Helicase Activity in DNA Repair of Saccharomyces Cerevisiae. *Curr. Genet.* **2000**, *37*, 75–78. [CrossRef]

45. Mullen, J.R.; Kaliraman, V.; Ibrahim, S.S.; Brill, S.J. Requirement for Three Novel Protein Complexes in the Absence of the Sgs1 DNA Helicase in Saccharomyces Cerevisiae. *Genetics* **2001**, *157*, 103–118.

46. Frei, C.; Gasser, S.M. The Yeast Sgs1p Helicase Acts Upstream of Rad53p in the DNA Replication Checkpoint and Colocalizes with Rad53p in S-Phase-Specific Foci. *Genes Dev.* **2000**, *14*, 81–96.

47. Gangloff, S.; Soustelle, C.; Fabre, F. Homologous Recombination Is Responsible for Cell Death in the Absence of the Sgs1 and Srs2 Helicases. *Nat. Genet.* **2000**, *25*, 192–194. [CrossRef]

48. Putnam, C.D.; Kolodner, R.D. Determination of Gross Chromosomal Rearrangement Rates. *Cold Spring Harb. Protoc.* **2010**, *2010*. [CrossRef]

49. Chen, C.; Kolodner, R.D. Gross Chromosomal Rearrangements in Saccharomyces Cerevisiae Replication and Recombination Defective Mutants. *Nat. Genet.* **1999**, *23*, 81–85. [CrossRef]

50. Hall, B.M.; Ma, C.X.; Liang, P.; Singh, K.K. Fluctuation Analysis Calculator: A Web Tool for the Determination of Mutation Rate Using Luria-Delbruck Fluctuation Analysis. *Bioinformatics* **2009**, *25*, 1564–1565. [CrossRef]

51. Bianchi, V.; Pontis, E.; Reichard, P. Changes of Deoxyribonucleoside Triphosphate Pools Induced by Hydroxyurea and Their Relation to DNA Synthesis. *J. Biol. Chem.* **1986**, *261*, 16037–16042.

52. Koc, A.; Wheeler, L.J.; Mathews, C.K.; Merrill, G.F. Hydroxyurea Arrests DNA Replication by a Mechanism That Preserves Basal Dntp Pools. *J. Biol. Chem.* **2004**, *279*, 223–230. [CrossRef]

53. Bax, R.; Raue, H.A.; Vos, J.C. Slx9p Facilitates Efficient Its1 Processing of Pre-Rrna in Saccharomyces Cerevisiae. *RNA* **2006**, *12*, 2005–2013. [CrossRef]

54. Kruisselbrink, E.; Guryev, V.; Brouwer, K.; Pontier, D.B.; Cuppen, E.; Tijsterman, M. Mutagenic Capacity of Endogenous G4 DNA Underlies Genome Instability in Fancj-Defective C. Elegans. *Curr. Biol.* **2008**, *18*, 900–905. [CrossRef]

55. Lopes, J.; Piazza, A.; Bermejo, R.; Kriegsman, B.; Colosio, A.; Teulade-Fichou, M.P.; Foiani, M.; Nicolas, A. G-Quadruplex-Induced Instability During Leading-Strand Replication. *EMBO J.* **2011**, *30*, 4033–4046. [CrossRef]

56. Lemmens, B.; van Schendel, R.; Tijsterman, M. Mutagenic Consequences of a Single G-Quadruplex Demonstrate Mitotic Inheritance of DNA Replication Fork Barriers. *Nat. Commun.* **2015**, *6*. [CrossRef]

57. London, T.B.; Barber, L.J.; Mosedale, G.; Kelly, G.P.; Balasubramanian, S.; Hickson, I.D.; Boulton, S.J.; Hiom, K. Fancj Is a Structure-Specific DNA Helicase Associated with the Maintenance of Genomic G/C Tracts. *J. Biol. Chem.* **2008**, *283*, 36132–36139. [CrossRef]

58. Maniatis, T.; Fritsch, E.F.; Sambrook, J. *Molecular Cloning: A Laboratory Manual*, 4th ed.; Cold Spring Harbor: New York, NY, USA, 1982.

59. Azvolinsky, A.; Giresi, P.G.; Lieb, J.D.; Zakian, V.A. Highly Transcribed Rna Polymerase Ii Genes Are Impediments to Replication Fork Progression in Saccharomyces Cerevisiae. *Mol. Cell* **2009**, *34*, 722–734. [CrossRef]

60.   Langmead, B.; Trapnell, C.; Pop, M.; Salzberg, S.L. Ultrafast and Memory-Efficient Alignment of Short DNA Sequences to the Human Genome. *Genome Biol.* **2009**, *10*, R25. [CrossRef]

61.   Zhang, Y.; Liu, T.; Meyer, C.A.; Eeckhoute, J.; Johnson, D.S.; Bernstein, B.E.; Nusbaum, C.; Myers, R.M.; Brown, M.; Li, W.; et al. Model-Based Analysis of Chip-Seq (Macs). *Genome Biol.* **2008**, *9*, R137. [CrossRef]

62.   Bailey, T.L.; Boden, M.; Buske, F.A.; Frith, M.; Grant, C.E.; Clementi, L.; Ren, J.; Li, W.W.; Noble, W.S. Meme Suite: Tools for Motif Discovery and Searching. *Nucleic Acids Res.* **2009**, W202–W208. [CrossRef] [PubMed]

63.   Longtine, M.S.; McKenzie, A., 3rd; Demarini, D.J.; Shah, N.G.; Wach, A.; Brachat, A.; Philippsen, P.; Pringle, J.R. Additional Modules for Versatile and Economical Pcr-Based Gene Deletion and Modification in Saccharomyces Cerevisiae. *Yeast* **1998**, *14*, 953–961. [CrossRef]

Sample Availability: Samples of the yeast strains are available from the authors on request.

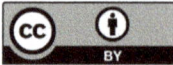

MDPI

Article

Bulged and Canonical G-Quadruplex Conformations Determine NDPK Binding Specificity

Mykhailo Kopylov [1,2], **Trevia M. Jackson** [1] **and M. Elizabeth Stroupe** [1,*]

1   Department of Biological Science and Institute of Molecular Biophysics, Florida State University, 91 Chieftain Way, Tallahassee, FL 32306, USA; mkopylov@nysbc.org (M.K.); tmj12b@my.fsu.edu (T.M.J.)
2   New York Structural Biology Center, 89 Convent Ave, New York, NY 10027, USA
*   Correspondence: mestroupe@bio.fsu.edu; Tel.: +1-850-644-1751

Academic Editor: Sara N. Richter
Received: 23 April 2019; Accepted: 22 May 2019; Published: 23 May 2019

Abstract: Guanine-rich DNA strands can adopt tertiary structures known as G-quadruplexes (G4s) that form when Hoogsteen base-paired guanines assemble as planar stacks, stabilized by a central cation like K^+. In this study, we investigated the conformational heterogeneity of a G-rich sequence from the 5' untranslated region of the *Zea mays hexokinase4* gene. This sequence adopted an extensively polymorphic G-quadruplex, including non-canonical bulged G-quadruplex folds that co-existed in solution. The nature of this polymorphism depended, in part, on the incorporation of different sets of adjacent guanines into a quadruplex core, which permitted the formation of the different conformations. Additionally, we showed that the maize homolog of the human nucleoside diphosphate kinase (NDPK) NM23-H2 protein—ZmNDPK1—specifically recognizes and promotes formation of a subset of these conformations. Heteromorphic G-quadruplexes play a role in microorganisms' ability to evade the host immune system, so we also discuss how the underlying properties that determine heterogeneity of this sequence could apply to microorganism G4s.

Keywords: G-quadruplex; G4; nucleoside diphosphate kinase; NDPK

---

1. Introduction

Traditionally, DNA is thought of as the genetic storage unit held in a double-stranded helical conformation. The famous double helix structure [1] falls short in light of the observations that guanine bases (Gs) in G-rich regions of DNA or RNA can form Hoogsteen base pairs with one another to create a planar G-quartet [2,3]. Sequential G-quartets can stack to form G-quadruplexes (G4s). In microorganisms, these secondary structures can play a role in antigenic variation to assist in evasion of the host immune response and in establishing viral latency [4]. G4s have been identified in eukaryotic nuclei using G4-specific antibody staining [5]. Further, functional roles in regulating transcription and replication continue to be identified from bacteria to mammals [6–11]. In short, DNA G4s are now a recognized structural form of DNA despite the initial controversy about their biological relevance.

G4s are identified throughout microorganisms—including viral, mammalian, and plant genomes— at similar, but not identical, loci. In bacteria, G4s are enriched in regulatory sequences as well as transfer, non-coding, and messenger RNAs [12]. In viruses, G4s that are conserved across viral classes are found in gene promoters and long terminal repeats, implicating them in gene expression regulation and viral latency [13,14]. In humans, G4s are enriched just upstream of transcription start sites (TSSs), as well as in introns near intron–exon boundaries, and are more commonly found in the sense strand and thus transcribed into mRNA [11]. Others are associated with telomeres [11] or oncogene promoters [15]. In the maize genome, G4s tend to occur just downstream of TSSs in the antisense strand (called "A5U"-type G4s for antisense 5'-untranslated region) and putative G4s are overrepresented in promoter regions of genes associated with energy status pathways, oxidative stress response, and hypoxia, suggesting a regulatory role for these elements [16]. For these reasons, G4 aptamer-based therapeutics that can inhibit bacteria-host cell interactions [17], override transcriptional [18] or epigenetic [19] signals, or regulate viral lifecycle [20] are an exciting avenue for drug discovery [21].

The analogy between these divergent genomes carries over into the surprising structural plasticity of the G4s and the protein factors that regulate G4 formation and dissolution in the nucleus and/or cytoplasm. For example, the ability for G4s in various pathogens to adopt protein-specific conformations suggests a role in those microorganisms to evade the host immune response [4,22]. Some viral genomes combine Watson–Crick base pairs with a G4 structure, perhaps influencing gene expression in HIV-1 [23]. Further, a number of mammalian proteins play a role in dissolving [24–29] or stabilizing [30–32] G4 interactions. Interestingly, we recently identified a nucleoside diphosphate kinase (NDPK) from maize, ZmNDPK1, that is analogous to the human NM23-H2, an NDPK homolog [33] (both bind the folded form of G4 DNA). However, the nature of their interaction is not completely understood because there is no reported three-dimensional structure of an NDPK–G4 DNA complex.

With accepting the importance of genic DNA G4s come questions about how they function. In this realm, biochemistry and biophysics shed light on the physical properties that lay the basis for defining these activities. To this end, various spectrophotometric and spectroscopic assays are available to assess the structure of model oligonucleotides in solution. Nonetheless, these techniques individually fall short of defining a single state of the oligonucleotide, and so must be used together to understand the G4 forming potential of any given G-rich stretch of nucleic acid. Structure determination is complicated by the innate polymorphism of even the simplest G4-forming sequences [34], formation of stable structures with bulges in G-tracts [35], topological interconversion [36,37], and G-tract slippage [38].

In this study, we combined UV spectrophotometry, CD spectrophotometry, and DMS footprinting to characterize the G4-forming DNA oligonucleotide *hex4_A5U*, which is derived from the 5′ untranslated region of the maize *hexokinase4* gene [16]. Each technique has different strengths in analyzing G4 structures, so we used them together to understand the biophysical properties of this sequence [39–41]. We then applied our analysis to characterizing the interaction between ZmNDPK1 and the G4 DNA, which form a high-affinity complex with a subset of the potential *hex4_A5U* G4 conformers [33]. Our analysis shows an unprecedented level of polymorphism in the *hex4_A5U* sequence that can be described by the topological isomers and G-register exchange concept [42], extended to include the non-canonical bulged G4 conformations. We further hypothesize that such polymorphism is a universal property of G4-forming sequences in eukaryotic as well as prokaryotic genomes.

2. Results

2.1. hex4_A5U Adopts a G4 Conformation in the Presence of Cations

We first tested the influence of different monovalent cations on the formation of G4 by the *hex4_A5U* sequence using UV-Vis and CD spectrophotometry. We will refer to the stretches of Gs as tracts I–IV, according to their order from the 56′ end of the DNA (Figure 1A). A characteristic G4 thermal difference spectrum (TDS) with a negative peak at 295 nm was obtained only in the presence of K^+ ions (Figure 1B). TDS spectra of oligonucleotides annealed with Na^+, Cs^+, and Li^+ ions were more negative at 295 nm than those determined in the absence of cations, but none had a prominent negative peak.

We next monitored the thermal denaturation of G4 structures by recording the change in absorbance at 295 nm (Figure 1C). A hypochromic shift at this wavelength with increasing temperature is associated with G4 melting [43,44]. In contrast, single-stranded DNA (ssDNA) experiences a hyperchromic shift at 295 nm upon increasing temperature due solely to denaturation of any transitory secondary structures such as ssDNA helix [45]. As expected, in the presence of K^+ we observed a sigmoidal decrease in absorbance at 295 nm with increasing temperature, revealing a midpoint of transition ($T_{1/2}$) at 58 °C. In the presence of Na^+, Li^+, or Cs^+ ions, we saw an initial decrease in absorbance at 295 nm that suggested melting of a G4-like structure, followed by an increase in absorbance that we attributed to ssDNA helix denaturation. In the absence of cations, the absorbance at 295 nm steadily increased with increasing temperature. Further supporting our assessment that *hex4_A5U* forms a quadruplex structure, CD spectra characteristic of a parallel G4 conformation [46] were visible in K$^+$, Na$^+$, Li$^+$, and Cs$^+$ (Figure 1D). In the absence of any small cation, CD spectra indicate that the oligonucleotide is disordered (Figure 1D). Finally, analytical ultracentrifugation (AUC) showed that the DNA was folded into a compact globular structure with an average molecular weight of 10.8 kDa (expected: 10.2 kDa) and an average f/f0 of 1.56, indicative of a monomeric G4 (Figure 2).

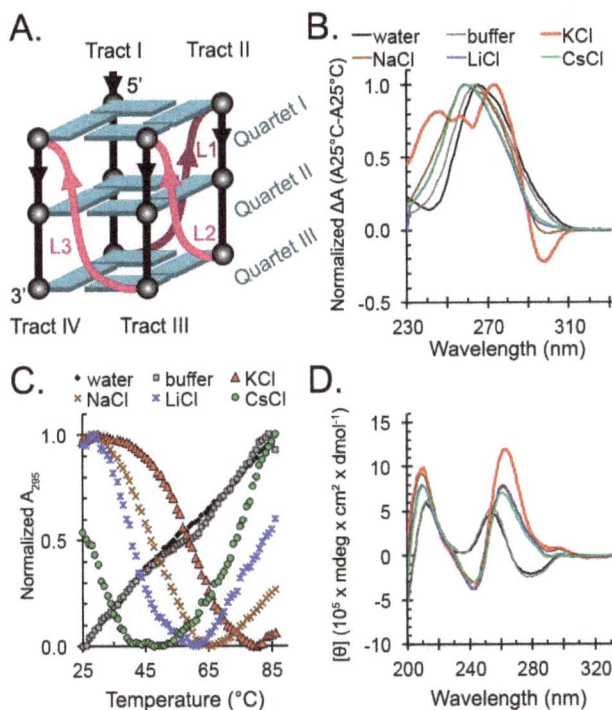

Figure 1. Spectroscopic analysis of a G-quadruplex (G4) formation by *hex4_A5U*. Oligonucleotides annealed in water (black), 10 mM tetrabutyl ammonium phosphate (TBA) buffer pH 7.5 (gray), or 10 mM TBA buffer supplemented with 100 mM of KCl (red), NaCl (brown), LiCl (blue), or CsCl (green). (**A**) Schematic representation of a canonical parallel unimolecular G4. Four tracts of three consecutive guanines (spheres) form three stacked G-quartets (cyan) stabilized by a monovalent cation. L1, L2, and L3 are lateral loops (magenta). (**B**) Normalized thermal difference spectra show formation of G4s, indicated by a negative peak at 295 nm. A prominent negative peak is observed only in KCl, and is absent in water or buffer, with intermediate values observed for NaCl, LiCl, and CsCl. (**C**) Thermal melting measured the cation-dependent stability of the G4 structures. G4s formed in KCl were the most stable, with a T$_{1/2}$ of 58 °C, followed by 50 °C for NaCl, 42 °C for LiCl, and <30 °C for CsCl. A linear increase in absorbance at 295 nm for oligonucleotides annealed in the absence of cation indicates that no G4 structures formed. (**D**) Circular Dichroism (CD) spectra show the formation of parallel G4s in the presence of cations. Peak maxima at 262 nm and minima at 242 nm were the hallmarks of the parallel G4s and were observed in KCl, NaCl, LiCl, and CsCl.

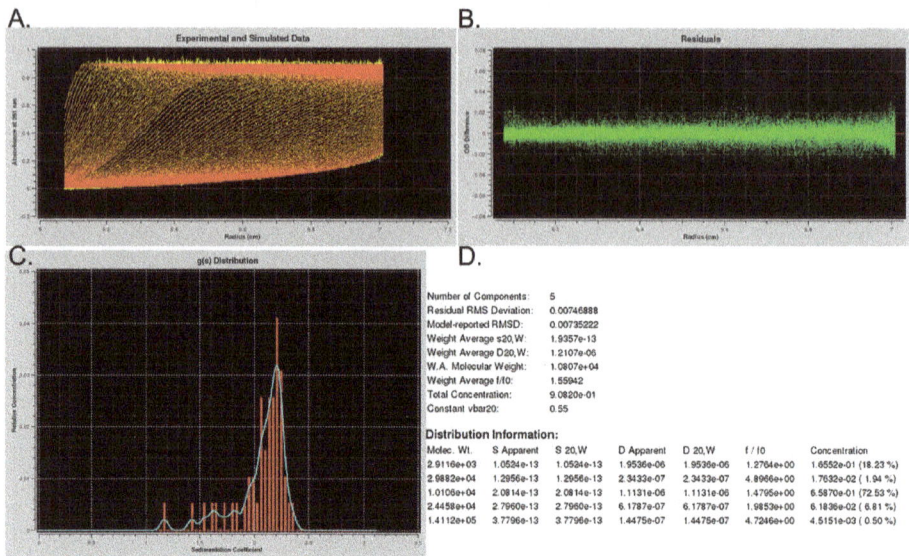

Figure 2. Analytical ultracentrifugation (AUC) of *hex4_A5U* annealed in KCl shows formation of a compact structure. (**A**) Raw sedimentation scans (yellow) overlaid with the calculated fit (red). (**B**) Residuals between the fit and the model plot showing their random nature. (**C**) Relative concentration and distribution of the species with different sedimentation coefficients. (**D**) Summary table of the contents of the solution after genetic algorithm analysis as implemented in Ultrascan 3 [47,48].

The formation of G4-like structures in the presence of cations other than K^+ was further evidenced by CD spectrophotometry. Samples annealed in the absence of cations had a positive peak maximum at 255 nm and did not undergo structural transitions with an increase in temperature (Figure 3A,B). At 25 °C, CD spectra of *hex4_A5U* annealed in the presence of any monovalent cation were similar to one another, whereas they were dramatically different from the spectra of *hex4_A5U* in the absence of cations. Negative ellipticity at 242 nm and positive ellipticity at 262 nm, as observed for cation-annealed samples, are the hallmarks of a parallel G4 [46]. K^+-annealed samples melted as a single species with an increase in temperature (Figure 3C), whereas samples annealed in Na^+, Li^+, and Cs^+ displayed a structural transition evidenced by a gradual shift of the maximum positive peak from 262 to 255 nm (Figure 3D–F).

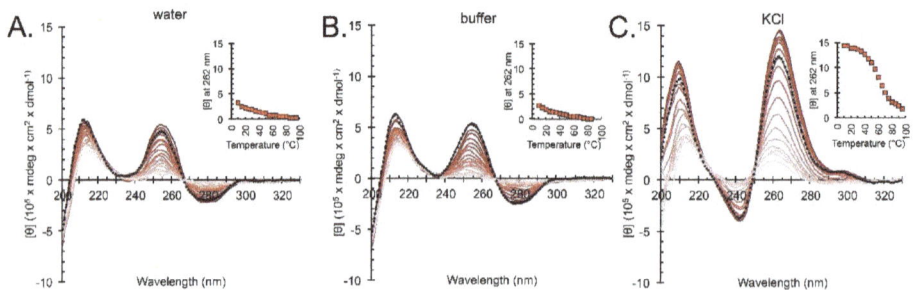

Figure 3. *Cont.*

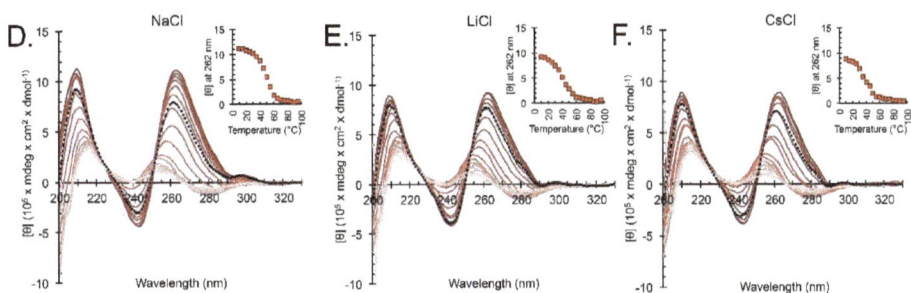

Figure 3. CD thermal denaturation shows reversible structural transition of a G4 formed by *hex4_A5U* with different cations. Oligonucleotides were annealed in 10 mM TBA buffer supplemented with 100 mM of KCl (**A**), NaCl (**B**), LiCl (**C**), CsCl (**D**), buffer alone (**E**), or water (**F**). In all conditions, we observed an overall decrease in CD signal intensity with an increase in temperature. Melting G4s annealed in KCl resulted in a sigmoidal curve with a $T_{1/2}$ of 58 °C. Melting in NaCl, LiCl, and CsCl revealed a two-state behavior indicative of a structural transition from a G4 to ssDNA in which a sigmoidal phase was followed by a linear phase. Melts for water and TBA buffer alone were linear and represented unstacking of the ssDNA bases. Thermal unfolding of the secondary structure was reversible, indicated by the dashed black line that corresponds to spectra collected immediately after the samples were cooled to 20 °C. Insets: plots of molar ellipticity at 262 nm versus temperature.

2.2. hex4_A5U Oligonucleotide is a Mix of G4 Conformations

We performed DMS footprinting followed by piperidine cleavage (Figure 4) to identify the Gs involved in G4 formation in K^+, and to characterize the G4-like structures that formed in the presence of non-K^+ cations. G4 prediction by the Quadparser algorithm [49] flagged G_4–G_6, G_{14}–G_{16}, G_{24}–G_{26}, and G_{28}–G_{30} as the four continuous G-tracts in the *hex4_A5U* sequence involved in G-tetrad formation [16]. A distinct footprinting pattern marked by missing products that correspond to Gs protected by G4 formation was seen only in K^+-annealed samples (Figure 4A, lane 1). Specifically, bands corresponding to cleavage at G_3–G_5 (G-tract I from the Quadparser model), G_{25}–G_{26} (partial G-tract III), and G_{28}–G_{30} (G-tract IV) were missing, indicating that those Gs were strongly protected from being DMS-labeled. Low intensity bands corresponding to cleavage at G_6 and G_{24} suggested weaker protection. In contrast, bands corresponding to cleavage at G_{14}–G_{16} (G-tract II) and other discontinuous Gs (G_8, G_{11}, G_{18}, G_{19}, G_{21} and G_{22}) were strong, indicating those Gs were not protected. Thus, we identified only two complete and one partial G-tract out of four G-tracts assigned by Quadparser for samples annealed in the presence of G4-inducing K^+.

There was a similar, but much less prominent, footprinting pattern in the Na^+, Li^+, and Cs^+-annealed samples (Figure 4A, lanes 2, 3, and 4) visible only in the 3′ region (compare intensity of the G_{31} band to G_{28}_G_{30}). In contrast, there was no protection in the absence of cations (Figure 4A, lane 5), and most of the oligonucleotide was degraded in the water alone (Figure 4A, lane 6). *hex4_A5U* DMS footprinting patterns in different cations agree with CD and UV-Vis melting experiments, which showed that K^+, and to a lesser degree Na^+, Li^+, and Cs^+, supported G4 formation, whereas no secondary structure was detectable in the absence of cations.

Despite unambiguous spectroscopic evidence of G4 formation in K^+, our DMS footprinting failed to assign all G-tract II or III Gs (Figure 4A). This raised a question about the role of the middle Gs in the G4 structure, as well as the possibility of heterogeneous G4 structures. We first created a shorter construct, trim_A5U, with a three-base truncation at the 5′ end and a one-base truncation at the 3′ end, to simplify our analysis and eliminate the structures that would arise due to the G-register exchange (Figure 4B). All further analysis was done in trim_A5U background.

DMS footprinting of trim_A5U construct showed a less complicated footprinting pattern, where G_{24}–G_{25} and G_{28}–G_{30} at the 3′ end were clearly protected. Some difference in the degree of digestion was observed for G_{25} versus G_{26}, G_{18} versus G_{19}, and G_{14} versus G_{15}–G_{16} (Figure 4B lane 2).

Additionally, G_4–G_6 were less digested in KCl versus LiCl, indicating their involvement in G4 formation (Figure 4B, lanes 1 and 2). To verify that canonical G4 can still form, we further modified trim_A5U construct by replacing G_8, G_{18}, G_{19}, G_{21}, and G_{22} with thymidines, giving rise to a "locked" canonical construct—A5U^{AH}. DMS footprinting of this locked variant clearly showed protection of 12 guanines in KCl but not LiCl. These guanines formed the G4 core, whereas overdigestion of G_{11} showed that it was not involved in core formation, as predicted.

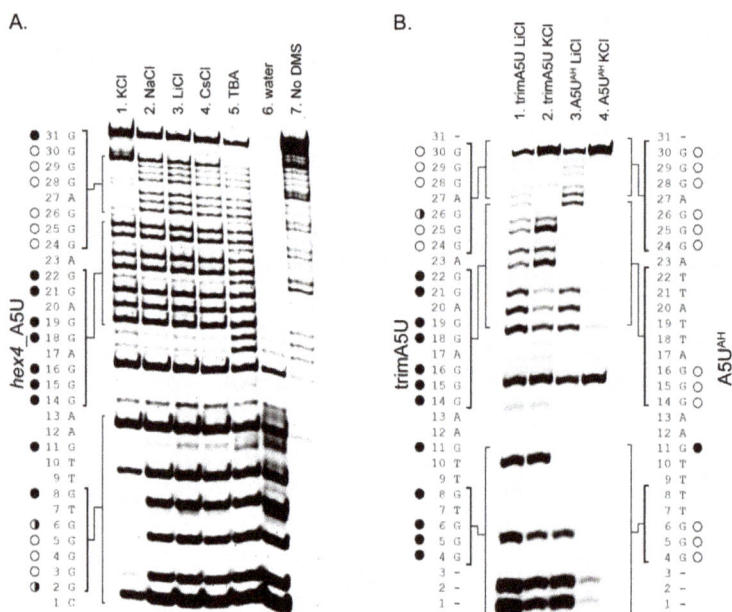

Figure 4. Dimethyl sulfate (DMS) footprinting of *hex4_A5U* and its variations reveal guanines involved in G4 core formation. (**A**) Missing bands on a gel indicate guanines protected from DMS labeling. A distinct footprinting pattern is observed only for the KCl sample (lane 1). In NaCl, LiCl, and CsCl, partial protection is observed for the GGGAGGG hairpin at the 5′ end of the oligonucleotide (lanes 2–4). In TBA, all guanines are digested evenly and in water alone the sample is overdigested. Circles (left) indicate guanines that are protected (○), partially protected (ɔ), or overdigested (●) when treated in KCl. (**B**) *hex4_A5U* was trimmed by removing bases 1, 2, 3, and 31, resulting in trimA5U construct. trimA5U was further altered by substituting G_8, G_{18}, G_{19}, G_{21}, and G_{22} with thymidines, resulting in A5U^{AH} construct. Both trim_A5U and A5U^{AH} oligonucleotides were subjected to DMS footprinting in KCl or LiCl.

Next, we employed rational mutagenesis to define the apparent heterogeneity of trim_A5U in G-tracts I, II, and III. Despite the predictions of middle G-tract involvement in G4 formation, deletion of the middle G-tract (G_{14}–G_{16}) or substitution of those Gs with adenines had no effect on G4 formation in the K$^+$ assessed by TDS (Figure 5A). We already established that G_{18}–G_{19} and G_{21}–G_{22} could not be exclusively involved as a bulged G-tract II, since their substitution by thymidines resulted in a sequence that was still capable of G4 formation (Figures 4B and 5A). Point mutations that simultaneously disrupted continuous G-tracts I, III, and IV (G_4, G_{25}, G_{30}) resulted in a sequence that did not form a G4 (Figure 5B). To test the possibility of intermolecular G4 formation from a two-G-tract containing oligonucleotide, we made an A5U^{R20} (random 20) construct where the 5′ sequence upstream of the GGGAGGG hairpin was replaced with 20 random non-G bases. This oligonucleotide did not form a stable G4 (Figure 5B), although it had a CD spectrum indicative of parallel G4s when annealed with K$^+$ or Li$^+$ (Figure 5B).

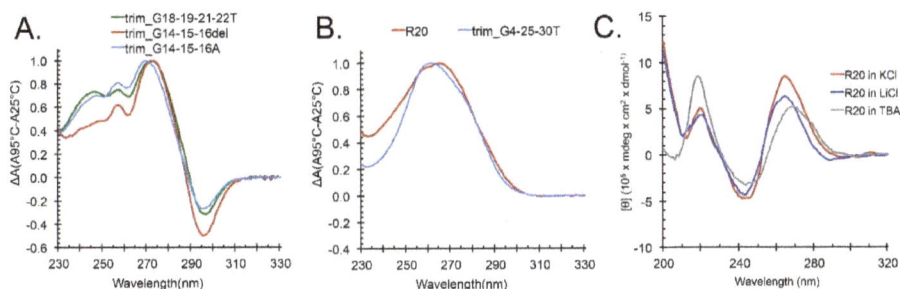

Figure 5. Preliminary mutagenesis of the trim_A5U oligonucleotide. Oligonucleotides were annealed in a buffer containing 10 mM TBA pH 7.5 supplemented with 100 mM KCl or LiCl. (**A**) trim_A5U variants with the deletion or substitution of tract II guanines with adenines form G4s. (**B**) trim_G4-25-30T oligonucleotide with point mutations in tracts I, III, and IV and A5U^{R20} oligonucleotide with a randomized sequence upstream of G-tract II did not form stable G4s. (**C**) G4-characteristic CD spectrum is observed only when A5U^{R20} oligonucleotides are annealed in the presence of cations, but not in the TBA buffer alone.

From this analysis, we further hypothesized that the trim_A5U sequence exists as a mix of G4 conformers in G-tracts II and III, including variants where continuous G-tracts were interrupted by non-G bases, forming a bulge [35]. We called this central stretch of non-continuous Gs a "G-slide" region, which defines the G4 heterogeneity. According to this extended model, G-tracts I and IV are fixed, but G-tracts II and III are formed by six bases from a G-slide region of 10 Gs with or without one-base bulges (Figure 6A). Based on these assumptions we identified 13 possible variants (Figure 6B), named according to the participating G triplets that form G-tract II and III (A–H). To test our model, we designed "locked" sequences that enforced a single conformation (Figure 6B, Table 1).

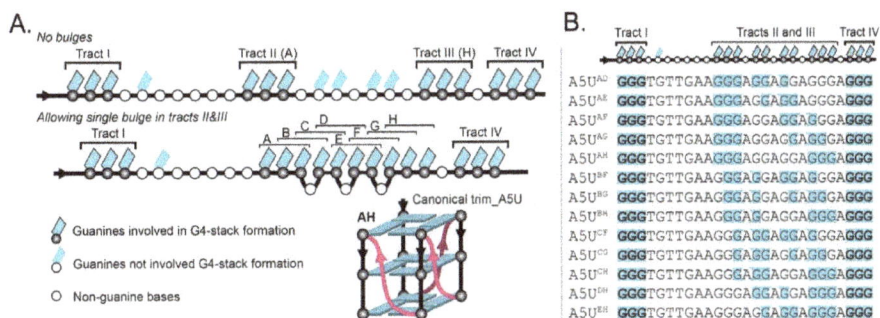

Figure 6. Extended model of G4 formation by trim_A5U allowing one bulge in G-tract. (**A**) Comparison between the canonical model and the extended G4 model. The extended model allows longer loops and a one-base-bulge interruption of G-tracts. Under the canonical model there is only one possible fold that can be adopted by trim_A5U to form a G4 core using tracts that do not contain bulges (i.e., tracts II (labeled A) and III (labeled H)). Under the extended model, trim_A5U can potentially form 13 different G4 core folds (including a canonical fold A5U^{AH}) with fixed tracts I and IV and the potential of one-base bulges in tracts II and III. (**B**) Guanines that can be involved in formation of the G4 core in the extended model are highlighted.

Table 1. Summary of the properties of trim_A5U-locked variants. Gs that participate in G4 formation are in bold and G-tracts are underlined and bold. Mutated residues are in lowercase.

Oligonucleotide	Sequence	CD	T_m	Competition %
A5U^{AD}	GGGTtTTGAAGGGAGGGAGGAGtAttAGGG	parallel	<30	73
A5U^{AE}	GGGTtTTGAAGGGAtGAGGGAtttAGGG	anti-h	37	16
A5U^{AF}	GGGTtTTGAAGGGAttAGGGAGtAGGG	anti-h	~30	15
A5U^{AG}	GGGTtTTGAAGGGAttAtGAGGtAGGG	anti-h	40	40
A5U^{AH} (canonical)	GGGTtTTGAAGGGAttAttAGGGAGGG	parallel	42	77
A5U^{BF}	GGGTtTTGAAtGGAGtAGGGAGtAGGG	anti-h	<30	23
A5U^{BG}	GGGTtTTGAAtGGAGtAtGAGGtAGGG	anti-h	<30	50
A5U^{BH}	GGGTtTTGAAtGGAGtAttAGGGAGGG	parallel	<30	85
A5U^{CF}	GGGTtTTGAAttGAGGAGGGAGtAGGG	parallel	<30	62
A5U^{CG}	GGGTtTTGAAttGAGGAtGAGGtAGGG	mixed	<30	36
A5U^{CH}	GGGTtTTGAAttGAGGAttAGGCGAGGG	parallel	~30	76
A5U^{DH}	GGGTtTTGAAtttAGGGAGGGAGGGAGGG	parallel	~30	77
A5U^{EH}	GGGTtTTGAAtttAtGAGGAGGGAGGG	parallel	35	81

2.3. Locked hex4_A5U Variants Form G4s with Distinct Properties

We proceeded to characterize the ability of locked trim_A5U variants to form G4s in K$^+$ through our series of spectroscopic assays. TDS showed that all locked variants A5U^{AD}–A5U^{EH} form G4s, albeit with variable amplitudes of the negative 295 nm peak (Figure 7A). CD spectra revealed additional differences between the variants (Figure 7B). Specifically, A5U^{AD}, A5U^{AH}, A5U^{BH}, A5U^{CF}, A5U^{CH}, A5U^{DH}, and A5U^{EH} had signatures of parallel G4s; A5U^{AE}, A5U^{AF}, A5U^{AG}, A5U^{BF}, and A5U^{BG} had signatures of antiparallel hybrid (anti-h) G4s; and A5U^{CG} had a mixed spectrum. Thermal denaturation experiments showed that A5U^{AD}, A5U^{CF}, and A5U^{CG} formed the weakest G4 structures, followed by A5U^{BF}, A5U^{BG}, and A5U^{BH}, which together formed a group of G4 variants with $T_{1/2}$ <30 °C (Figure 7C). The remaining seven variants—A5U^{AE}, A5U^{AF}, A5U^{AG}, A5U^{AH}, A5U^{CH}, A5U^{DH}, and A5U^{EH}—formed G4s that were stable at room temperature. All but A5U^{AH} contained one or two bulged G-tracts. Taken together, these data show that all 13 locked trim_A5U variants formed G4s but varied in their topology and thermal stability (Table 1).

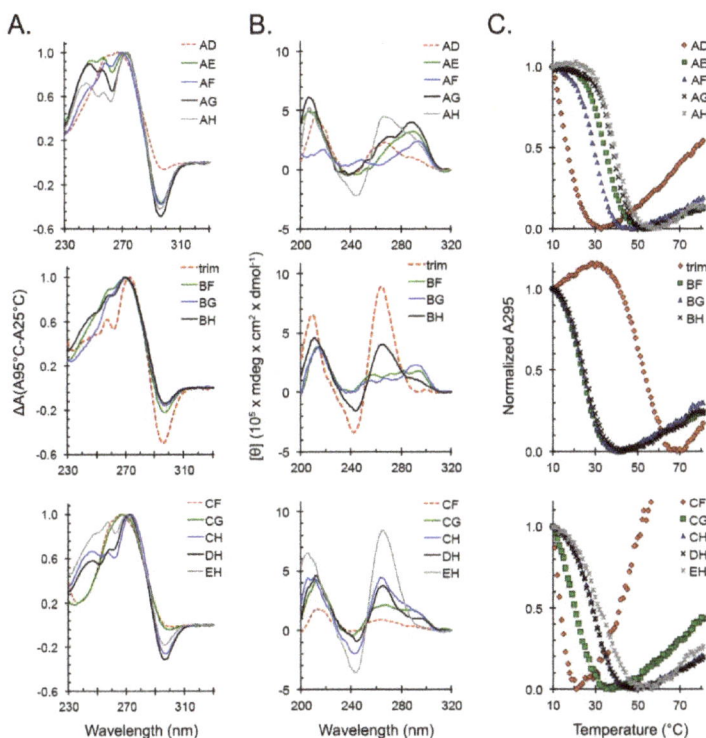

Figure 7. Spectroscopic analysis of a G-quadruplex (G4) formation by trim_A5U-locked variants. trim_A5U variants based on the extended model (derived from Figure 6B) were tested for their ability to form G4s. Guanines were substituted with thymidines to preclude their involvement in G4 core formation. (**A**) With the exception of A5U^{AD}, A5U^{CF}, and A5U^{CG}, all trim_A5U variants have a prominent negative peak at 295 nm, indicating G4 formation. (**B**) Thermal meltings monitored at 295 nm show that all locked variants formed G4s with different stabilities; however, A5U^{AD}, A5U^{BF}, A5U^{BG}, A5U^{BH}, A5U^{CF}, A5U^{CG}, formed weak G4s with $T_{1/2}$ < 30 °C. (**C**) CD spectra show that locked variants formed G4s with different topologies. Variants A5U^{AD}, A5U^{AH}, A5U^{BH}, A5U^{CF}, A5U^{CH}, A5U^{DH}, and A5U^{EH} formed parallel G4s with a major peak at 262 nm. A5U^{AE}, A5U^{AF}, A5U^{AG}, A5U^{BF}, and A5U^{BG} formed antiparallel hybrid G4s with a major peak at 292 nm. A5U^{CG} has a mixed spectra with similar ellipticity at 262 and 292 nm.

2.4. ZmNDPK1 Requires Two Consecutive G-Tracts with a Single One-Base Loop for Efficient Binding

Previously, we demonstrated that ZmNDPK1 binds to wild-type *hex4_A5U* G4 DNA with high affinity [22]. We determined that ZmNDPK1 also binds with high affinity to trim_A5U (K_d = 16.6 nM), as well as to the locked canonical variant A5U^{AH} (K_d = 14.4 nM), but not to another locked variant A5U^{AE} (K_d = 194 nM) (Figure 8A–C). We further tested which locked variant competed with wild-type *hex4_A5U* for binding to ZmNDPK1 to assess its binding specificity. At a 100-fold excess of the competitor, locked variants showed varying degrees of competition efficiency (Figure 8D, Table 1). Although each of the 13 variants competed for binding, only those classified as parallel according to CD measurements competed with greater than 50% efficiency (Figure 8D). The common feature shared by the strong competitors (A5U^{AD}, A5U^{AH}, A5U^{BH}, A5U^{CF}, A5U^{CH}, A5U^{DH}, and A5U^{EH}) was the presence of two G-tracts connected by a single adenosine: GGGAGGG (or GGGAG$_A$GG with a bulge in the second G-tract as in A5U^{AD}) (Table 1).

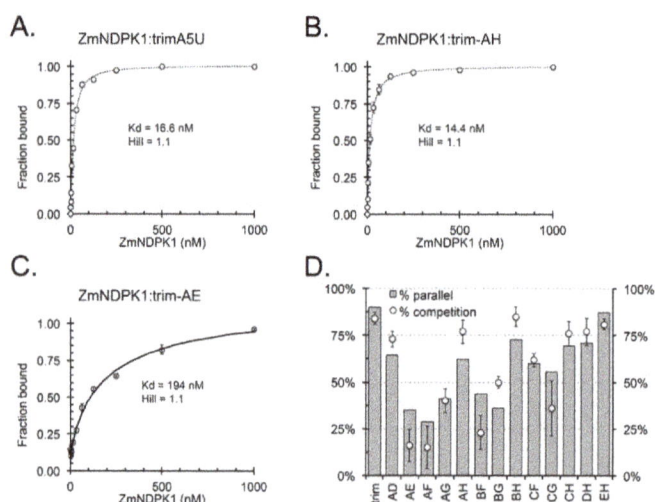

Figure 8. G4-binding protein ZmNDPK1 preferentially binds to the parallel locked variants of trim_A5U. (**A**) Binding of ZmNDPK1 to the trim_A5U caused the retention of the fluorescently labeled oligonucleotide on the nitrocellulose. (**B**) Binding of ZmNDPK1 to the trim_AH caused the retention of the fluorescently labeled oligonucleotide on the nitrocellulose. (**C**) Binding of ZmNDPK1 to the trim_AE caused the retention of the fluorescently labeled oligonucleotide on the nitrocellulose. (**D**) Competition efficiency was calculated as the amount of the probe retained on the nitrocellulose compared to the no-competitor control. Only parallel G4-locked variants competed with high efficiency: A5U^{AD}, A5U^{AH}, A5U^{BH}, A5U^{CF}, A5U^{CH}, A5U^{DH}, and A5U^{EH}.

2.5. ZmNDPK1 Binds Intermolecular and Intramolecular G4s

ZmNDPK1 binds to G4s that are annealed in Li$^+$ with 40-fold weaker affinity [33], but promotes G4 folding upon binding (Figure 9A). To further explore the binding properties of ZmNDPK1 with G-rich DNA that is not pre-formed into an intramolecular G4 conformation, we tested whether or not ZmNDPK1 could bring together two separate DNA strands. When equimolar amounts of 5′ fluorescein (FAM)-labeled *hex4_A5U* and 3′ TAMRA-labeled *hex4_A5U* oligonucleotides were mixed and then annealed either in K$^+$ or Li$^+$, neither sample exhibited Förster resonance energy transfer (FRET) in the absence of protein (Figure 9B). When ZmNDPK1 was added to the K$^+$-annealed oligonucleotide there was no change to the FRET signal. In contrast, the single-labeled oligonucleotides pre-annealed in Li$^+$ exhibited FRET when mixed with ZmNDPK1 (Figure 9B). Interestingly, when A5U^{R20} oligonucleotide

(20 random bases ending with the 3′ GGGAGGG hairpin) was used instead of *hex4_A5U*, no FRET was observed despite A5U^R20′s signature of parallel G4 in CD experiments

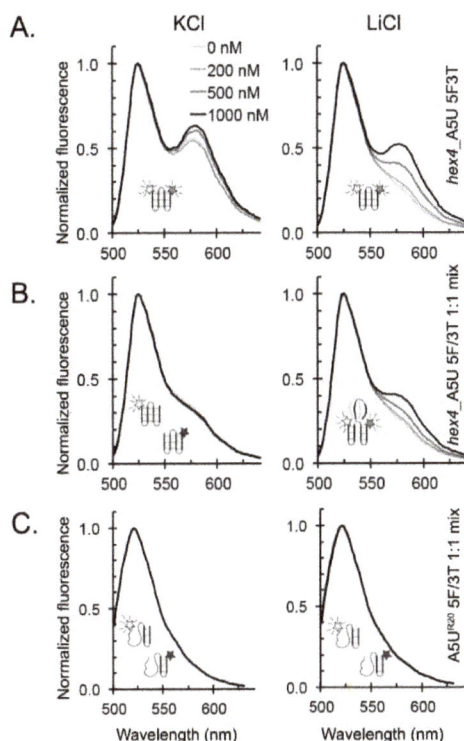

Figure 9. ZmNDPK1 binds to intermolecular and intramolecular G4s. Fluorescence emission data were collected by exciting the FAM fluorophore, and resulting plots were normalized to the peak maxima of 1 to better visualize the changes. (**A**) *hex4_A5U_5F3T*: dual-labeled oligonucleotides. When annealed in KCl, the FRET signal changed little with increasing protein concentration. When annealed in LiCl, the FRET signal increased with increasing protein concentration. (**B**) *hex4_A5U_5F/3T*: two single-labeled oligonucleotides. When annealed in KCl, FRET did not change with added protein. When annealed in LiCl, the FRET signal increased with increasing in protein concentration. (**C**) A5UR20 5F/3T: two single-labeled oligonucleotides, with 20 random non-G bases ending with a GGGAGGG hairpin. When annealed in either KCl or LiCl, the FRET signal did not change with added protein.

2.6. ZmNDPK1 and Trim_A5U form a Heterogeneous Protein: Nucleic Acid Complex

To gain insight into the mechanism of complex formation between ZmNDPK1 and trim_A5U, we used electron microscopy to visualize the protein alone and in the presence of the G4 oligonucleotide (Figure 10). For ZmNDPK1 alone, we saw uniformly distributed globular protein molecules of the expected size (Figure 10A). After ZmNDPK1 was incubated with trim_A5U we saw the formation of filamentous structures of uniform thickness but various lengths and shapes (Figure 10B). ZmNDPK–trim_A5U complex was then plunge-frozen and images were collected in vitrified ice under the cryogenic conditions (Figure 10C). We saw that filaments were well preserved in ice and uniformly distributed. 2D classification of the particles picked from cryogenic electron microscopy (cryo-EM) images confirmed that the complex had a distinct structure over short distances but was too heterogeneous for further 3D analysis (Figure 10D).

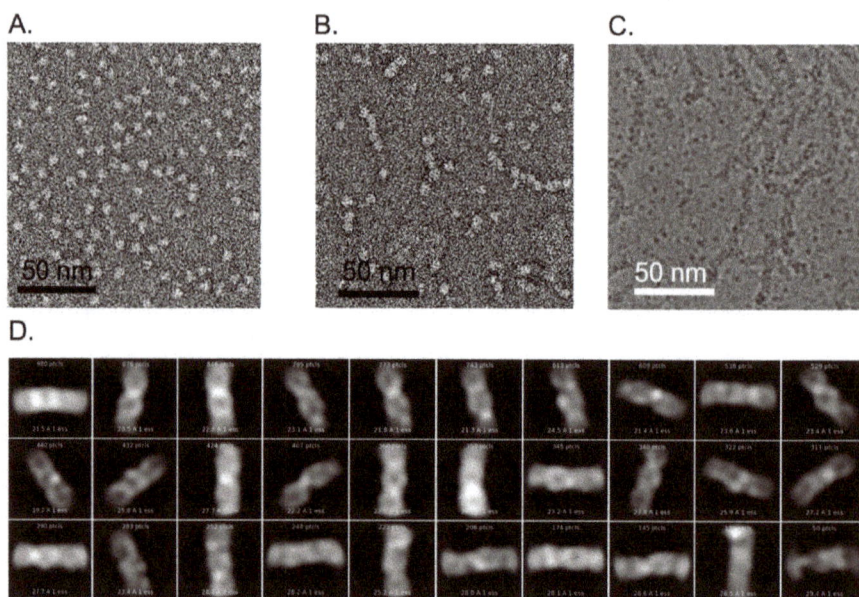

Figure 10. Electron microscopy of the complex between ZmNDPK1 and trim_A5U. (**A**) Image of a negatively stained ZmNDPK1 alone. (**B**) Image of the negatively stained ZmNDPK1 in complex with trim_A5U. (**C**) CryoEM image of ZmNDPK1 in complex with trim_A5U stain in vitreous ice. (**D**) Results of 2D classification of 30.000 filament segments picked from the cryoEM images.

3. Discussion

3.1. G4s in the Stress Response

G4s are now recognized as important elements in the regulation of intracellular processes related to replication, transcription, translation, splicing, and telomere maintenance [50]. In fact, G4 formation in the promoter of a gene can either inhibit [51,52] or facilitate its transcription [6,53]. In vivo, G4s exist in the context of the double-stranded genome and are regulated through interaction with G4-binding proteins like XPB and telomere end-binding proteins [50,54–56]. In vitro, G4 formation is largely driven by the presence of K^+ or Na^+, so in addition to possible coordination by proteins, G4 formation is also sensitive to the ionic environment of the cell. In this study, we investigated the properties of the *hex4_A5U* oligonucleotide derived from the G-rich sequence located on the template strand in the 5′ untranslated region of the maize *hexokinase4* gene. This gene is particularly interesting because it has three putative G4s—two on the template strand and one on the coding strand of DNA [16].

3.2. Limitations in G4 Characterization Affect Analysis of hex4_A5U

UV-Vis spectrophotometry, CD spectrophotometry, and DMS footprinting are commonly used techniques to verify G4 formation by a given nucleotide sequence. Each has unique strengths, but none is able to unambiguously assess the G4 conformation, and so they must be used together to understand the possible G4 variations of even the simplest G-rich sequence. TDS is a qualitative technique based on UV-Vis spectrophotometry that relies on the hyperchromicity of G4s at 295 nm, but the signal changes qualitatively with the base composition of the nucleic acid [57]. *hex4_A5U* shows a distinct G4 TDS profile only in the presence of K^+ ions (Figure 1B), whereas the TDS profile of *hex4_A5U* in Na^+, Li^+, and Cs^+ is intermediate between K^+ and the absence of cations, suggesting formation of a weak G4. Aside from TDS, UV-Vis spectrophotometry can be used to monitor the stability of the G4 by measuring the change in absorbance at 295 nm with increasing temperature [6]. In 100 mM K^+, *hex4_A5U* had a

$T_{1/2}$ of 58 C, showing that it is stable at physiologically relevant temperatures (Figure 1C). We also observed an initial decrease in absorbance at 295 nm for all other cations, suggesting melting of a transient G4, but not in the absence of cations. Overall, these observations show that *hex4_A5U*, expectedly, forms a G4 only if stabilized by a cation, where $K^+ >> Na^+ > Li^+ > Cs^+$.

CD spectrophotometry is commonly used to assess the properties of oligonucleotides to give clues about secondary structure. *hex4_A5U* has CD spectra characteristic of a parallel G4 conformation [46] in K^+, Na^+, Li^+, and Cs^+ (Figure 1D). In the absence of any small cation, CD spectra indicate that the oligonucleotide is disordered (Figure 1D). Interestingly, CD thermal denaturation experiments show that G4s in K^+ melt as a single species, whereas in Na^+, Li^+, and Cs^+ there is a structural transition evidenced by the shift of the peak maxima from 262 to 255 nm (Figure 3). After the transition, melting profiles for Na^+, Li^+, and Cs^+ resemble that of the oligonucleotides annealed in the absence of cations. The temperature at which this transition occurs is cation-dependent and matches the G4 stability order for cations determined in UV-Vis thermal denaturation experiments: $K^+ >> Na^+ > Li^+ > Cs^+$.

Lastly, DMS footprinting provides an additional insight into G4 topology by analyzing solvent-accessible Gs. DMS footprinting showed strong protection of Gs only in K^+ (Figure 4A, lane 1), whereas protection in Na^+, Li^+, and Cs^+ was limited to the GGGAGGG hairpin at the 3′ end of the sequence (Figure 4A, lanes 2–4). All Gs were completely unprotected in absence of cations, representing a fully unfolded state. We attribute the partial protection in Na^+, Li^+, and Cs^+ to the formation of a weak intermolecular G4 that forms by cation stabilization of the 3′ GGGAGGG hairpins from two DNA molecules. Indeed, the A5U^{R20} oligonucleotide, which has 20 random non-G bases followed by a GGGAGGG hairpin on the 3′ end, does not have a characteristic G4 TDS spectrum (Figure 5B), but does have a parallel G4 CD spectrum in the presence of cations (Figure 5C). We conclude that *hex4_A5U* forms an intramolecular parallel G4 only in the presence of K^+, whereas it forms a weak intermolecular G4 in the presence of Na^+, Li^+, or Cs^+

3.3. hex4_A5U and its Truncated Variant trim_A5U are Highly Polymorphic G4-Forming Sequences

G4 polymorphism is a common, complicating predicting their structures based on sequence alone. Examples of polymorphism include extra G-tracts that can act as a "spare tire" [58]; formation of an ensemble of structures with different topologies [59,60]; variation in number of strands (one, two, or four) and tetrads (two or more); presence of bulges [35]; and loops longer than seven nucleotides [60]. *hex4_A5U* was initially predicted to form from four uninterrupted G-tracts of three sequential Gs (Figure 6A). Instead, DMS footprinting revealed that only two G-tracts were fully protected, whereas G-tract II was not protected and G-tract III was only partially protected (Figure 4A, lane 1). Further, G-tract II was not strictly required for G4 formation in K^+ (Figure 4A, Figure 5A). To explain this mismatch, we hypothesize that adjacent Gs can be substituted into G-tract II, forming a series of structures with bulged G-tracts that co-exist in solution (Figure 6A). Such a polymorphic system combines G-register exchange [42] with the formation of bulged variants and leads to the apparent absence of protection in G-tract II and only partial protection in G-tract III over the course of DMS labeling. DMS footprinting of trim_A5U revealed that, in this truncated construct, the strong protection of guanines was only for tracts III and IV (Figure 6B, lane 2). The only sequence variant in which we observed complete protection of all 12 guanines involved in G4 core formation was in DMS footprinting of A5U^{AH} construct (Figure 6B, lane 4), in which all extra guanines were substituted by thymidines. In this case, the locked variants described only one possibility of the variations that the native DNA sequence might adopt. We interpreted the data measured on the locked variants to inform us about the ensemble of structures that can possibly form by the native sequence, but it could also be that no single mutation exactly mimics the behavior of the oligonucleotide with the full-length, native *hex4_A5U* sequence

An expanded definition of G4-forming sequences emerges that allows G-tracts to be interrupted by a one-base bulge connected into a continuous region that we call a "G-slide" (Figure 6A). This guanine-rich region can also be mathematically described as a 10-choose-6 combinatorics problem that results in 260 combinations, of which we explored only 13 variants by limiting ourselves to single-bulge interruptions of G-tracts. From our formulation, trim_A5U can form at least 13 different conformers, isolated structurally by point mutagenesis (Figure 6B, Table 1). By all measurements, each resulting variant behaves in a sequence-specific manner that is ultimately predictive of its fold and determines its interaction with the G4-binding protein ZmNDPK1 (Figures 7 and 8). The CD spectrum of the trim_A5U sequence has a minor contribution to the anti-parallel signal when compared to the locked variants (Figures 7B and 8B). This suggests that predominantly antiparallel hybrids (A5U^{AE}, A5U^{AF}, A5U^{AG}, A5U^{BF}, and A5U^{BG}) as well as unstable variants (A5U^{AD}, A5U^{CF}, and A5U^{CG}) constitute a small fraction of solution conformations. Therefore, the co-existence of parallel G4s with variable G-slide picks (A5U^{AH}, A5U^{BH}, A5U^{CH}, A5U^{DH}, and A5U^{EH}) represent the majority of conformational states of trim_A5U. Overall, the wild-type conformation is likely determined by the relative stability of the fold and the presence of a GGGAGGG hairpin that favors the formation of a parallel G4 (Figure 7B, Table 1) [61].

3.4. The G4-Binding Protein ZmNDPK1 Recognizes a Subset of Conformations Adopted by hex4_A5U DNA and Forms Filamentous Structures upon Binding

DNA is associated with protein binding partners within the nucleus. ZmNDPK1, a plant homolog of human NM23-H2, interacts with *hex4*_A5U with high affinity and specificity [33]. Despite the analogy between plant and human NDPKs binding to G-rich DNA sequences [62–64], we do not know how they interact or, until now, what structural motifs direct binding. ZmNDPK1 does not have a single preferred G4 conformation, but binds more specifically to parallel G4s that contain the GGGAGGG motif with or without bulges (Figure 8, Table 1). Additionally, ZmNDPK1 recognizes the structural element that gives rise to weak G4 signals in sub-optimal G4-promoting ions (i.e., Li$^+$), perhaps a transitory guanine hairpin [65], and then facilitates bimolecular G4 formation (Figure 9A,B).

Electron microscopy of the ZmNDPK1–trim_A5U complex revealed its assembly into filamentous structures (Figure 10B,C). These structures differed in their lengths, but not thickness. 2D classification of particles from cryoEM images provided a low-resolution look into organization of this complex (Figure 10D). We can see that the complex is highly flexible, and poorly resolved, which made it not possible to distinguish between protein and DNA densities in our 2D classes. One thing was clear—the complex of Z4sNDPK1–trim_A5U was not as simple as two G4s per one hexamer as we predicted from the stoichiometry determined biochemically in solution.

3.5. Generalization of G4 Heterogeneity across Domains of Life

The ability for G4 DNA to form multiple conformations with protein-binding specificity is not unique to maize, so characterizing the range of morphologies that long, non-continuous G-rich stretches can adopt is relevant in possibly exploiting the phenomenon for anti-microbial or anti-viral therapies. For example, a common bacterial (G$_4$CT)$_3$G$_4$ motif associated with antigenic variation exhibits cation-stabilizing, concentration-dependent conformational variability that is sequence dependent [66]. The striking similarity to the phenomenon we observed with the *hex4*_A5U motif suggests that this conformational variability may well influence how the sequence interacts with its protein partners in microorganisms. This idea is supported by the observation that in *Neisseria gonorrhoeae*, a monomeric—but not dimeric—parallel, G4 binds RecA to direct recombination at the pilin expression locus during antigenic switching [67]. Further, the ability for a G4 linked to nitrate assimilation in *Paracoccus denitrificans* to form inter- or intramolecular G4s (i.e., G4's insensitivity to NH$_4$$^+$) and a mix of parallel and anti-parallel conformations in solution suggests plasticity could also play a role in this microorganism [68]. This feature is not limited to microorganisms—the G-rich proviral HIV-1 U3 DNA forms polymorphic G4 structures that have different Sp1-binding capabilities that are proposed to fine-tune transcription [69]. Human G4s including c-myc [38], RET [70–72], VEGF [73], and BCL-2 [74] also have the ability to form multiple conformations. Indeed, a minimal version composed of four Gs in a single G-tract where the 5′ or 3′ G can swap into the three-G stretch of the slide region has been described as a slippage of the G-tract in *c-myc* [38]. Similarly, a specific instance of the slide can be seen in the oxidative protection mechanism described as the spare tire, where a fifth terminal G-tract can slide into place, positioning the fourth G-tract in a long loop that allows repair of oxidatively damaged Gs [58]. Here, we have generalized these specific examples into a model that allows Gs from long, non-continuous G stretches to slide into the G4 stack, creating a range of G4 conformations that have unique properties and specific responses to a G4-binding protein (Figure 11). Such heterogeneity in G4 formation is an innate biophysical property of G4s that is likely conserved from prokaryotes to eukaryotes.

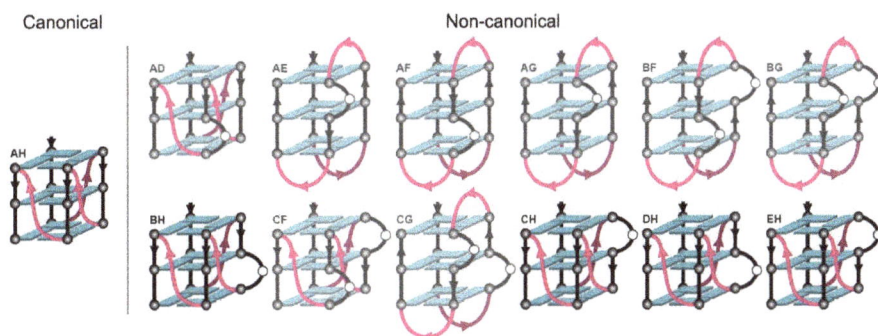

Figure 11. Possible topologies that can be adopted by the trim_A5U oligonucleotides. Out of 13 conformation possibilities predicted by the extended model, only one is canonical (A5U^A), while 12 others contain a bulge in G-tract II, III, or in both G-tracts. ZmNDPK1 binds to the variants with the conserved GGGAGGG hairpin (contrasted models).

4. Materials and Methods

4.1. Oligonucleotide and Protein Preparation

All oligonucleotides were purchased from Eurofins MWG Operon LLC (Huntsville, AL, USA) as salt-free (non-labeled oligonucleotides) or HPLC-purified (fluorescently labeled oligonucleotides) and used without further purification. Base positions in oligonucleotide variants were numbered according to the positions in the *hex4*_A5U sequence [33]. Unless indicated otherwise, oligonucleotides were annealed by heating to 95 °C, then slowly cooled overnight to room temperature in 10 mM tetrabutyl ammonium phosphate (TBA, pH 7.5) buffer with or without 100 mM salt (KCl, LiCl, CsCl, or NaCl), or in water alone. Recombinant ZmNDPK1 protein was purified as previously described [33].

4.2. Absorption Spectrophotometry

Non-labeled oligonucleotides were annealed at 10 μM concentration and diluted to 2.5 μM before data collection. All UV-Vis experiments were performed on a Cary 300 Bio UV/Vis spectrophotometer equipped with a Peltier temperature controller (Agilent Technology, Santa Clara, CA, USA). For thermal difference spectroscopy (TDS), a first spectrum was collected at 25 °C, samples were heated to 95 °C, and a second spectrum was collected. TDS was calculated by subtracting the 25 °C spectrum from the 95 °C spectrum and normalizing the maximum peak to an absorbance of 1 and the absorbance at 330 nm to 0. For thermal denaturation experiments, the absorbance at 295 nm was monitored in the temperature range from 25 to 95 °C at a heating rate of 0.5 °C/min. Data were normalized to a maximum of 1.

4.3. Circular Dichroism Spectrophotometry

Non-labeled oligonucleotides were annealed at 10 μM concentration and used without further dilution. Circular dichroism (CD) spectra were collected on an Aviv 202 CD spectrometer (Aviv

Biomedical, Lakewood, NJ, USA). Single temperature experiments were performed at 25 °C over a 200–330 nm range with a 3-s average time. The same parameters were used for thermal denaturation experiments in which measurements were made between 10 and 95 °C with a 5 °C increment between measurements after a 10-min equilibration. All spectra were background corrected against blank buffer and normalized to have zero ellipticity at 330 nm.

4.4. Dimethyl Sulfate (DMS) Footprinting

Oligonucleotides with a 5′ 6-carboxyfluorescein (FAM) modification were annealed at 10 μM concentration and diluted to 500 nM concentration prior to DMS treatment. Samples were treated with 1% DMS for 5 min at 25 °C and stopped by adding 25 μL of quench solution (1.5 M sodium acetate pH 7.0, 1 M β-mercaptoethanol and 100 μg/mL calf thymus DNA). DNA was ethanol-precipitated and pellets were resuspended in 100 μL of 1 M piperidine, incubated for 15 min at 95 °C, and dried in a rotary centrifuge. Dried samples were washed with distilled water, resuspended in alkaline sequencing dye (80% formamide, 10 mM NaOH, 0.005% bromophenol blue), and heated to 95 °C for 3 min. Cleavage products were resolved on a 17.5% polyacrylamide denaturing gel (4 M urea, 0.5x tris-borate-EDTA, 0.4 mm thick, 33 × 39 cm, 29:1 acrylamide/bisacrylamide) run for 1.5 h at a constant 50 W power. Glass plates were separated and the gel was imaged on a GE Typhoon scanner (GE Healthcare Bio-Sciences, Pittsburg, PA, USA) in fluorescence mode using a 488-nm excitation wavelength and a 520-nm band pass filter.

4.5. Nitrocellulose Filter Binding Assays for ZmNDPK1/G4 DNA Binding Affinity Analysis

For binding-affinity determination, we used a modified slot-blot binding assay as previously described [33], substituting a 5′ biotin label with a 5′ carboxyfluorescein. We used the same approach to determine the efficiency of ZmNDPK1 binding to labeled oligonucleotides in the presence of competitor oligonucleotides. All oligonucleotides were annealed in 10 mM TBA (pH 7.5) + 20 mM KCl. Labeled oligonucleotide at 1 nM was mixed with 100 nM competitor oligonucleotide and 5 nM ZmNDPK1. Reactions were incubated for 60 min and applied to the slot-blot apparatus, where the solution first passes through a negatively charged nitrocellulose membrane (Hybond-C Exatra 0.45 μM pore size, GE Healthcare Life Sciences, Piscataway, NJ, USA) that retains protein and protein–DNA complex. Unbound DNA was then captured by a positively charged nylon membrane (Nytran N 0.45 μM pore size, GE Healthcare Life Sciences, Piscataway, NJ, USA). Membranes were dried and scanned on a GE Typhoon scanner in fluorescence mode using a 488-nm excitation wavelength and a 520-nm band pass filter. Images were background corrected and the intensities of the bands were determined in ImageJ. Competition efficiency was calculated from the retention percentage of the fluorescent probe on nitrocellulose against zero competitor control.

4.6. Analytical Ultracentrifugation (AUC)

Sedimentation experiments were carried out in a Beckman Coulter ProteomeLab XL-1 analytical ultracentrifuge using an AN60-Ti rotor and double-sector quartz cells. We loaded 420 μL of annealed oligonucleotides at 1 μm into sample sectors and 430 μL of corresponding annealing buffers into reference sectors. Initial scans and rotor calibrations were performed at 3000 rpm and a 260-nm wavelength. Data were collected at 58,000 rpm and analyzed using Ultrascan III software [48].

4.7. Fluorescence Resonance Energy Transfer (FRET)

*hex4*_A5U oligonucleotides were labeled with either 5′ 6-carboxyfluorescein (*hex4*_A5U-5F) or 3′ carboxytetramethylrhodamine (*hex4*_A5U-3T) or both fluorophores (*hex4*_A5U-5F3T). Reactions were set up in triplicate in 96-well Nunclon plates (Thermo Fisher Scientific, Waltham, MA) containing 200 nM of either *hex4*_A5U-5F3T or a mix of 100 nM *hex4*_A5U-5F + 100 nM *hex4*_A5U-3T annealed in 10 mM TBA (pH 7.5) + 100 mM KCl or 100 mM LiCl. Protein was added at 0, 200 nM, 500 nM, or 1000 nM concentrations and incubated for 1 h at 4 °C before data collection. Data were collected on a Spectramax M5^e Multi-Mode Microplate Reader (Molecular Devices, Sunnyvale, CA, USA) and processing was performed as previously described [33]. Labeling and data collection for A5U^{R20} oligonucleotides were done as described for *hex4_A5U*.

4.8. Electron Microscopy (EM)

NDPK–G4 complex was assembled by mixing 3 μM ZmNDPK1 and 6 μM *hex4_A5U* in a buffer containing 10 mM Hepes pH 7.5 and 50 mM KCl. For negative staining, the mixture was applied to plasma-cleaned CF200-Cu carbon-coated copper grids (Electron Microscopy Sciences, Hatfield, PA, USA), incubated for 60 s, washed 3x with distilled water, and stained for 60 s with 1% uranyl-acetate. Images were collected on a FEI/Philips CM120 Biotwin electron microscope (Thermo Fisher Scientific, Waltham, MA, USA) at 40,000 magnification (2.8 Å/px). For cryo-electron microscopy (cryoEM) the mixture was applied to the carbon side of the plasma-cleaned Quantifoil R2/2 grids (Electron Microscopy Sciences, Hatfield, PA, USA) and plunged into liquid ethane using FEI Vitrobot (Thermo Fisher Scientific, Waltham, MA, USA). Plunge-frozen grids were imaged on an FEI Titan Krios (Thermo Fisher Scientific, Waltham, MA, USA) equipped with a DE20 direct electron detector camera (Direct Electron, San Diego, CA, USA) at 37,000 magnification and 0.99 Å pixel size. Automatic data acquisition was set up using Leginon software [75]. Images were collected with a 1.5–3.5 μm defocus range. Particles were manually picked from the images using a Leginon particle picker. Particle coordinates were used to create a particle stack of ~30.000 particles. Particle stack was 2D classified in cryoSPARC [76] into 30 classes.

Author Contributions: Conceptualization, M.K. and M.E.S.; Funding acquisition, M.E.S.; Investigation, M.K. and T.J.; Supervision, M.E.S.; Writing—original draft, M.K.; Writing—review and editing, M.E.S.

Funding: This research was funded by the National Science Foundation, grant number MCB1149763, and a Florida State University Planning Grant. The authors acknowledge the use of instruments at the Biological Science Imaging Resource supported by Florida State University and NIH grants S10 RR025080 and S10 OD018142.

Acknowledgments: The authors would like to thank Jay Rai and Joseph Pennington for helpful discussions.

Conflicts of Interest: The authors declare no conflict of interest.

References

1. Watson, J.D.; Crick, F.H. Genetical implications of the structure of deoxyribonucleic acid. *Nature* **1953**, *171*, 964–967. [CrossRef]
2. Gellert, M.; Lipsett, M.N.; Davies, D.R. Helix formation by guanylic acid. *Proc. Natl. Acad. Sci. USA* **1962**, *48*, 2013–2018. [PubMed]
3. Zimmerman, S.B.; Cohen, G.H.; Davies, D.R. X-ray fiber diffraction and model-building study of polyguanylic acid and polyinosinic acid. *J. Mol. Biol.* **1975**, *92*, 181–192. [PubMed]
4. Harris, L.M.; Merrick, C.J. G-quadruplexes in pathogens: A common route to virulence control? *PLoS Pathog.* **2015**, *11*, e1004562. [CrossRef]
5. Biffi, G.; Tannahill, D.; McCafferty, J.; Balasubramanian, S. Quantitative visualization of DNA G-quadruplex structures in human cells. *Nat. Chem.* **2013**, *5*, 182–186. [CrossRef] [PubMed]
6. Farhath, M.M.; Thompson, M.; Ray, S.; Sewell, A.; Balci, H.; Basu, S. G-Quadruplex-Enabling Sequence within the Human Tyrosine Hydroxylase Promoter Differentially Regulates Transcription. *Biochemistry* **2015**, *54*, 5533–5545. [PubMed]
7. Lemmens, B.; van Schendel, R.; Tijsterman, M. Mutagenic consequences of a single G-quadruplex demonstrate mitotic inheritance of DNA replication fork barriers. *Nat. Commun.* **2015**, *6*, 8909.
8. Kanoh, Y.; Matsumoto, S.; Fukatsu, R.; Kakusho, N.; Kono, N.; Renard-Guillet, C.; Masuda, K.; Iida, K.; Nagasawa, K.; Shirahige, K.; et al. Rif1 binds to G quadruplexes and suppresses replication over long distances. *Nat. Struct. Mol. Biol.* **2015**, *22*, 889–897. [CrossRef] [PubMed]
9. Wu, Y.; Shin-ya, K.; Brosh, R.M. FANCJ Helicase Defective in Fanconia Anemia and Breast Cancer Unwinds G-Quadruplex DNA To Defend Genomic Stability. *Mol. Cell. Biol.* **2008**, *28*, 4116–4128. [CrossRef] [PubMed]

10. Paeschke, K.; Capra, J.A.; Zakian, V.A. DNA Replication through G-Quadruplex Motifs Is Promoted by the Saccharomyces cerevisiae Pif1 DNA Helicase. *Cell* **2011**, *145*, 678–691.

11. Smestad, J.A.; Maher, L.J. Relationships between putative G-quadruplex-forming sequences, RecQ helicases, and transcription. *BMC Med. Genet.* **2015**, *16*, 91. [CrossRef] [PubMed]

12. Bartas, M.; Čutová, M.; Brázda, V.; Kaura, P.; Šťastný, J.; Kolomazník, J.; Coufal, J.; Goswami, P.; Červeň, J.; Pečinka, P. The Presence and Localization of G-Quadruplex Forming Sequences in the Domain of Bacteria. *Molecules* **2019**, *24*, 1711. [CrossRef] [PubMed]

13. Ruggiero, E.; Tassinari, M.; Perrone, R.; Nadai, M.; Richter, S.N. The Long Terminal Repeat promoter of Retroviruses contains stable and conserved G-quadruplexes. *ACS Infect. Dis.* **2019**. [CrossRef]

14. Scalabrin, M.; Frasson, I.; Ruggiero, E.; Perrone, R.; Tosoni, E.; Lago, S.; Tassinari, M.; Palù, G.; Richter, S.N. The cellular protein hnRNP A2/B1 enhances HIV-1 transcription by unfolding LTR promoter G-quadruplexes. *Sci. Rep.* **2017**, *7*, 45244. [CrossRef] [PubMed]

15. Eddy, J.; Maizels, N. Gene function correlates with potential for G4 DNA formation in the human genome. *Nucleic Acids Res.* **2006**, *34*, 3887–3896. [CrossRef] [PubMed]

16. Andorf, C.M.; Kopylov, M.; Dobbs, D.; Koch, K.E.; Stroupe, M.E.; Lawrence, C.J.; Bass, H.W. G-quadruplex (G4) motifs in the maize (Zea mays L.) genome are enriched at specific locations in thousands of genes coupled to energy status, hypoxia, low sugar, and nutrient deprivation. *J. Genet. Genom.* **2014**, *41*, 627–647. [CrossRef]

17. Kalra, P.; Mishra, S.K.; Kaur, S.; Kumar, A.; Prasad, H.K.; Sharma, T.K.; Tyagi, J.S. G-Quadruplex-Forming DNA Aptamers Inhibit the DNA-Binding Function of HupB and Mycobacterium tuberculosis Entry into Host Cells. *Mol. Ther. Nucleic Acids* **2018**, *13*, 99–109. [CrossRef]

18. Verma, A.; Yadav, V.K.; Basundra, R.; Kumar, A.; Chowdhury, S. Evidence of genome-wide G4 DNA-mediated gene expression in human cancer cells. *Nucleic Acids Res* **2009**, *37*, 4194–4204. [CrossRef]

19. Sengupta, A.; Ganguly, A.; Chowdhury, S. Promise of G-Quadruplex Structure Binding Ligands as Epigenetic Modifiers with Anti-Cancer Effects. *Molecules* **2019**, *24*, 582. [CrossRef]

20. Métifiot, M.; Amrane, S.; Litvak, S.; Andreola, M.L. G-quadruplexes in viruses: Function and potential therapeutic applications. *Nucleic Acids Res.* **2014**, *42*, 12352–12366.

21. Ruggiero, E.; Richter, S.N. G-quadruplexes and G-quadruplex ligands: Targets and tools in antiviral therapy. *Nucleic Acids Res.* **2018**, *46*, 3270–3283. [CrossRef]

22. Saranathan, N.; Vivekanandan, P. G-Quadruplexes: More Than Just a Kink in Microbial Genomes. *Trends Microbiol.* **2019**, *27*, 148–163. [CrossRef] [PubMed]

23. Amrane, S.; Kerkour, A.; Bedrat, A.; Vialet, B.; Andreola, M.L.; Mergny, J.L. Topology of a DNA G-quadruplex structure formed in the HIV-1 promoter: A potential target for anti-HIV drug development. *J. Am. Chem. Soc.* **2014**, *136*, 5249–5252. [CrossRef]

24. Hudson, J.S.; Ding, L.; Le, V.; Lewis, E.; Graves, D. Recognition and binding of human telomeric G-quadruplex DNA by unfolding protein 1. *Biochemistry* **2014**, *53*, 3347–3356. [CrossRef]

25. Johnson, J.E.; Cao, K.; Ryvkin, P.; Wang, L.S.; Johnson, F.B. Altered gene expression in the Werner and Bloom syndromes is associated with sequences having G-quadruplex forming potential. *Nucleic Acids Res.* **2010**, *38*, 1114–1122. [CrossRef] [PubMed]

26. Khateb, S.; Weisman-Shomer, P.; Hershco, I.; Loeb, L.A.; Fry, M. Destabilization of tetraplex structures of the fragile X repeat sequence (CGG)n is mediated by homolog-conserved domains in three members of the hnRNP family. *Nucleic Acids Res.* **2004**, *32*, 4145–4154. [CrossRef] [PubMed]

27. London, T.B.C.; Barber, L.J.; Mosedale, G.; Kelly, G.P.; Balasubramanian, S.; Hickson, I.D.; Boulton, S.J.; Hiom, K. FANCJ is a structure-specific DNA helicase associated with the maintenance of genomic G/C tracts. *J. Biol. Chem.* **2008**, *283*, 36132–36139. [CrossRef] [PubMed]

28. Qureshi, M.H.; Ray, S.; Sewell, A.L.; Basu, S.; Balci, H. Replication protein A unfolds G-quadruplex structures with varying degrees of efficiency. *J. Phys. Chem. B* **2012**, *116*, 5588–5594. [CrossRef] [PubMed]

29. Safa, L.; Delagoutte, E.; Petruseva, I.; Alberti, P.; Lavrik, O.; Riou, J.-F.; Saintomé, C. Binding polarity of RPA to telomeric sequences and influence of G-quadruplex stability. *Biochimie* **2014**, *103*, 80–88. [CrossRef]

30. Dempsey, L.A.; Sun, H.; Hanakahi, L.A.; Maizels, N. G4 DNA binding by LR1 and its subunits, nucleolin and hnRNP D, A role for G-G pairing in immunoglobulin switch recombination. *J. Biol. Chem.* **1999**, *274*, 1066–1071. [CrossRef]

31. Hanakahi, L.A.; Sun, H.; Maizels, N. High affinity interactions of nucleolin with G-G-paired rDNA. *J. Biol. Chem.* **1999**, *274*, 15908–15912. [CrossRef]

32. Quante, T.; Otto, B.; Brázdová, M.; Kejnovská, I.; Deppert, W.; Tolstonog, G.V. Mutant p53 is a transcriptional co-factor that binds to G-rich regulatory regions of active genes and generates transcriptional plasticity. *Cell Cycle* **2012**, *11*, 3290–3303. [CrossRef] [PubMed]

33. Kopylov, M.; Bass, H.W.; Stroupe, M.E. The maize (Zea mays L.) nucleoside diphosphate kinase1 (ZmNDPK1) gene encodes a human NM23-H2 homologue that binds and stabilizes G-quadruplex DNA. *Biochemistry* **2015**, *54*, 1743–1757. [CrossRef]

34. Webba da Silva, M. Geometric formalism for DNA quadruplex folding. *Chemistry* **2007**, *13*, 9738–9745. [CrossRef] [PubMed]

35. Mukundan, V.T.; Phan, A.T. Bulges in G-quadruplexes: Broadening the definition of G-quadruplex-forming sequences. *J. Am. Chem. Soc.* **2013**, *135*, 5017–5028. [CrossRef] [PubMed]

36. Li, J.; Correia, J.J.; Wang, L.; Trent, J.O.; Chaires, J.B. Not so crystal clear: The structure of the human telomere G-quadruplex in solution differs from that present in a crystal. *Nucleic Acids Res.* **2005**, *33*, 4649–4659. [CrossRef] [PubMed]

37. Dailey, M.M.; Miller, M.C.; Bates, P.J.; Lane, A.N.; Trent, J.O. Resolution and characterization of the structural polymorphism of a single quadruplex-forming sequence. *Nucleic Acids Res.* **2010**, *38*, 4877–4888. [CrossRef] [PubMed]

38. Seenisamy, J.; Rezler, E.M.; Powell, T.J.; Tye, D.; Gokhale, V.; Joshi, C.S.; Siddiqui-Jain, A.; Hurley, L.H. The dynamic character of the G-quadruplex element in the c-MYC promoter and modification by TMPyP4. *J. Am. Chem Soc.* **2004**, *126*, 8702–8709. [CrossRef]

39. Miannay, F.; Banyasz, A.; Gustavsson, T.; Markovitsi, S. Excited States and Energy Transfer in G-Quadruplexes. *J. Phys. Chem. C* **2009**, *113*, 11760–11765. [CrossRef]

40. Randazzo, A.; Spada, G.P.; da Silva, M.W. Circular dichroism of quadruplex structures. *Top. Currr. Chem.* **2013**, *330*, 67–86.

41. Sun, D.; Jurley, L.H. Biochemical techniques for the characterization of G-quadruplex structures: EMSA, DMS footprinting, and DNA polymerase stop assay. *Methods Mol. Bio.* **2010**, *608*, 65–79.

42. Harkness, R.W.t.; Mittermaier, A.K. G-register exchange dynamics in guanine quadruplexes. *Nucleic Acids Res.* **2016**, *44*, 3481–3494. [CrossRef]

43. Mergny, J.-L.; Lacroix, L. Analysis of thermal melting curves. *Oligonucleotides* **2003**, *13*, 515–537. [CrossRef] [PubMed]

44. Mergny, J.L.; Phan, A.T.; Lacroix, L. Following G-quartet formation by UV-spectroscopy. *FEBS Lett.* **1998**, *435*, 74–78. [CrossRef]

45. Uzman, A. Molecular Cell Biology (4th edition) Harvey Lodish, Arnold Berk, S. Lawrence Zipursky, Paul Matsudaira, David Baltimore and James Darnell; Freeman & Co., New York, NY, 2000, 1084 pp., list price $102.25, ISBN 0-7167-3136-3. *Biochem. Mol. Biol. Educ.* **2001**, *29*, 126–128.

46. Balagurumoorthy, P.; Brahmachari, S.K.; Mohanty, D.; Bansal, M.; Sasisekharan, V. Hairpin and parallel quartet structures for telomeric sequences. *Nucleic Acids Res.* **1992**, *20*, 4061–4067. [CrossRef]

47. Cao, W.; Demeler, B. Modeling analytical ultracentrifugation experiments with an adaptive space-time finite element solution for multicomponent reacting systems. *Biophys. J.* **2008**, *95*, 54–65. [CrossRef]

48. Demeler, B. *UltraScan—A Comprehensive Data Analysis Software Package for Analytical Ultracentrifugation Experiments*; Scott, D.J., Harding, S.E., Rowe, A.J., Eds.; Royal Society of Chemistry: Cambridge, UK, 2005; pp. 210–230.

49. Huppert, J.L.; Balasubramanian, S. Prevalence of quadruplexes in the human genome. *Nucleic Acids Res.* **2005**, *33*, 2908–2916. [CrossRef]

50. Rhodes, D.; Lipps, H.J. G-quadruplexes and their regulatory roles in biology. *Nucleic Acids Res.* **2015**, *43*, 8627–8637. [CrossRef]

51. Balasubramanian, S.; Hurley, L.H.; Neidle, S. Targeting G-quadruplexes in gene promoters: A novel anticancer strategy? *Nat. Rev. Drug Discov.* **2011**, *10*, 261–275. [CrossRef]

52. Cogoi, S.; Xodo, L.E. G-quadruplex formation within the promoter of the KRAS proto-oncogene and its effect on transcription. *Nucleic Acids Res.* **2006**, *34*, 2536–2549. [CrossRef]

53. Catasti, P.; Chen, X.; Moyzis, R.K.; Bradbury, E.M.; Gupta, G. Structure-function correlations of the insulin-linked polymorphic region. *J. Mol. Biol.* **1996**, *264*, 534–545. [CrossRef] [PubMed]

54. Brázda, V.; Hároníková, L.; Liao, J.C.C.; Fojta, M. DNA and RNA quadruplex-binding proteins. *Int. J. Mol. Sci.* **2014**, *15*, 17493–17517. [CrossRef]

55. Gray, L.T.; Vallur, A.C.; Eddy, J.; Maizels, N. G quadruplexes are genomewide targets of transcriptional helicases XPB and XPD. *Nat. Chem. Biol.* **2014**, *10*, 313–318. [CrossRef]
56. Paeschke, K.; Simonsson, T.; Postberg, J.; Rhodes, D.; Lipps, H.J. Telomere end-binding proteins control the formation of G-quadruplex DNA structures in vivo. *Nat. Struct. Mol. Biol.* **2005**, *12*, 847–854. [CrossRef] [PubMed]
57. Mergny, J.-L.; Li, J.; Lacroix, L.; Amrane, S.; Chaires, J.B. Thermal difference spectra: A specific signature for nucleic acid structures. *Nucleic Acids Res.* **2005**, *33*, e138. [CrossRef]
58. Fleming, A.M.; Zhou, J.; Wallace, S.S.; Burrows, C.J. A Role for the Fifth G-Track in G-Quadruplex Forming Oncogene Promoter Sequences during Oxidative Stress: Do These "Spare Tires" Have an Evolved Function? *ACS Cent. Sci.* **2015**, *1*, 226–233. [CrossRef] [PubMed]
59. Dai, J.; Carver, M.; Punchihewa, C.; Jones, R.A.; Yang, D. Structure of the Hybrid-2 type intramolecular human telomeric G-quadruplex in K+ solution: Insights into structure polymorphism of the human telomeric sequence. *Nucleic Acids Res.* **2007**, *35*, 4927–4940. [CrossRef]
60. Guédin, A.; Gros, J.; Alberti, P.; Mergny, J.-L. How long is too long? Effects of loop size on G-quadruplex stability. *Nucleic Acids Res.* **2010**, *38*, 7858–7868. [CrossRef]
61. Tippana, R.; Xiao, W.; Myong, S. G-quadruplex conformation and dynamics are determined by loop length and sequence. *Nucleic Acids Res.* **2014**, *42*, 8106–8114. [CrossRef]
62. Hildebrandt, M.; Lacombe, M.L.; Mesnildrey, S.; Véron, M. A human NDP-kinase B specifically binds single-stranded poly-pyrimidine sequences. *Nucleic Acids Res.* **1995**, *23*, 3858–3864. [CrossRef]
63. Postel, E.H.; Berberich, S.J.; Flint, S.J.; Ferrone, C.A. Human c-myc transcription factor PuF identified as nm23-H2 nucleoside diphosphate kinase, a candidate suppressor of tumor metastasis. *Science* **1993**, *261*, 478–480. [CrossRef]
64. Boissan, M.; Lacombe, M.L. Learning about the functions of NME/NM23: Lessons from knockout mice to silencing strategies. *Naunyn-Schmiedeberg's Arch. Pharmacol.* **2011**, *384*, 421–431. [CrossRef]
65. Yafe, A.; Etzioni, S.; Weisman-Shomer, P.; Fry, M. Formation and properties of hairpin and tetraplex structures of guanine-rich regulatory sequences of muscle-specific genes. *Nucleic Acids Res.* **2005**, *33*, 2887–2900. [CrossRef]
66. Rehm, C.; Holder, I.T.; Groß, A.; Wojciechowski, F.; Urban, M.; Sinn, M.; Drescher, M.; Hartig, J.S. A bacterial DNA quadruplex with exceptional K + selectivity and unique structural polymorphism. *Chem. Sci.* **2014**, *5*, 2809–2818. [CrossRef]
67. Kuryavyi, V.; Cahoon, L.A.; Seifert, H.S.; Patel, D.J. RecA-binding pilE G4 sequence essential for pilin antigenic variation forms monomeric and 5' end-stacked dimeric parallel G-quadruplexes. *Structure* **2012**, *20*, 2090–2102. [CrossRef] [PubMed]
68. Waller, Z.A.; Pinchbeck, B.J.; Buguth, B.S.; Meadows, T.G.; Richardson, D.J.; Gates, A.J. Control of bacterial nitrate assimilation by stabilization of G-quadruplex DNA. *Chem. Commun. (Camb)* **2016**, *52*, 13511–13514. [CrossRef] [PubMed]
69. Piekna-Przybylska, D.; Sullivan, M.A.; Sharma, G.; Bambara, R.A. U3 region in the HIV-1 genome adopts a G-quadruplex structure in its RNA and DNA sequence. *Biochemistry* **2014**, *53*, 2581–2593. [CrossRef] [PubMed]
70. Shin, Y.J.; Kumarasamy, V.; Camacho, D.; Sun, D. Involvement of G-quadruplex structures in regulation of human RET gene expression by small molecules in human medullary thyroid carcinoma TT cells. *Oncogene* **2015**, *34*, 1292–1299. [CrossRef]
71. Kumarasamy, V.M.; Shin, Y.-J.; White, J.; Sun, D. Selective repression of RET proto-oncogene in medullary thyroid carcinoma by a natural alkaloid berberine. *BMC Cancer* **2015**, *15*, 599. [CrossRef]
72. Guo, K.; Pourpak, A.; Beetz-Rogers, K.; Gokhale, V.; Sun, D.; Hurley, L.H. Formation of pseudosymmetrical G-quadruplex and i-motif structures in the proximal promoter region of the RET oncogene. *J. Am. Chem. Soc.* **2007**, *129*, 10220–10228. [CrossRef] [PubMed]
73. Sun, D.; Liu, W.-J.; Guo, K.; Rusche, J.J.; Ebbinghaus, S.; Gokhale, V.; Hurley, L.H. The proximal promoter region of the human vascular endothelial growth factor gene has a G-quadruplex structure that can be targeted by G-quadruplex-interactive agents. *Mol. Cancer Ther.* **2008**, *7*, 880–889. [CrossRef]
74. Dexheimer, T.S.; Sun, D.; Hurley, L.H. Deconvoluting the structural and drug-recognition complexity of the G-quadruplex-forming region upstream of the bcl-2 P1 promoter. *J. Am. Chem. Soc.* **2006**, *128*, 5404–5415. [CrossRef] [PubMed]
75. Suloway, C.; Pulokas, J.; Fellmann, D.; Cheng, A.; Guerra, F.; Quispe, J.; Stagg, S.; Potter, C.S.; Carragher, B. Automated molecular microscopy: The new Leginon system. *J. Struct. Biol.* **2005**, *151*, 41–60. [CrossRef]

76. Punjani, A.; Rubinstein, J.L.; Fleet, D.J.; Brubaker, M.A. cryoSPARC: Algorithms for rapid unsupervised cryo-EM structure determination. *Nat. Methods* **2017**, *14*, 290–296. [CrossRef]

Sample Availability: Samples of ZmNDPK expression plasmid is available upon request from the authors.

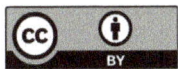

molecules

MDPI

Review

Parasitic Protozoa: Unusual Roles for G-Quadruplexes in Early-Diverging Eukaryotes

Franck Dumetz and Catherine J. Merrick *

Department of Pathology, University of Cambridge, Cambridge CB2 1QP, UK; fd353@cam.ac.uk
* Correspondence: cjm48@cam.ac.uk

Academic Editor: Sara N. Richter
Received: 19 March 2019; Accepted: 3 April 2019; Published: 5 April 2019

Abstract: Guanine-quadruplex (G4) motifs, at both the DNA and RNA levels, have assumed an important place in our understanding of the biology of eukaryotes, bacteria and viruses. However, it is generally little known that their very first description, as well as the foundational work on G4s, was performed on protozoans: unicellular life forms that are often parasitic. In this review, we provide a historical perspective on the discovery of G4s, intertwined with their biological significance across the protozoan kingdom. This is a history in three parts: first, a period of discovery including the first characterisation of a G4 motif at the DNA level in ciliates (environmental protozoa); second, a period less dense in publications concerning protozoa, during which DNA G4s were discovered in both humans and viruses; and third, a period of renewed interest in protozoa, including more mechanistic work in ciliates but also in pathogenic protozoa. This last period has opened an exciting prospect of finding new anti-parasitic drugs to interfere with parasite biology, thus adding new compounds to the therapeutic arsenal.

Keywords: G-quadruplex; G4; protozoa

1. Introduction

Traditionally DNA is viewed by the public, and indeed by the vast majority of scientists, as a double helical structure composed of four nucleotides, pairing adenine-thymine (A-T) and cytosine-guanine (C-G) [1], as observed by Watson and Crick in 1953. However, numerous publications have now demonstrated that DNA can be arranged to form different secondary structures, including secondary motifs based on non-Watson and Crick pairing. Such pairing is notable in two motifs, the guanine-quadruplex (G4) and the i-motif composed of cytosine residues [2,3]. These structures can form when the DNA is single stranded, thus primarily during replication, and potentially also during transcription [4].

The G4 motif is a family of structurally-diverse four-stranded secondary structures composed of stacks of planar guanine tetrads connected by intervening loop sequences following the general sequence $G_{(>2)}N_xG_{(>2)}N_xG_{(>2)}N_xG_{(>2)}$ [5] (Figure 1). This motif is stabilised in the presence of K^+, or to a lesser extent Na^+, and destabilised in the presence of Li^+ [6]. In the human genome, G4s are enriched in key regulatory sites, including oncogene promoters and telomeres, as well as appearing more generally in gene sequences and 5'UTRs [7]. Studies carried out on the functionality of G4 motifs have implicated them in oncogenesis, telomere structure and gene expression regulation [8]. A previous review from our group summarised the implications of G4s for the biology of many micro-organisms, mainly viruses and bacteria as well as a few protozoans of clinical interest. It highlighted a strong role for these motifs in immune evasion and virulence [9]. In this present review we focus first on the historical perspective brought by the fact that G4s were originally characterised in environmental protozoans. Then, after the first demonstration that G4s were also present in human cells, the field shifted towards research on human cells and viruses. It was only in the mid-2000s that G4 research again took an interest in protozoans and began to examine their biological significance, mostly with the idea to generate new anti-parasitic drugs (Figure 2).

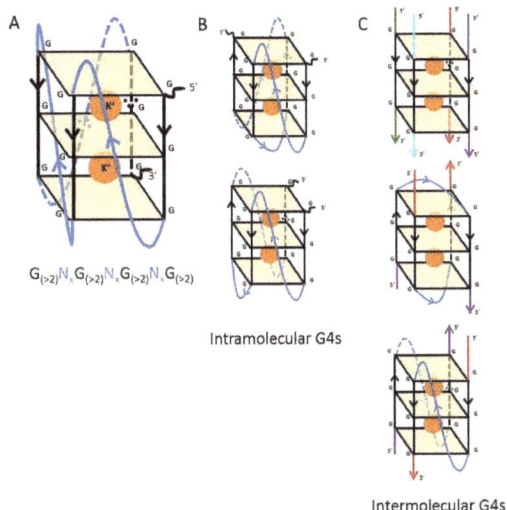

$$G_{(>2)}N_xG_{(>2)}N_xG_{(>2)}N_xG_{(>2)}$$

Intramolecular G4s

Intermolecular G4s

Figure 1. Schematic representations of G-quadruplex structures. (**A**) Schematic representation of a parallel G-quadruplex: the three planar G-stacks are represented in yellow, the T-loops or polypurine tracks are represented in blue and stabilising potassium cations, in orange. (**B**) Intramolecular G4s in two antiparallel configurations. (**C**) Intermolecular G4s in both parallel and antiparallel configurations: structures involving four DNA molecules (red, purple, blue and green) or two DNA molecules (red and purple) are shown.

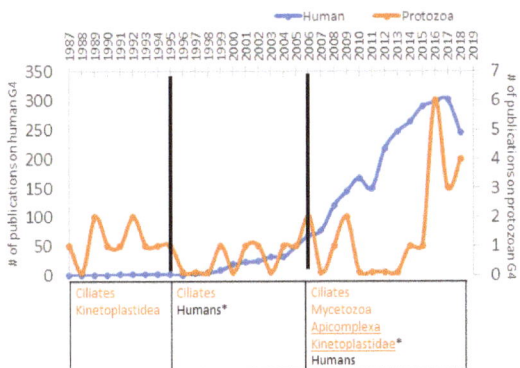

Figure 2. Compared evolution of the number of G4 publications related to protozoa and humans across time. Data were extracted from PubMed on 20/02/19 using the search terms "G-quadruplex human", "G4 humans" and "Guanine quadruplex humans", then compared to eliminate duplicates. The protozoan literature count is derived from the publications reviewed here, which represent the totality of the work available so far in the field. Orange line and taxa represent the protozoan data and the blue ones represent the human data. Underlined taxa include studies of human pathogens. * represents clades where rG4 work is available.

2. To Begin at the Beginning: A Free-Living Protozoan

Protozoans are ancient forms of eukaryotic life, now considered as early-diverging from more "classical" eukaryotes. However, the original observation of the different forms of G4s, as well as their further characterisation, was made on environmental protozoans of the Ciliophora phylum, like *Oxytricha* and *Tetrahymena*. This was due to two genomic particularities in these organisms: (1) the multiplicity of their genomic fragments (~16,000 different molecules of DNA for the former [10] and more than 200 for the latter [11]), and (2) the presence of a highly guanine-rich telomeric repeat, T_4G_4, on each fragment [12]. These two features rendered the investigation of GC-rich sequences much easier. In 1987, Oka et al. demonstrated the DNA/DNA interaction of the telomeric guanine clusters using macromolecular genomic DNA from *Oxytricha nova*. They hypothesised three different spatial conformations for this arrangement: antiparallel triplex, antiparallel quadruplex and parallel quadruplex [6]. It was in 1989 that Williamson et al. proposed clearly "the G-quartet model" based on their investigation of telomeric shape in *Oxytricha* and *Tetrahymena*. Using synthetic oligos of the telomere sequence in various salt conditions they demonstrated that in the presence of K^+, Na^+ and Cs^+, telomeres had an increase in electrophoretic mobility compared to telomeric sequences in presence of Li^+ or no salt [13]. Further characterisation of the G4 motif was pursued using dimethylsulfate (DMS), a chemical that methylates guanine residues on N7 or O6. Thus, the G-G bonding in position N7 was characterised and the first model of an anti-parallel G4 was proposed, using two telomeric sequences of *Tetrahymena* with four stacks of guanine [14].

At this time a fraction of the research turned to investigate the biological function of G4s in telomeric sequences. Investigating the kinetics of dissociation of K^+- and Na^+-stabilised G4s, Raghuraman et al. defined for the first time the period required to unfold these structures at 37 °C. The G4s had a lengthy half-life of 4 h for the Na^+-stabilised and 18 h for the K^+-stabilised version, suggesting that there might be an active, protein-mediated unfolding mechanism in vivo. They also compared the ability of *Oxytricha* telomere-binding-protein to bind to three different states of DNA: fully-folded G4, intermediate G4 and non-folded DNA. Protein-binding was not observed in the fully-folded structure, whereas the two latter structures were a good substrate for *Oxytricha*'s telomere-binding protein [15]. Finally, K^+ was also confirmed to be the most stabilising monovalent cation via biochemical rather than biophysical methods [16]. All this information implied the likelihood of G4 folding in cellulo, since potassium is the most abundant cation inside the cell. It also highlighted the high stability of the G4 structure and the need for an active unfolding mechanism allowing the access of DNA binding proteins.

After the discovery and primary characterisation of G4 formation, the next step, from 1992 to 1994, was to characterise the G4 at the atomic level. Several teams then either used crystallography or nucleic magnetic resonance spectroscopy of the telomeric G4 from *Oxytricha*. From a modern perspective, all this work could theoretically have been conducted on any G4-forming oligonucleotide, but since G4s were primarily recognised at this time in ciliate telomere sequences, these remained the model system of choice. First, using K^+ as the stabilising cation, the spatial organisation of the arrangement between the different guanine residues of the quadruplex was characterised, showing that both *syn-* and *anti-* bonding of the different guanine residues is possible [17]. This work was further supported and deepened by the additional structures of two different forms of G4, the intermolecular G4, and the intramolecular G4 (in which a single DNA strand encoding a canonical G4 sequence forms the secondary structure within itself) [13]. At the same time, four different topologies of the G4 were described, all depending on the charge, and thus the sequence, of the so-called T-loop [18,19] (Figure 1). Later work would show that the type of conformation is also defined by the length of the T-loop [20]. The work of Schultze et al. also paved the way to the structural description of parallel and antiparallel G4s. Firstly, two different conformations were described for the G4 formed from two single-stranded DNA molecules: (1) the two molecules are oriented in the same direction (5' to 3' // 5' to 3'), thus forming a parallel conformation, and (2) the two molecules are oriented in the opposite direction (5' to 3' // 3' to 5') making an anti-parallel conformation [18]. Concomitantly, Lu et al. in 1993 unravelled the difference in thermodynamics between parallel and anti-parallel G4s, measuring a higher stability of the parallel G4 in the presence of Na$^+$ [21].

Finally, this flourishing period for G4 discovery and characterisation was brought to a close with a publication on a so-far unexplored protozoan from the class of *Kinetoplastida*—the plant pathogen *Phytomonas serpens*, a Trypanosomatid. *P. serpens* has a nucleus and also a kinetoplast, which is a *Kinetoplastidea*-specific organelle functioning like a mitochondrion and containing the kDNA. The kDNA is a made up of two different families of circles, the maxi- and the mini-circles [22]. Based on oligonucleotide sequences of the minicircles exposed to DMS in G4-forming conditions, the authors described the potential for parts of the minicircles to form intramolecular G4s [23]. This was the first description of G4s in a protozoan outside of the *Ciliophora* family and it would be another 20 years before G4s were further investigated in *Kinetoplastid* parasites, including those that are important human pathogens.

3. Increased Interest in G4s in Humans Correlates with the Diminution of Attention to Protozoa

For more than ten years (1995 to 2006), only a few papers were published on G4s in protozoans. However, after the first period of description and characterisation, a series of articles began to appear related to the biological relevance of G4s, and some of these again took advantage of ciliate protozoa. First, some G4 structure-specific antibodies were produced: an important new research tool for the field. Using another *Ciliophora* telomeric sequence, that of *Stylonychia lemnae*, Schaffitzel et al. produced two different antibodies using ribosome display: Sty3 that binds to parallel and antiparallel G4s and Sty49 with higher specificity for antiparallel G4s. Two very interesting biological observations were made: (1) there is no trace of staining of the replication band, indicating that, in ciliates, G4s are resolved during replication, and (2) that G4 motifs were only present in the macronucleus of *Stylonychia* and not in the micronucleus, suggesting a difference of DNA organisation between the two nuclei [24]. This observation highlights a very unusual feature of these ciliates: *Stylonychia* has two nuclei assuring two different biological functions. The macronucleus is the centre of the metabolic activity and undergoes drastic remodelling during the reproductive life cycle, while the micronucleus codes for the germline genetic material [25]. It is notable, however, that although Sty49 was the first antibody to detect G4 motifs, it was not used subsequently to study G4s outside of ciliates. This fact has some potential explanations: the number of telomeres in ciliates creates a very high density of G4s, and the G4 sequence of the ciliate telomeres is more stable than the human one, having one more stack of guanine. It was only in 2013 that Biffi et al. produced an antibody, BG4, binding to human G4 motifs [2].

A few years later, using the Sty49 antibody, Paeschke et al. published the first functional study on the regulatory role of telomeric G4s in *S. lemnae*. They reported the essentiality of the two Telomere End Binding Proteins, TEBPa and TEBPb, for the formation of G4s in vitro and in vivo, and further demonstrated that TEBPb phosphorylation was necessary for G4 formation [26]. Meanwhile, working on the interaction between telomere-associated proteins and G4 motifs, Oganesian et al. focused their investigation on telomerase activity in two ciliates, *Tetrahymena* and *Euplotes*. In a primer extension assay using Na$^+$-stabilised intermolecular G4s and telomerase from both organisms, they described the intermolecular G4 as being an excellent substrate for the enzyme, suggesting that, at least in vitro, telomere extension is mediated by the presence of the G4 motifs [27].

Secondly during this period, more structural work was performed using NMR and crystallography on *Oxytricha* and *Tetrahymena* sequences, changing the stabilising cations in G4s in crystal form or in solution [28–31]. The first crystal of a G4 structure from a protozoan interacting with a G4-binding protein was reported: Horvath and Schultz described the interaction between *Oxytricha nova* TEBP and Na$^+$-stabilised G4 telomeric sequence [32]. Thus, as widespread interest in the G4s in human cells, and particularly in cancer cells, began its exponential growth, some important work did continue to use protozoa as tractable model systems for the study of G4s.

4. Biological Significance of G4s in Environmental and Pathogenic Protozoans

The third period of the history between G4s and protozoa saw the research expand to pathogenic protozoa as well. This period can be split into two different paths. First, the characterisation of the motif and its various biological functions was further pursued in ciliates and then extended to eukaryotic pathogens. Second, G4s began to be pursued as a potential target for anti-parasitic drugs.

4.1. G4 Structures and Functions in Protozoa

This period opened with the discovery of a previously-undescribed form of G4: the V4-motif introduced by Nielsen et al. To achieve this, they used the *Oxytrichia* T_4G_4 telomere repeat with the addition of locked nucleic acids, which are analogues of nucleic acids with a locked ribose in C3'-*endo*, forbidding a *syn* or *anti* conformation depending on the pre-existing chemical arrangement [33]. The authors speculated that V4 structures could form in certain conditions; however, it is yet to be demonstrated that this fold is actually physiological, either in *Oxytrichia* or elsewhere. In fact, the G4 research community remains preoccupied to this day with the question of whether all motifs observed in vitro can actually exist in vivo as well.

Secondly, the importance of sequence diversity within the G4 motif itself, which had thus far been largely neglected, was now studied, with ciliate telomeres again being the model sequences of choice. For this work, the highly homogenous T_4G_4 repeat was clearly an ideal model. First, Abu-Ghazalah et al. in 2009 looked at the composition of the G-track and the T-loop of *Oxytricha* G4s. Using oligonucleotide sequences of *Oxytricha* telomere repeats with the addition or deletion of a G in the G-track or a T in the T-loop, they showed that stability correlates with the number of guanine residues. They then demonstrated an effect of the T-loop length on the global conformation. Lastly, they ran stability experiments with all residues of the T-loop replaced by adenosine, showing different behaviours of G4s with T-loops versus A-loops [20]. Enforcing the first statement that stability increases when more guanines are present in the motif, Demkovičová et al. "humanised" the G4 sequence of *Tetrahymena* by changing the first guanine of the G-track to an adenine (T_2G_4 -> T_2AG_3). They showed that the substitution does not impair G4 formation but may change the topology of the G4 and also reduce its stability [34]. This work highlights an important transition away from studies of highly homogenous ciliate telomere sequences (which were originally chosen for their very homogeneity), towards studies of a greater diversity of G4-forming sequences.

Indeed, the second conclusion of the work done by Abu-Ghazalah et al. opened the perspective to study diverse, non-telomeric G4 motifs, which also occur in ciliate genomes. Ciliates like *Oxytricha* and *Tetrahymena* restructure their somatic genome during sexual differentiation and during this process up to a third of the genetic material is excised and lost. The lost fragments, also called internal eliminated sequences (IES), have the particularity to be outside of the telomeric regions and flanked by cis-acting sequences, one of the most studied being the polypurine tract (A_5G_5) [25,35,36]. While confirming that A_5G_5 is a G4 forming sequence, Carle et al. demonstrated that the protein Lia3 was binding to parallel G4s, as well as ensuring DNA cleavage. When the *LIA3* gene was knocked out, excision of the IES was prevented and the presence of the G4 was also essential for the binding of Lia3 [37]. Thus, G4s in ciliates evidently play specific biological roles beyond those in telomere maintenance. Over the past decade, as work on G4s has extended to pathogenic protozoa which also have unusual basic biology, it has become increasingly clear that this is a common theme: G4s can play interesting species-specific roles in the biology of many different protozoan parasites.

4.2. G4 Motifs in an AT-Rich Genome: The Example of Plasmodium Falciparum

Using bioinformatic tools, it was reported in 2007 that 40% of human gene promoters are carrying a Putative G-Quadruplex Sequence (PQS), and that PQSs appear on average approximately every kilobase in this genome [38]. This, therefore, is the PQS distribution that might be 'expected' in similarly G-C/A-T balanced genomes. However, not all eukaryotes have such genomes and nucleotide imbalance is a particularly striking feature of some protozoan parasites: certain malaria parasites, for example, have A-T content exceeding 80%, while *Leishmania* parasites are G-C-biased.

In 2009, Smargiasso et al. published the first bioinformatic PQS screen of the genome of the malaria parasite *Plasmodium falciparum*, which is extremely A-T-biased. They identified only 63 PQSs in non-telomeric sequences and, interestingly, these were concentrated in the upstream regions of a subset of the *var* virulence genes (the 'group B' *var* genes). This gene family encodes the major variant antigen of this parasite, *P. falciparum* Erythrocyte Membrane Protein 1 (PfEMP1), which is expressed at the surface of the infected erythrocytes. Each parasite genome has ~60 *var* variants; their expression is mutually exclusive and is regulated by epigenetic silencing and switching [39]. The authors demonstrated that G4s can indeed form within the *var* B upstream sequence, leading to a new hypothesis that *var* gene expression might be regulated via structure-specific helicases that can target G4s [40]. Two recent papers have now addressed this idea by knocking out one of the two RecQ helicase homologs found in *P. falciparum*, called *Pf*BLM [41,42]. Both papers reported changes in *var* gene expression, but curiously Claessens et al. found that *var* gene expression increased in their knockout, whereas Li et al. found that expression of the gene family was completely shut down. The reason for this difference remains, at present, unclear.

In order for *P. falciparum* parasites to continually evade the immune system, antigenic switching amongst a ~60-gene family is not enough: *var* genes must also recombine to create new variants [43]. In 2016, Stanton et al. implicated G4s in this process of recombination, in addition to the regulation of *var* gene expression. Stanton et al. found 80 PQSs in an updated version of the *P. falciparum* reference genome and reported a strong spatial association between PQSs and *var* gene recombination events. Furthermore, it was again suggested that G4-targetting DNA helicases could regulate this process in the parasite [44]. Indeed, the same group subsequently demonstrated the importance of a *P. falciparum* RecQ helicase in *var* gene recombination. This time, the *Pf*WRN helicase was knocked down, and recombination events in the *var* gene family dramatically increased (whereas knockout of the parasite's only other RecQ homolog, *Pf*BLM, had no such effect) [41]. Overall, the *P. falciparum* parasite has evidently evolved to retain G4-forming sequences in a highly A-T-rich genome for a very specific purpose: regulating both the expression and the evolution of a key virulence gene family.

Finally, in 2016, Bhartiya et al. performed another bioinformatic G4 screening on 6 different species of *Plasmodium*. They included 2-quartet as well as 3-quartet motifs and therefore described a higher number of PQSs (conventionally, three quartets are considered necessary for a stable DNA G4, but two may be sufficient for an RNA G4 (rG4)). Concentrating on these potential rG4s, they then re-analysed various RNA-seq datasets and ribosome footprinting studies and concluded that translation efficiency was reduced at certain lifecycle stages in PQS-harbouring genes [45]. A mechanistic basis for this observation has yet to emerge, but this was the first report to focus on rG4s in *P. falciparum*, and the first to suggest a G4-based expression-regulating system in a protozoan.

P. falciparum has the most A-T-rich genome yet sequenced, but other protozoa do exist with similarly biased genomes. One such organism is the environmental Mycetozoa *Distyostelium discoideum*. Bedrat et al. recently developed a bioinformatic program, G4Hunter, which uses a new and more sophisticated algorithm to detect the presence of G4 motifs based on genome sequences: they included two A-T-rich protozoa in their analysis, *D. discoideum* and *P. falciparum*. The number of predicted G4s from this new algorithm remained low, depending on the parameters: between 249 and 1055 for *D. discoideum* (and even lower for *P. falciparum*), but the authors hypothesised that the few PQSs retained in the *D. discoideum* genome could be informative to study [7]. Therefore, the same team solved the crystal structure of a non-telomeric G4-forming sequence (A_5G_5) located in a putative promoter of two divergent *D. discoideum* genes [46]. A biological function for this G4 has yet to be established, but this last publication at least physically confirmed the presence of G4 motifs outside of non-telomeric regions in this protozoan.

4.3. G4 Motifs in Transcription Control and RNA Editing in Trypanosomatids

After the demonstration of G4 formation in *P. serpens* kDNA [23], the field remained unexplored in the *Trypanosomatid* family. However, interest was raised again in *Trypanosomatidae* with the study of human pathogens such as *Trypanosoma brucei*, two subspecies of which cause human sleeping sickness; *Trypanosoma cruzi*, causing Chagas disease; and *Leishmania spp*, responsible for the complex of diseases called leishmaniasis [47]. It was only in 2015 that Genest et al. performed the first SMRT sequencing of *L. tarentolae*, revealing DNA sequence together with epigenetic base modifications. They demonstrated the presence of PQSs surrounding regions of β-D-glucosyl-hydroxymethyluracil, or 'base J', a *Trypanosomatid*-specific epigenetic modification of thymine. The *Trypanosomatidae* group of protozoa is characterised by unusual poly-cistronic transcription: base J is a marker of transcriptional strand-switching between poly-cistrons and it is also present in abundance in the telomeres (99%). They verified their discovery using a plasmid carrying the detected PQS, $(GGGTTA)_{10}$, and found that even plasmids carrying only this sequence without any coding sequence were modified to harbour base J. This result suggests that the presence of a G4 is a hallmark for base J positioning [48]. Again, it implies that G4s have evolved to play a highly specific role in this group of organisms relating to their unique biology – in this instance, their use of polycistronic transcription and base J.

Regarding the same family of parasites, and after the discovery of G4 formation at the RNA level in humans [49], Leeder et al., in a series of two articles, paved the road for rG4 studies in kinetoplastids. Kinetoplastids, as previously stated, carry a kinetoplast that contains the mitochondrial DNA. The RNA molecules transcribed from the kDNA are called kRNA and undergo a unique, complex and drastic editing process (uracil insertion/deletion). This mechanism is driven by a mitochondrial multienzyme complex, the editosome, guided by guide RNA encrypted on the minicircles. The editosome edits the pre-kRNA molecule where the gRNA binds [50]. In 2015, it was demonstrated, using selective 2′-hydroxyl acylation primer extension (SHAPE) on kRNA in different stages of maturation, that pre-kRNA molecules can form several rG4s (up to four rG4s in certain pre-kRNA). In the presence of the editosome, up to fifty percent of the rG4 structures unwound, favouring the formation of pre-kRNA:gRNA hybrid RNAs for maturation into fully functional kRNA [51]. In the second article, where they included the in silico structure of the kRNA of two other species, *T. cruzi* and *L. tarentolae*, they made the same conclusion as previously, and finally hypothesised that kDNA replication versus kDNA transcription is directly linked to the presence of intra-molecular G4 structures in the pre-kRNA. When the rG4 is formed on the neo-synthetised pre-kRNA, it cannot recognise PQSs on the maxicircle, leading to active transcription and inactive maxicircle replication. On the contrary, when the rG4 in the pre-kRNA molecule is unwound, it allows the formation of a kDNA/kRNA hybrid, preventing transcription and activating kDNA replication [52]. Yet again, G4s are evidently being used in sophisticated ways to modulate a highly specific aspect of *Trypanosomatidae* biology.

Overall, G4 motifs have been shown to play several different roles in the biology of protozoa. They either organise the genome, as in ciliates with germline formation or in *P. falciparum* with *var* gene recombination, or they regulate gene expression, as in Trypanosomatids with the placement of base J. Furthermore, the first demonstration of G4 presence at the RNA level—now reported in *T. brucei*—gives a role to the rG4 in regulating transcript editing. Regarding the pathogenic species, most of these mechanisms are essential for parasite survival and this makes G4s potential targets for anti-parasitic drugs.

4.4. Targeting the G4 Motifs In Pathogenic Protozoan: A New Strategy in the Design of Anti-Parasitic Drugs

The second path of G4-related research that remains very active today is represented by the discovery of new anti-protozoan drugs to fight pathogenic species. In the era of drug-resistant pathogens, new pharmaceutical compounds are necessary to complete the pharmacopeia. In this regard, non-pathogenic protozoa can be useful as well – before directly working on pathogenic organisms, which require a specialised biosafety level of confinement, ciliates have sometimes been used as models to test anti-G4 drugs [53]. In pathogenic protozoa, meanwhile, there are exciting prospects for the development of G4-targetting drugs, some of which are described below, or alternatively, G4-based aptamers [54], which are as yet little-explored for protozoan parasites but are fast becoming an established research avenue for anti-virals [55].

The very first report of compounds binding to G4s in *P. falciparum* telomeres was made in 2008 by De Cian et al., at the same time as the description of the structure and characteristics of *P. falciparum* G4s. They showed that known G4-binding compounds, developed primarily for human G4s, also bound to *P. falciparum* G4s more effectively than to duplex DNA. However, none of the 12 compounds tested showed a particular discrimination between *Plasmodium* and human G4 structures in vitro [56]. Nevertheless, as for many good drugs, pathogen-over-host specificity isn't always required, particularly if the pathogen replicates faster than the host cell. Therefore, Calvo et al. tested the telomerase activity and parasite growth of *P. falciparum* when exposed to two drugs previously tested by De Cian et al., TMPyP4 and telomestatin. While the first showed the highest reduction in telomerase activity, the second showed the highest parasite growth inhibition. It is important to note that G4-targetting was not proven and telomestatin activity could interfere with other pathways inside the parasite [57]. However, three other G4-binding compounds were subsequently tested by another research group, and showed significant *P. falciparum* telomere erosion, suggesting a common mode of interference with telomerase activity [58].

While the first compound screens focused entirely on molecules capable of inhibiting telomerase activity, others focused on molecules capable of interfering with the G4s scattered across the genome and regulating different biological functions, as described earlier in this review. Belmonte-Reche et al. recently published a screen of seven carboxy-NDI derivatives against *T. b. brucei*, *L. major* and *P. falciparum*. Amongst the seven, two derivatives showed a particular action against *T. b. brucei* and a limited toxicity in human cells, making them potential drug candidates against the *T. brucei* subspecies responsible for sleeping sickness [59]. Focusing on *P. falciparum*, Harris et al. demonstrated G4-related anti-parasitic activity of a candidate anticancer drug, a fluoroquinolone called quarfloxin. Quarfloxin showed rapid killing activity against the erythrocytic forms of the malaria parasite in culture and could represent a good drug for repurposing against malaria. Unlike telomestatin, quarfloxin did not apparently cause telomere erosion: it may instead exert its toxicity via genes encoding non-telomeric G4s [60].

5. Conclusions

As can be observed throughout this review, the history of G4 discovery is intertwined with protozoan biology, from the understanding of genome organisation to drug development. Looking at the large diversity of biological systems that represent the protozoan phylum, it is safe to assume that we still have a lot to learn from these small but far-from-simple organisms. Furthermore, the presence of G4s within the telomeres, regulatory elements and coding regions of many pathogenic protozoa makes them a structure of choice to develop new compounds or repurpose or modify existing ones, thus opening new perspectives for the treatment of major parasitic diseases.

Author Contributions: Conceptualization, F.D. and C.J.M.; Writing—Original Draft Preparation, F.D.; Writing—Review & Editing, C.J.M.; Funding Acquisition, C.J.M.

Funding: This work was supported by the UK Medical Research Council [grant MR/P010873 to C.J.M.].

Acknowledgments: The authors would like to thank Jennifer McDonald and Francis Totanes for their critical reading of the manuscript.

Conflicts of Interest: The authors declare no conflict of interest associated with this manuscript.

References

1.   Watson, J.D.; Crick, F.H.C. Molecular structure of nucleic acids: A structure for deoxyribose nucleic acid. *Nature* **1953**, *171*, 737–738. [CrossRef] [PubMed]

2. Biffi, G.; Tannahill, D.; McCafferty, J.; Balasubramanian, S. Quantitative visualization of DNA G-quadruplex structures in human cells. *Nat. Chem.* **2013**, *5*, 182–186. [CrossRef] [PubMed]
3. Zeraati, M.; Langley, D.B.; Schofield, P.; Moye, A.L.; Rouet, R.; Hughes, W.E.; Bryan, T.M.; Dinger, M.E.; Christ, D. I-motif DNA structures are formed in the nuclei of human cells. *Nat. Chem.* **2018**, *10*, 631–637. [CrossRef] [PubMed]
4. Lopes, J.; Piazza, A.; Le Bermejo, R.; Kriegsman, B.; Colosio, A.; Teulade-Fichou, M.P.; Foiani, M.; Nicolas, A. G-quadruplex-induced instability during leading-strand replication. *EMBO J.* **2011**, *30*, 4033–4046. [CrossRef] [PubMed]
5. Smargiasso, N.; Rosu, F.; Hsia, W.; Colson, P.; Baker, E.S.; Bowers, M.T.; De Pauw, E.; Gabelica, V. G-quadruplex DNA assemblies: Loop length, cation identity, and multimer formation. *J. Am. Chem. Soc.* **2008**, *130*, 10208–10216. [CrossRef] [PubMed]
6. Oka, Y.; Thomas, C.A. The cohering telomeres of Oxytricha. *Nucleic Acids Res.* **1987**, *15*, 8877–8898. [CrossRef] [PubMed]
7. Bedrat, A.; Lacroix, L.; Mergny, J.-L. Re-evaluation of G-quadruplex propensity with G4Hunter. *Nucleic Acids Res.* **2016**, *44*, 1746–1759. [CrossRef]
8. Murat, P.; Balasubramanian, S. Existence and consequences of G-quadruplex structures in DNA. *Curr. Opin. Genet. Dev.* **2014**, *25*, 22–29. [CrossRef] [PubMed]
9. Harris, L.M.; Merrick, C.J. G-quadruplexes in pathogens: A common route to virulence control? *PLoS Pathog.* **2015**, *11*, 1–15. [CrossRef]
10. Swart, E.C.; Bracht, J.R.; Magrini, V.; Minx, P.; Chen, X.; Zhou, Y.; Khurana, J.S.; Goldman, A.D.; Nowacki, M.; Schotanus, K.; et al. The *Oxytricha trifallax* macronuclear genome: A complex eukaryotic genome with 16,000 tiny chromosomes. *PLoS Biol.* **2013**, *11*, e1001473. [CrossRef]
11. Eisen, J.A.; Coyne, R.S.; Wu, M.; Wu, D.; Thiagarajan, M.; Wortman, J.R.; Badger, J.H.; Ren, Q.; Amedeo, P.; Jones, K.M.; et al. Macronuclear genome sequence of the ciliate *Tetrahymena thermophila*, a model eukaryote. *PLoS Biol.* **2006**, *4*, 1620–1642. [CrossRef]
12. Price, C.M.; Cech, T.R. Telomeric DNA-protein interactions of Oxytricha macronuclear DNA. *Genes Dev.* **1987**, *1*, 783–793. [CrossRef]
13. Williamson, J.R.; Raghuraman, M.K.; Cech, T.R. Monovalent cation-induced structure of telomeric DNA: The G-quartet model. *Cell* **1989**, *59*, 871–880. [CrossRef]
14. Sundquist, W.I.; Klug, A. Telomeric DNA dimerizes by formation of guanine tetrads between hairpin loops. *Nature* **1989**, *342*, 825–829. [CrossRef]
15. Raghuraman, M.K.; Cech, T.R. Effect of monovalent cation-induced telomeric DNA structure on the binding of Oxytricha telomeric protein. *Nucleic Acids Res.* **1990**, *18*, 4543–4552. [CrossRef]
16. Hardin, C.C.; Henderson, E.; Watson, T.; Prosser, J.K. Monovalent cation induced structural transitions in telomeric DNAs: G-DNA folding intermediates. *Biochemistry* **1991**, *30*, 4460–4472. [CrossRef]
17. Kang, C.; Zhang, X.; Ratliff, R.; Moyzis, R.; Rich, A. Crystal structure of four-stranded Oxytricha telomeric DNA. *Nature* **1992**, *356*, 126–131. [CrossRef]
18. Schultze, P.; Smith, F.W.; Feigon, J. Refined solution structure of the dimeric quadruplex formed from the Oxytricha telomeric oligonucleotide d(GGGGTTTTGGGG). *Structure* **1994**, *2*, 221–233. [CrossRef]
19. Smith, F.W.; Feigon, J. Quadruplex structure of Oxytricha telomeric DNA oligonucleotides. *Nature* **1992**, *356*, 164–168. [CrossRef]
20. Abu-Ghazalah, R.M.; Macgregor, R.B. Structural polymorphism of the four-repeat *Oxytricha nova* telomeric DNA sequences. *Biophys. Chem.* **2009**, *141*, 180–185. [CrossRef]
21. Lu, M.; Guo, Q.; Kallenbach, N.R. Thermodynamics of G-tetraplex formation by telomeric DNAs. *Biochemistry* **1993**, *32*, 598–601. [CrossRef]
22. Lukes, J.; Hashimi, H.; Zíková, A. Unexplained complexity of the mitochondrial genome and transcriptome in Kinetoplastid flagellates. *Curr. Genet.* **2005**, *48*, 277–299. [CrossRef]
23. Sá-Carvalho, D.; Traub-Cseko, Y.M. Sequences with high propensity to form G-quartet structures in Kinetoplast DNA from *Phytomonas Serpens*. *Mol. Biochem. Parasitol.* **1995**, *72*, 103–109. [CrossRef]
24. Schaffitzel, C.; Berger, I.; Postberg, J.; Hanes, J.; Lipps, H.J.; Pluckthun, A. In vitro generated antibodies specific for telomeric guanine-quadruplex DNA react with *Stylonychia Lemnae* macronuclei. *Proc. Natl. Acad. Sci. USA* **2001**, *98*, 8572–8577. [CrossRef]

25. Prescott, D.M. Restructuring of DNA sequences in the germline genome of Oxytricha. *Curr. Opin. Genet. Dev.* **1993**, *3*, 726–729. [CrossRef]
26. Paeschke, K.; Simonsson, T.; Postberg, J.; Rhodes, D.; Lipps, H.J. Telomere End-Binding Proteins control the formation of G-quadruplex DNA structures *in vivo*. *Nat. Struct. Mol. Biol.* **2005**, *12*, 847–854. [CrossRef]
27. Oganesian, L.; Moon, I.K.; Bryan, T.M.; Jarstfer, M.B. Extension of G-quadruplex DNA by ciliate telomerase. *EMBO J.* **2006**, *25*, 1148–1159. [CrossRef]
28. Schultze, P.; Hud, N.V.; Smith, F.W.; Feigon, J. The effect of sodium, potassium and ammonium ions on the conformation of the dimeric quadruplex formed by the *Oxytricha nova* telomere repeat oligonucleotide d(G(4)T(4)G(4)). *Nucleic Acids Res.* **1999**, *27*, 3018–3028. [CrossRef]
29. Haider, S.; Parkinson, G.N.; Neidle, S. Crystal structure of the potassium form of an *Oxytricha nova* G-quadruplex. *J. Mol. Biol.* **2002**, *320*, 189–200. [CrossRef]
30. Phan, A.T.; Modi, Y.S.; Patel, D.J. Two-repeat Tetrahymena telomeric d(TGGGGTTGGGGT) sequence interconverts between asymmetric dimeric G-quadruplexes in solution. *J. Mol. Biol.* **2004**, *338*, 93–102. [CrossRef]
31. Gill, M.L.; Strobel, S.A.; Loria, J.P. Crystallization and characterization of the thallium form of the *Oxytricha nova* G-quadruplex. *Nucleic Acids Res.* **2006**, *34*, 4506–4514. [CrossRef] [PubMed]
32. Horvath, M.P.; Schultz, S.C. DNA G-quartets in a 1.86 Å resolution structure of an *Oxytricha nova* telomeric protein-DNA complex. *J. Mol. Biol.* **2001**, *310*, 367–377. [CrossRef] [PubMed]
33. Nielsen, J.T.; Arar, K.; Petersen, M. Solution structure of a locked nucleic acid modified quadruplex: Introducing the V4 folding topology. *Angew. Chemie Int. Ed.* **2009**, *48*, 3099–3103. [CrossRef] [PubMed]
34. Demkovičová, E.; Bauer, Ľ.; Krafčíková, P.; Tlučková, K.; Tóthova, P.; Halaganová, A.; Valušová, E.; Víglaský, V. Telomeric G-quadruplexes: From human to Tetrahymena repeats. *J. Nucleic Acids* **2017**, *2017*. [CrossRef] [PubMed]
35. Godiska, R.; Yao, M.C. A Programmed Site-specific DNA rearrangement in *Tetrahymena thermophila* requires flanking polypurine tracts. *Cell* **1990**, *61*, 1237–1246. [CrossRef]
36. Fass, J.N.; Joshi, N.A.; Couvillion, M.T.; Bowen, J.; Gorovsky, M.A.; Hamilton, E.P.; Orias, E.; Hong, K.; Coyne, R.S.; Eisen, J.A.; et al. Genome-scale analysis of programmed DNA elimination sites in *Tetrahymena thermophila*. *G3 (Bethesda)*. **2011**, *1*, 515–522. [CrossRef]
37. Carle, C.M.; Zaher, H.S.; Chalker, D.L. A Parallel G-quadruplex-binding protein regulates the boundaries of DNA elimination events of *Tetrahymena thermophila*. *PLoS Genet.* **2016**, *12*, 1–22. [CrossRef]
38. Huppert, J.L.; Balasubramanian, S. G-quadruplexes in promoters throughout the human genome. *Nucleic Acids Res.* **2007**, *35*, 406–413. [CrossRef]
39. Scherf, A.; Hernandez-Rivas, R.; Buffet, P.; Bottius, E.; Benatar, C.; Pouvelle, B.; Gysin, J.; Lanzer, M. Antigenic variation in malaria: In situ switching, relaxed and mutually exclusive transcription of *var* genes during intra-erythrocytic development in *Plasmodium falciparum*. *EMBO J.* **1998**, *17*, 5418–5426. [CrossRef]
40. Smargiasso, N.; Gabelica, V.; Damblon, C.; Rosu, F.; De Pauw, E.; Teulade-Fichou, M.P.; Rowe, J.A.; Claessens, A. Putative DNA G-quadruplex formation within the promoters of *Plasmodium falciparum var* genes. *BMC Genom.* **2009**, *10*, 1–12. [CrossRef]
41. Claessens, A.; Harris, L.M.; Stanojcic, S.; Chappell, L.; Stanton, A.; Kuk, N.; Veneziano-Broccia, P.; Sterkers, Y.; Rayner, J.C.; Merrick, C.J. RecQ helicases in the malaria parasite *Plasmodium falciparum* affect genome stability, gene expression patterns and DNA replication dynamics. *PLoS Genet.* **2018**, *14*, e1007490. [CrossRef]
42. Li, Z.; Yin, S.; Sun, M.; Cheng, X.; Wei, J.; Gilbert, N.; Miao, J.; Cui, L.; Huang, Z.; Dai, X.; et al. DNA helicase RecQ1 regulates mutually exclusive expression of virulence genes in *Plasmodium falciparum* via heterochromatin alteration. *Proc. Natl. Acad. Sci. USA* **2019**, *116*, 3177–3182. [CrossRef]
43. Claessens, A.; Hamilton, W.L.; Kekre, M.; Otto, T.D.; Faizullabhoy, A.; Rayner, J.C.; Kwiatkowski, D. Generation of antigenic diversity in *Plasmodium falciparum* by structured rearrangement of *var* genes during mitosis. *PLoS Genet.* **2014**, *10*, e1004812. [CrossRef] [PubMed]
44. Stanton, A.; Harris, L.M.; Graham, G.; Merrick, C.J. Recombination events among virulence genes in malaria parasites are associated with G-quadruplex-forming DNA motifs. *BMC Genom.* **2016**, *17*, 1–16. [CrossRef]
45. Bhartiya, D.; Chawla, V.; Ghosh, S.; Shankar, R.; Kumar, N. Genome-wide regulatory dynamics of G-quadruplexes in human malaria parasite *Plasmodium falciparum*. *Genomics* **2016**, *108*, 224–231. [CrossRef]

46. Guédin, A.; Lin, L.Y.; Armane, S.; Lacroix, L.; Mergny, J.-L.; Thore, S.; Yatsunyk, L.A. Quadruplexes in 'Dicty': Crystal structure of a four-quartet G-quadruplex formed by G-rich motif found in the *Dictyostelium discoideum* genome. *Nucleic Acids Res.* **2018**, *46*, 5297–5307. [CrossRef]

47. Kaufer, A.; Ellis, J.; Stark, D.; Barratt, J. The evolution of Trypanosomatid taxonomy. *Parasites and Vectors* **2017**, *10*, 1–17. [CrossRef]

48. Genest, P.-A.; Baugh, L.; Taipale, A.; Zhao, W.; Jan, S.; van Luenen, H.G.A.M.; Korlach, J.; Clark, T.; Luong, K.; Boitano, M.; et al. Defining the sequence requirements for the positioning of base J in DNA using SMRT sequencing. *Nucleic Acids Res.* **2015**, *43*, 2102–2115. [CrossRef]

49. Biffi, G.; Di Antonio, M.; Tannahill, D.; Balasubramanian, S. Visualization and selective chemical targeting of RNA G-quadruplex structures in the cytoplasm of human cells. *Nat. Chem.* **2014**, *6*, 75–80. [CrossRef]

50. Aphasizhev, R.; Aphasizheva, I. Mitochondrial RNA editing in Trypanosomes: Small RNAs in control. *Biochimie* **2014**, *100*, 125–131. [CrossRef]

51. Leeder, W.M.; Voigt, C.; Brecht, M.; Göringer, H.U. The RNA chaperone activity of the *Trypanosoma brucei* editosome raises the dynamic of bound pre-mRNAs. *Sci. Rep.* **2016**, *6*, 1–11. [CrossRef]

52. Leeder, W.-M.; Hummel, N.F.C.; Göringer, H.U. Multiple G-quartet structures in pre-edited mRNAs suggest evolutionary driving force for RNA editing in Trypanosomes. *Sci. Rep.* **2016**, *6*, 29810. [CrossRef]

53. Barthwal, R.; Tariq, Z. Molecular recognition of parallel G-quadruplex [d-(TTGGGGT)]4 containing Tetrahymena telomeric DNA sequence by anticancer drug daunomycin: NMR-based structure and thermal stability. *Molecules* **2018**, *23*, 2266. [CrossRef]

54. Platella, C.; Riccardi, C.; Montesarchio, D.; Roviello, G.N.; Musumeci, D. G-quadruplex-based aptamers against protein targets in therapy and diagnostics. *Biochim. Biophys. Acta Gen. Subj.* **2017**, *1861*, 1429–1447. [CrossRef]

55. Musumeci, D.; Riccardi, C.; Montesarchio, D. G-Quadruplex forming oligonucleotides as anti-HIV agents. *Molecules* **2015**, *20*, 17511–17532. [CrossRef]

56. De Cian, A.; Grellier, P.; Mouray, E.; Depoix, D.; Bertrand, H.; Monchaud, D.; Teulade-Fichou, M.P.; Mergny, J.L.; Alberti, P. Plasmodium telomeric sequences: Structure, stability and quadruplex targeting by small compounds. *Chembiochem* **2008**, *9*, 2730–2739. [CrossRef]

57. Calvo, E.P.; Wasserman, M. G-quadruplex ligands: Potent inhibitors of telomerase activity and cell proliferation in *Plasmodium falciparum*. *Mol. Biochem. Parasitol.* **2016**, *207*, 33–38. [CrossRef]

58. Anas, M.; Sharma, R.; Dhamodharan, V.; Pradeepkumar, P.I.; Manhas, A.; Srivastava, K.; Ahmed, S.; Kumar, N. Investigating pharmacological targeting of G-quadruplexes in the human malaria parasite. *Biochemistry* **2017**, *56*, 6691–6699. [CrossRef] [PubMed]

59. Belmonte-Reche, E.; Martínez-García, M.; Guédin, A.; Zuffo, M.; Arévalo-Ruiz, M.; Doria, F.; Campos-Salinas, J.; Maynadier, M.; López-Rubio, J.J.; Freccero, M.; et al. G-quadruplex identification in the genome of protozoan parasites points to naphthalene diimide ligands as new antiparasitic agents. *J. Med. Chem.* **2018**, *61*, 1231–1240. [CrossRef]

60. Harris, L.M.; Monsell, K.R.; Noulin, F.; Famodimu, M.T.; Smargiasso, N.; Damblon, C.; Horrocks, P.; Merrick, C.J. G-Quadruplex DNA motifs in the malaria parasite *Plasmodium falciparum* and their potential as novel antimalarial drug targets. *Antimicrob. Agents Chemother.* **2018**, *62*, 1–14. [CrossRef]

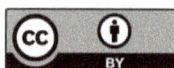

molecules

MDPI

Review

G-Quadruplex-Based Fluorescent Turn-On Ligands and Aptamers: From Development to Applications

Mubarak I. Umar [†], Danyang Ji [†], Chun-Yin Chan [†] and Chun Kit Kwok *

Department of Chemistry, City University of Hong Kong, Kowloon Tong, Hong Kong SAR, China
* Correspondence: ckkwok42@cityu.edu.hk; Tel.: +852-3442-6858
† These authors contributed equally to this work.

Academic Editor: Sara N. Richter
Received: 27 April 2019; Accepted: 24 June 2019; Published: 30 June 2019

Abstract: Guanine (G)-quadruplexes (G4s) are unique nucleic acid structures that are formed by stacked G-tetrads in G-rich DNA or RNA sequences. G4s have been reported to play significant roles in various cellular events in both macro- and micro-organisms. The identification and characterization of G4s can help to understand their different biological roles and potential applications in diagnosis and therapy. In addition to biophysical and biochemical methods to interrogate G4 formation, G4 fluorescent turn-on ligands can be used to target and visualize G4 formation both in vitro and in cells. Here, we review several representative classes of G4 fluorescent turn-on ligands in terms of their interaction mechanism and application perspectives. Interestingly, G4 structures are commonly identified in DNA and RNA aptamers against targets that include proteins and small molecules, which can be utilized as G4 tools for diverse applications. We therefore also summarize the recent development of G4-containing aptamers and highlight their applications in biosensing, bioimaging, and therapy. Moreover, we discuss the current challenges and future perspectives of G4 fluorescent turn-on ligands and G4-containing aptamers.

Keywords: nucleic acids; G-quadruplex; aptamers; turn-on ligands; fluorescence; microbes

1. Introduction

Guanine (G)-rich sequences in nucleic acids have the potential to fold into structural motifs referred to as G-quadruplexes (G4s). G4s can be intra- or inter-molecularly folded, and they are formed by the stacking of G-quartets to form planar 2D structures between four guanosines by hydrogen bond interactions at their Watson–Crick and Hoogsteen edges (Figure 1A). Furthermore, a monovalent cation occupies the central cavity of the G-quartet to stabilize the structure, with a strength of stabilization in the order of $K^+ > Na^+ > NH_4^+ > Li^+$ [1,2]. The formation of intra-molecular canonical G4s requires at least four regions of three consecutive Gs in a single strand, which are separated by 1–7 linking nucleotides known as loops [3]. Inter-molecular G4s are formed by G-interactions among multiple strands, from bimolecular (two strands) to tetramolecular (four strands). Generally, the stability of the G4 structure decreases as loop length increases [4,5]; therefore, it was generally thought that sequences that obey the consensus of $(G_{3+}N_{1-7}G_{3+}N_{1-7}G_{3+}N_{1-7}G_{3+})$ can form G4s in the genome and transcriptome [3]. More recently, non-canonical G4s were discovered [6], such as G4s with long loops [5], bulges [7,8], 2-quartets [9], G-vacancies [10,11], duplexes [12], and triplexes [13], which broaden the sequence definition and the structural diversity of G4s. G4s are polymorphic, meaning that the G-tracts can be arranged into parallel, anti-parallel, or hybrid topologies [14,15] (Figure 1B). Guanosines can also be oriented as anti- or syn- conformations based on whether the purine rings are flipped outward or inwards with respect to the pentose sugar [14,15] (Figure 1C). Such conformational variety leads to wide, medium, and narrow grooves that describe the spatial availability of the corresponding edge of the G-quartet [14,15] (Figure 1A).

G4s play significant roles in almost every cellular event, including but not limited to DNA replication, transcription, translation, RNA metabolism, and epigenetic remodeling [16,17]. Recent studies have also suggested that G4 structures can serve as promising cancer and anti-microbe targets [18,19]. To identify such potential G4 targets, various computational methods such as QGRS Mapper [20], quadparser [3], G4 Hunter [21], G4NN [22], and Quadron [23] have been developed to predict G4 formations. Spectroscopic techniques such as circular dichroism (CD) [24], UV melting [25], mass spectrometry [26], nuclear magnetic resonance (NMR) [27], and intrinsic fluorescence [28] can also detect G4 formation based on its physical properties in a label-free manner. In addition to these biophysical methods, biochemical methods such as polymerase stop assay [29] and dimethyl sulfate (DMS) footprinting [30] can interrogate DNA G4 formation by template extension stalling and measuring the guanine nucleotide's resistance to the attachment of a chemical probe, respectively. More recently, in vitro methods that utilize rG4-mediated reverse transcriptase stalling have been developed to interrogate rG4 in low-abundance transcripts [31], and selective 2'-hydroxyl acylation analyzed by a lithium ion-mediated primer extension (SHALiPE), and DMSLiPE [32] have been developed to map distinctive structural patterns of rG4. Several next-generation sequencing-based approaches such as G4-seq [33], G4-Chip [34], rG4-seq [35], DMS-seq [36], and G4RP [37] enable the genome-wide and transcriptome-wide profiling of G4s. Another key category for G4 detection is to use fluorogenic G4 ligands whose fluorescence is selectively enhanced when interacting with G4s. These fluorescent turn-on ligands can be used to track G4 formation both in vitro and in cells, and they are discussed in detail in this review.

Besides acting as potential targets, G4s can be used as molecular tools for diverse applications. It is worth noting that the structure of G4s has been identified in studies using combinatorial methods and the systematic evolution of ligands by exponential enrichment (SELEX) technique with the aim of developing aptamers for therapeutic and diagnostic purposes [38–40]. G4s provide extra chemical and thermal stability for aptamer-based therapeutics, and such aptamers have been successfully designed to target a number of HIV proteins [41,42], prion proteins [43], and anti-cancer targets [44,45]. In diagnostics, G4-containing aptamers have been widely applied to target a wide range of pathogenic proteins and small molecules to emit a fluorescence-like signal [40]. In this review, we summarize the recent development of fluorogenic G4 ligands and G4-containing aptamers, and highlight their latest applications in vitro and in cells (Figure 1D). We will also discuss current challenges and future perspectives for better detection and targeting of G4s in diverse organisms, as well as for designing and developing G4-related tools for various biological applications.

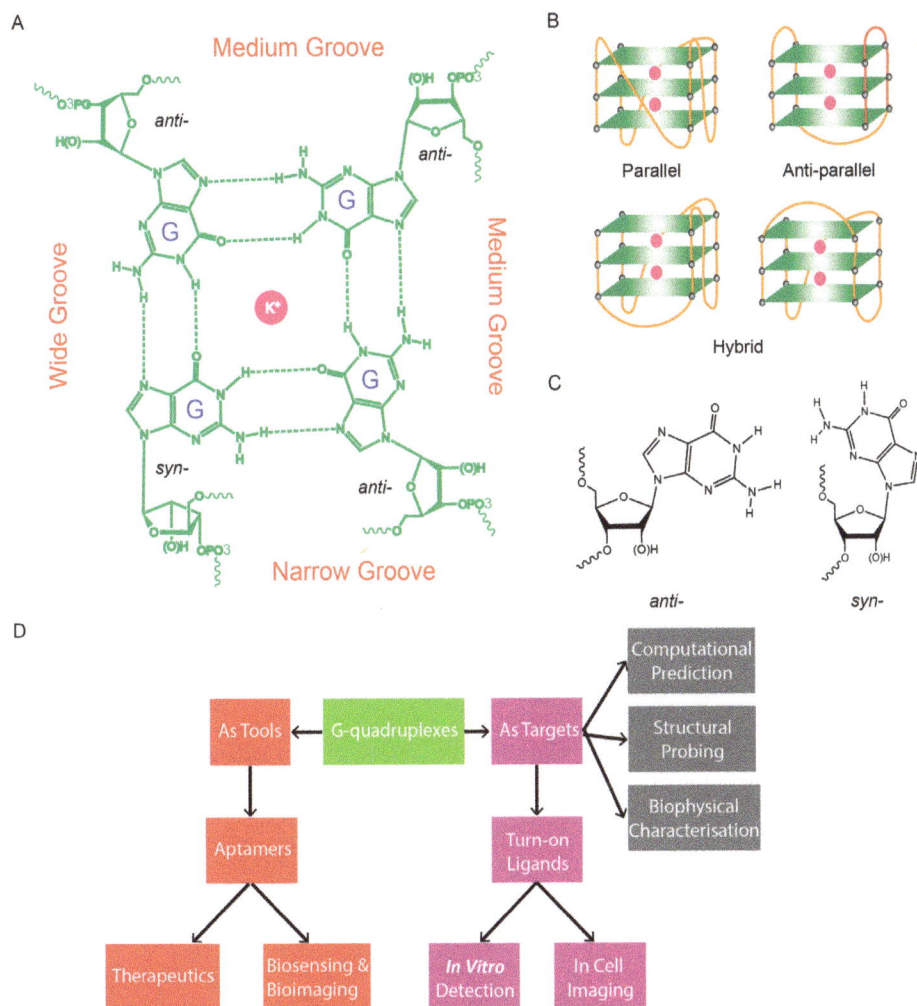

Figure 1. Overview of G4 structure, detection, and application. (**A**) Chemical structure of a G-quartet, showing the interactions between H-bond donors and acceptors at the Watson–Crick and Hoogsteen edges. K^+ is located at the core of G-quartet, which can provide further stabilization. (**B**) Parallel, anti-parallel and hybrid topologies of G4, demonstrating its polymorphism. (**C**) Anti- and syn-conformations of guanosine in a G-quartet that leads to wide, narrow, and medium grooves in (A). (**D**) Review overview. Red or purple boxes are topics that will be covered, while topics in the grey boxes were reviewed elsewhere. (see references for computational prediction [46,47], structural probing [48,49], and biophysical characterization [46,50]).

2. Fluorescent Turn-on G-Quadruplex Ligand

The biological significance of G4s in cells has led to a quest to develop diverse ligands that could help researchers understand their different cellular roles. On the one hand, some of these ligands are designed as fluorescent/imaging probes to verify G4 formation. On the other hand, some ligands can stabilize G4s and serve as chemical tools to challenge and alter G4-dependent processes. Also, it is possible that some ligands can perform both functions. In this review, we mainly focus on the organic G4 probes that is fluorogenic for in vitro and in cell detection of G4. As shown in Figure 2, these organic ligands in aqueous solvents have low fluorescence intensities; however, upon interacting with G4, an increased fluorescence intensity is observed, making fluorescence detection and imaging of G4 in vitro and in cells possible [51,52]. It should also be of note that there are also large repertoires of inorganic G4 probes that are luminogenic, and they have been extensively studied and several excellent reviews can be found elsewhere [53–56]. One representative example includes iridium (III) complex based G4s sensing methods; luminescent G4 switch-on probe for highly selective and tunable detection of cysteine and glutathione based on iridium (III) complex [57]. This method showed an enhanced intensity in the presence of desired metabolites [57]. Other examples of iridium (III) complex G4s based methods have also been reported, for instance, detection method for nicking endonuclease Nb.BsmI activity [58], for prostate specific antigen detection [59], thymine DNA glycosylase activity detection [60], for the detection of Siglec – 5 [61] and for ribonuclease H detection [62]. Platinum (II) complexes are another representative example of inorganic G4 ligand; Ma et al [63] reported the synthesis of platinum (II) complexes containing dipyridophenazine ligand as a highly sensitive luminescence probe for the detection of G4s and also showed to inhibit human telomerase enzyme (property also seen with organic ligands) and occur via an end stacking approach with a binding affinity of ~10^7 dm^3 mol^{-1} [63]. Other examples of platinum (II) complexes reported includes the detection of nanomolar silver (I) ion in solution [64], as luminescence probe for G4 and c-myc downregulation [65]. Also, terpyridine ligand containing platinum (II) complexes have been shown by Sunthaaralingam et al. [66] to strongly binds to G4s of hTelo and c-myc through π-π stacking [66], which binding affinity and selectivity influenced by their aromatic surface [67]. Additionally, Ruthenium (II) complexes have been also reported as a selective luminescence probe for G4 detection, and occur via stacking of the ligand onto the G-tetrad and also based on insertion of the complex into the groove [68]. Other examples of ruthenium (II) complexes were also reported; for instance for sensing and methylation of duplex and G4s using Ruthenium (II) complexes containing dipyridylphenazine (dppz) ligand [69] for selective binding to various G4s using a bromo-substituent to the dipyridylphenazine [70]. Some advantages of inorganic fluorogenic ligands include their tunability, distinct properties (like anticancer drug development and their ability to induce G4s), and structures [66,68,71].

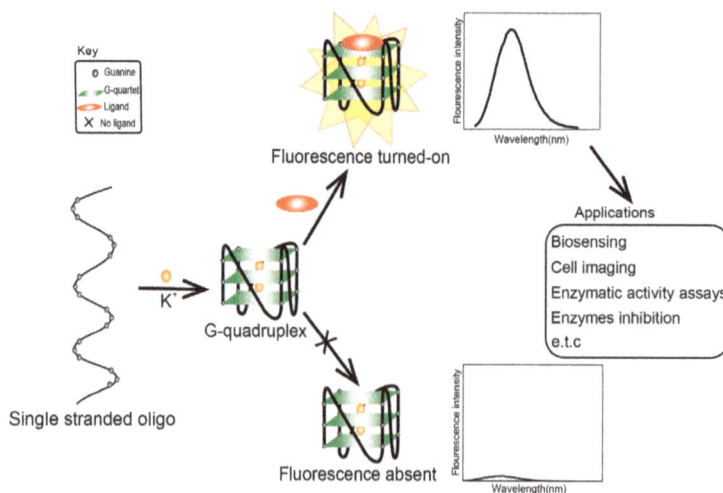

Figure 2. Schematic representation of ligand-enhanced fluorescence of G4. In the presence of ligand (top), it binds to G4 and results in enhancement in fluorescence. While in the absence of ligand (bottom), there is no such G4-ligand interaction, and hence no enhancement in fluorescence. This approach has been applied in different areas including but not limited to biosensing [72], cell imaging [51,52,73], enzymatic activity assay [74], and detecting G4 ligand inhibition of some enzymes [75,76] such as telomerase and ferrochelatase.

In the following, we will focus on the organic fluorogenic ligands/probes. Several representative classes and examples of each class are highlighted below:

2.1. Porphyrins

Porphyrins exist in nature and are utilized by living organisms as co-factors in different enzymatic processes [77]. Ligands in this class inhibit telomerase via stacking with the G-quartet of G4 and its subsequent stabilization [78]. As shown in Table 1, *N*-methyl meso porphyrin IX (NMM) is an asymmetric anionic porphyrin and a major example of the porphyrin class of ligands. It has fluorescence excitation and emission wavelengths of 393 nm and 610 nm, respectively. It shows favorable binding to parallel G4s compared with anti-parallel G4s [79,80], and thus has the potential to discriminate between different strand orientations based on its fluorescence fold enhancement [81].

2.1.1. Application of NMM and its Derivatives (TMPyP4 and TMPipEOPP)

NMM ligands have been applied in diverse applications, including enzyme activity and inhibition, cell imaging, and microbial detection, which are discussed below.

The NMM inhibitory effect was demonstrated by Huber et al. [75], in which NMM was applied as an inhibitor of G4 unwinding by stabilizing and preventing helicase from accessing the desired G4 strand [75]. In 2010, Hu and coworkers [76] demonstrated a G4-based fluorescence assay that allowed both real-time monitoring and inhibition of RNase H. This method required an RNA–DNA substrate (with the DNA strand containing G4-forming sequences). In the presence of RNase H, the RNA strand gets cleaved and the DNA strand gets released, which then folds into G4 and subsequently binds with NMM and produces an enhanced fluorescence intensity [76]. Ren et al. [82] reported the use of NMM with tetrakis(diisopropylguanidino)-zinc-phthalocyanine (Zn-DIGP) to develop a dual fluorescent probe for the detection of nucleic acids. This approach was shown to be applicable with urines and serum samples [82]. NMM was also applied in a live-cell imaging study. When added to the cells, a large Stokes shift and a red-shift emission were observed, both of which were higher than the emissions seen with a different class of ligand, thioflavin T (ThT) [83]. This could be due to the green fluorescence emission of ThT, which can easily coincide with the intrinsic fluorescence of the cell's other components [83].

Interestingly, NMM was also applied to microbial pathogen detection using integrated quaternized magnetic nanoparticles and a DNA amplification assay coupled with NMM. This method was based on the conformational transition from hairpin to G4 (assisted by Exo III nuclease) and subsequent specific interaction of the G4 with NMM. The method was able to detect as few as 50 cells mL^{-1} and 80 cells mL^{-1} of *E. coli* and *S. aureus*, respectively [84]. In 2016, Waller et al. [85] demonstrated ligand-specific regulation of nitrate assimilation in *Paracoccus denitrificans* (a Gram-negative soil bacterium). This method was based on stabilization of the *nasT* gene (which contains G4) by the 5,10,-15,20-tetra-(*N*-methyl-4-pyridyl)porphine (TMPyP4) ligand. Although NMM is an asymmetric porphyrin, cationic derivatives such as 5,10,15,20-tetra-4-[2-(1-methyl-1-piperidinyl)ethoxy]phenyl porphyrin (TMPipEOPP) and TMPyP4 were also applied as significant G4 binding ligands [86]. Notably, the TMPipEOPP ligand was shown to allow visual discrimination between G4s, duplexes and single-stranded DNA [86]. Limitation of some of these derivatives include off-target effects that lead to cell cytotoxicity [87] and they were not shown to have inhibitory properties like NMM [87]. More studies into these aspects are needed to fast track and improve the potentials of these ligands in live-cell investigations at both the macro- and micro-organism level.

2.1.2. Mechanism of NMM and its Derivatives (TMPyP4 and TMPipEOPP)

The mechanisms of interaction by this class of ligand were demonstrated to occur through both direct interaction with G4 and indirect interactions such as partial charge neutralization [88]. It was hypothesized that the interaction of porphyrin and G4s is based on intercalation with the adjacent G-quartets [77]. It was later shown that, when bound to G4, NMM fine-tuned its shape to fit the end face of the G4, resulting in enhanced fluorescence [76,89,90]. Another insight into the interactions was demonstrated in a triplet excited and decay study of zinc cationic porphyrin [5,10,15,20-tetrakis (1-methyl-4-pyridyl)-21H, 23H-porphine] (ZnTMPyP4). The interaction was demonstrated to occur via π–π stacking of the G4s ([AG3(T2AG3)3, (G4T4G4)2, and (TG4T)4]) and the macrocycle of ZnTMPyP4 [91]. The parent ligand, TMPyP4, from which ZnTMPyP4 was derived, was also shown to inhibit telomerase via external stacking on the G-tetrads [92]. However, the mechanism of interaction for the TMPipEOPP ligand was demonstrated to be dependent on the concentration of either the ligand or the targeted G4. At lower concentrations, one G4 binds two TMPipEOPP ligands via an 'end stacking and outside binding' approach [86]. Wheelhouse et al. previously demonstrated a similar effect [92]. At higher concentrations, two G4s bind one TMPipEOPP ligand via a 'sandwich end-stacking' approach [86].

2.2. Benzothiozole

Thioflavin T (ThT), a 3,6-dimethyl-2-(4-dimethylaminophenyl) benzothiazolium cation, is also a commercially available dye like NMM, but unlike NMM, ThT is cationic (benzothiozole). ThT has excitation and emission wavelengths of 425 nm and 490 nm, respectively. It also has the advantage of low background fluorescence intensity, which translates to a high signal-to-noise ratio [6,87]. Prior to 2013, ThT was mainly used to bind other structures such as protein fibrils and amyloids through extensive π-stacking with tyrosine and tryptophan amino acids [93]. ThT was also demonstrated to inhibit interactions between fibrils and proteins [94].

2.2.1. Application of ThT, its Derivatives (ThT-DB, ThT-HE, & ThT-NE), and IMT

Because of its high sensitivity, ThT attracts the attention of chemists and has been applied in diverse applications, including biosensing, G4-specific probes, toxin detection, cell imaging, and microbial detection, among others, which are discussed below.

ThT was first reported in 2013 as a G4 ligand to study the human telomere G4 22AG [dAGGG(TTAGGG)3], and it was demonstrated to differentiate between G4, duplexes and single strands with high fluorescence intensity [87,95]. This fluorescence turn-on ligand has been widely applied as a sensor, for instance, for Ag^+ [96] and Hg^+ [97] detection, based on the interaction between the ligand and G4. ThT has also been applied as a label-free fluorescent turn-on ligand for sensing bio-thiols based on its ability to induce unique G4 structures [72], and it was demonstrated as a probing method for structural changes in i-motif (four stranded DNA secondary structures that consist of hemi-protonated and intercalated cytosine base pairs (C:C$^+$)) [98]. It was applied as a highly sensitive sensor for thrombin detection using Förster resonance energy transfer (FRET). This method is based on the ability of ThT to induce G4, which is then used as an energy acceptor, with a conjugated polymer on the other side as the energy donor [99]. More recently, ThT was applied as a G4-based aptasensor for the detection of adenosine deaminase activity and inhibition [74]. ThT was also applied in toxin detection, as demonstrated using a G4-based aptasensor that selectively quantified the amount of toxins in food materials. This method was based on an aptamer (selected against a toxin) binding to ThT to form a G4–ThT complex (in the absence of the target toxin). When the toxin is present, it binds to the G4-based aptamer, which leads to the release of ThT, and a subsequent change in fluorescence is observed [100]. As shown in Table 1, unlike NMM, some G4 studies have indicated that ThT-induced G4s can potentially cause topological changes [101], producing false positive and false negative results [97]. It was also shown to bind tightly to non-G4 G–A-rich containing sequences and dimerise them into a parallel double-stranded modes [96]. Furthermore, ThT was found to be difficult to use for effective monitoring of G4s in the chromatin of live cells because of its inability to stain the nuclei [102]. This led to the synthesis of some ThT derivatives.

Some derivatives of ThT have been reported, such as ethyl-substituted ThT, which was applied as a fluorescence probe with high specificity for G4 structure detection and discrimination from other nucleic acid forms [103]. Interestingly, this method allows naked-eye visualization of G4 in solution under ultraviolet light. In a similar study, Kataoka and coworkers [101] synthesized two derivatives of ThT by replacing the N3 methyl on the benzothiozole ring with either a ((*p*-(dimethylamino)-benzoyl)-oxy)-ethyl group (ThT-DB) or a hydroxyethyl group (ThT-HE) and applied them as parallel G4 probes. Their results showed over 200-fold enhancement in fluorescence intensity compared with normal ThT, and also great specificity to parallel G4s. Other benzothiazoles have been reported, such as IMT, which can selectively bind G4s in a cell's chromatin (with negligible cytotoxicity). It can be applied in vivo to demonstrate the changing response of G4s to different chemicals in real time [51]. This method is simpler than the triangulenium method reported earlier [52], which requires a longer acquisition time and specialized equipment.

Lastly, ThT has also been applied in studies of G4 prevalence in micro-organisms. For example, in 2016, Burrows and coworkers [104] applied ThT as a fluorescence probe to study the prevalence of G4s in the zika virus. Two years later, the same group applied ThT as a fluorescence probe for the detection of G4s in *Chlamydomonas reinhardtii* [105]. That same year, Zahin et al. [106] applied ThT for the identification of G4-forming sequences in papillomaviruses (using ThT as a fluorescence probe to screen for G4-forming sequences). Similarly, ThT derivatives have been applied in viral RNA genome detection and monitoring. This was demonstrated very recently by Luo et al. [107], who developed the ligand ThT–NE, with the excitation and emission wavelengths shown in Table 1 (ThT derivative). The ligand was a cell permeable and highly specific G4-based fluorescence turn-on probe for real-time imaging of native viral RNA in the hepatitis C virus (HCV). This method was shown to allow subcellular monitoring and continuous live-cell monitoring of infected cells [107]. However, the limitation of this ligand class include the fact that only few were shown to penetrate the cells [107] and reach their desired target. The possible reasons could be due to their physical size, non-selectivity in complex samples or conditions or the potential to form aggregates in cells [108]. Some of the other imperative factors in designing novel fluorescence G4 probes include permeability, affinity, selectivity, and cytotoxicity. Some G4-containing aptamers (such as Mango) have been shown to discriminate between this class of ligands via a concerted mechanism, whereas others (such as Spinach) enhance the fluorescence intensities of many ligands with no discriminating properties between them [109]. Hence, there is a need for G4 ligand with higher specificity, affinity, and low toxicity for live cell application.

2.2.2. Mechanism of ThT, ThT-NE, and IMT

The mechanism of interaction between ThT and G4s was demonstrated to be ligand concentration dependent, in which several ThT ligands bound cooperatively to the 5′-G4 unit [87]. Unlike the NMM derivative TMPipEOPP (which also depends on ligand concentration), in this case, the fluorescence enhancement was higher when a single ThT ligand was bound to G4. The enhanced fluorescence intensity was demonstrated to be a result of the restriction in circular movement and subsequent conformational changes between the benzothiazole and dimethylaminobenzene rings [87]. However, the fluorescence intensity diminished when more than one ThT ligand was bound to the rearranged/changed G4 structure [87]. It was also demonstrated that the interaction between ThT and G4 may be due to end stacking with the upper G-tetrad of RNA G4; that is, the benzothiazole unit stacks onto the upper G-quartet of the G4, thereby donating most of the π-stacking force in its binding [110]. Similarly, the mechanism of interaction for ThT-NE was demonstrated to occur via pi–pi stacking of the ligand and the ending G-quartet of the G4, resulting in rotational restriction of the ligand. Likewise, the mechanism of IMT interaction with G4s was shown to occur via stacking to the terminal (5′-end) G-quartet [51].

2.3. Triphenylmethane (TPM)

The TPM class of ligands has many members, including methyl violet (MV), ethyl violet (EV), methyl green (MEG), malachite green (MG), and crystal violet (CV). This class was shown to distinguish intramolecular from intermolecular G4s and single DNA strands from duplex DNAs [111]. For this review, we focus on CV and MG. Prior to its application in G4 detection, CV was widely used as a dye for staining papers, textiles, drugs, and food materials [112]. It then began to attract enormous attention as a stain for biological studies. It has fluorescence excitation and emission wavelengths of 540 nm and 640 nm, respectively, as shown in Table 1.

2.3.1. Application of CV and MG

Like NMM and ThT, CV has been widely applied in diverse areas, including sensing that can distinguish single strand and duplex structures from G4 [113–115], and it preferentially binds to intramolecular rather than intermolecular G4 [113]. It is also applied in biosensing and thrombin detection. Other applications are discussed below.

G4-based aptasensors (discussed in detail in Section 3 of this review) are attracting enormous scientific interest. Nonetheless, in this section, we touch on the G4 ligand-based fluorescence turn-on aspect of some representative aptasensors. One example is an aptasensor selected through modified-affinity chromatography to replace G4 binding [116] and subsequent detection of CV. CV was also applied as a biosensor for the detection of Pb^{2+} based on the electrochemical current of a G4–CV complex [114]. He et al. [117] developed a label-free G4-based aptamer probe for the selective detection of ATP in aqueous solution using CV as a G4 fluorescent probe. In this method, the ATP aptamer is in a duplex format (i.e., hybridized to its complementary sequence); in the absence of ATP, it gives a weak fluorescence intensity. However, in the presence of ATP, the duplex dissociates, resulting in an aptamer–G4 complex via a 'population shift mechanism'. The presence of CV results in its specific binding to the G4 complex, thus enhancing the fluorescence (depicted in Figure 2). CV was demonstrated to distinguish between parallel and anti-parallel topologies [118]; it preferentially binds to anti-parallel G4 and produces enhanced fluorescence intensity due to the shielding effect of the G4 end-loop on CV against the solvent, whereas the parallel G4 cannot provide CV with such a shield due to the lack of the end-loop.

Jin et al. [119] reported another G4-based aptasensor and demonstrated its ability to detect human thrombin protein. This method was based on the enhanced fluorescence of CV as a result of its binding to a thrombin–G4 aptamer complex. In 2009, Kong et al. [113] demonstrated a simple and sensitive method for discriminating between G4s, single strands and duplexes based on the fluorescence enhancement of CV or CV energy transfer fluorescence. Interestingly, in the presence of C-rich sequences (complementary strands to G-rich), this method was shown to measure the amount of G-rich sequences that partake in G4 formation based on the fluorescence enrichment of G4–CV complexes. That same year, a novel biosensor for the homogenous sensing of K^+ was also reported. This biosensor was based on increasing and decreasing fluorescence intensity with increasing K^+ [120]. A similar approach (of decreased fluorescence with increasing K^+) for the determination of K^+ was reported. However, this method was based on the interaction between G4 containing a thrombin-binding aptamer (TBA) and CV. The interaction of TBA with CV (in the absence K^+) produces enhanced fluorescence. However, in the presence of K^+, TBA-based G4 is formed, and when it interacts with CV, the difference in fluorescence intensity is measured (depending on the K^+ concentration) [121]. Thus, the amount of K^+ can be determined. MG has also been applied as fluorescence G4-based aptasensors for binding recognition to MG ligands. However, the limitation of this class includes the fact that it does not allow naked-eye visualization of G4s in solution. Also, they have different binding modes such as the stacking and end loop protection modes (as discussed in Section 2.3.2 below), and G4 and other nucleic acid structural motifs and topologies can sometimes significantly influence the ligand's fluorescence enhancement [122].

2.3.2. Mechanism of CV and MG

In 2009, the mechanism of interaction was demonstrated to occur via stacking of CV to the two outside G-quartets of G4 [118] and the binding of two CVs per one G4. This stacking increased the rigidity of the ligand and subsequently the fluorescence intensity. In the same year, Kong et al.

demonstrated the end-loop protection mechanism of bound ligands in an antiparallel topology [120]. The stacking mechanism was also reported for CV interactions with i-motif [123].

2.4. Other Ligands Reported in the Literature as G4 Fluorescence Turn-On Ligands

As summarized in Table 1, several fluorescence turn-on ligands were also demonstrated to recognize G4. However, acridine-based ligands are largely used as efficient G4 stabilizers, such as trisubstituted acridines. N,N'-[9-[[4-(Dimethylamino)phenyl]amino]-3,6-acridinediyl]bis [1-pyrrolidinepropanamide], known as BRACO-19, has attracted much scientific interest due to its G4 stabilization and inhibition of telomerase enzyme activity [37,124,125]. It also shows antiviral activity as it impairs HIV-1 long terminal repeats promoter activity, which controls the viral gene transcription [126]. Pyridostatin (PDS) was also reported to bind to G4 with high specificity through an end-stacking approach [127–129], but it did not fluoresce. Later they synthesized a PDS analogue which allows the evaluation of the cellular localization of the drug ("by promoting telomere dysfunction and long-term growth inhibition in human cancer cells") [130], more so, they explored how PDS interferes with the roles of proteins that operates on G4s and how that in turn affects targeting of G4s by small molecules [131]. This changed with the very first fluorogenic acridine dyes containing cyanine, which allowed a wide spectrum ranging from orange to the near infrared region, as demonstrated by Mahmood and coworkers [132]. Later on, the same group (motivated again by the incredible potential of BRACO-19) demonstrated the development of a tri-substituted (3,6,9-trisubstituted acridine; cyanine dye 1) water-soluble acridine-based dual probe, a pH-sensitive and G4 fluorescence probe containing monomethine cyanine dye (which has fluorescence excitation and emission wavelengths of 400 nm and 475 nm, respectively) [133]. Cellular pH is an essential factor in cell activities, and the probe was demonstrated to be sensitive to a pH range of 5–9. In acidic conditions, the probe showed enhanced fluorescence due to the protonation of acridine. A positive charge delocalises between the acridine and indole moieties and fluorescence is reduced at higher pH values (as the acridine can no longer be protonated). The system was reported to operate based on a 'push–pull mechanism' [133]. The limitation of this ligand is that its application was not demonstrated in vivo. BRACO-19 was shown to bind to G4 via three modes of interaction: stacking to the top quartet, intercalation on the lower quartet and groove binding [124,134].

Other reports on G4 fluorescence turn-on ligands include that of Jin et al. [135]. In 2014, they applied a BPBC ligand composed of benzimidazole and carbazole groups as a fluorescence turn-on probe for parallel G4 detection. The ligand was shown to bind parallel G4s via an end-stacking approach. It was also shown to have incredible selectivity towards parallel G4s due to its possession of a 'crescent-shaped pi-conjugated planar core', which is bigger than the G4 plane dimension. Likewise, Yang et al. [136] reported a new class of bis(4-aminobenzylidene)acetone derivative called GD3 as an effective red-emitting fluorescence turn-on ligand for parallel G4s. They demonstrated the biological application of this ligand in fixed cells and showed that it allows the visualization and monitoring of G4 structures. The mechanism of interaction was the dipole moment created in the microenvironment of the ligand and the restriction of the fluorophores, resulting in altered charge transfer in the system and hence enhanced fluorescence [136]. However, the limitation of this ligand is that it can only allow monitoring of G4s in fixed cells. Other parallel G4 binding ligands were reported by Chen and coworkers [137], who demonstrated the use of 2,4,5-triaryl-substituted imidazole (IZCM-1) as an effective ligand that binds specifically to parallel G4s without affecting their topology or thermal stability. Later, the same team [138] synthesized another G4 fluorescence turn-on triaryl-substituted imidazole ligand called [2-(4-(4,5-bis(4-(4-methylpiperazin-1-yl)phenyl)-1H-imidazol-2-yl)phenyl)-6-(4-methylpiperazin-1-yl)-1H-benzo[de]isoquinoline-1,3(2H)-dione] (IZNP-1) and demonstrated its application to highly and specifically target telomeric multimeric G4 structures (i.e., it can discriminate between telomeric multimeric G4s and monomeric G4s) through intercalation of the ligand into the 'pocket' of two G-quartet units of G4. This ligand was demonstrated to induce apoptosis and senescence in cancer cells as result of telomeric DNA damage and telomere functional disruption due to the ligand intercalation into the G4 structure [138]. Shavalingam et al. [52] applied a triaryl methyl carbocation (triangulenium) derivative called DAOTA-M2 that localizes in the nuclei (with low toxicity) and interact with G4. Also, a "one-to-one G4-specific sensor", IZFL-2, that can distinguish between different G4s was demonstrated [139]. This method allows the visualization of interactions between ligands and G4s by fluorescence lifetime microscopy. The binding mechanism of this ligand occurred via π–π stacking between the guanine moieties of the outer G-quartet and core of the ligand [140].

Most of the fluorescence turn-on probes can only accommodate one output. In 2014, Yan et al. [141] developed a multifunctional probe called (*E*)-3-((7-(diethylamino)-2-oxo-2*H*-chromen-3-yl)methylene)-6,7-difluoro-4-methyl-9-oxo-1,2,3,9-tetrahydropyrrolo [2,1-*b*]quinazolin-4-ium iodide (ISCH-1) that utilized two different outputs (i.e., colorimetric and fluorescence). These types of probes are reliable and applicable to diverse applications. The ligand was designed based on an isaindigotone framework that incorporated coumarin–hemicyanine to achieve a multifunctional probe. The application of this probe to detect G4s was demonstrated [141]. The limitation of this ligand is that it cannot allow specific targeting of G4s at a given RNA region (such as the 5′ UTR). To address this issue, Chen et al., refined ISCH-1 by attaching an oligonucleotide (which had a complementary sequence to an adjacent sequence of the G4 sequence of interest) that would allow subsequent fluorescence in situ hybridization (FISH) to be performed. Hence, the probe consisted of two distinct segments, the fluorescence turn-on and oligonucleotide hybridization segments. They referred to the probe as a G4-triggered fluorogenic hybridization (GTFH) probe [142]. The refined ISCH-1 ligand was called (*E*)-3-((7-(diethylamino)-2-oxo-2*H*-chromen-3-yl)methylene)-7-fluoro-4-methyl-9-oxo-6-(prop-2-yn-1-yloxy)-1,2,3,9-tetrahydropyrrolo[2,1-*b*]quinazolin-4-ium (ISCH-oa1) [142]. The application of this ligand was demonstrated with 5′ UTR of *NRAS* mRNA by incorporating an oligonucleotide complimentary to the adjacent sequence of the *NRAS* G4 sequence to form ISCH-nras1 ligand that can selectively bind and uniquely allow the visualization of G4s in this region both in vitro and in cells [142], however, this ligand has limitations of not able to detect the 'in-situ spots' of a given RNA in single cell and also requires RNAs to be transfected into cells to increase their concentration. Amazingly, the same team developed yet another ligand that was also based on an isaindigoton framework, but it contained coumarin aldehyde and an *N*-methylated quinoline moiety, this ligand was named (*E*)-2-(2-(7-(diethylamino)-2-oxo-2*H*-chromen-3-yl)vinyl)-6-fluoro-1-methyl-7-(4-methylpiperazin-1-yl)quinolin-1-ium iodide (QUMA-1). Unlike GD3 ligand that was only shown in fixed cells, QUMA-1 was demonstrated through live-cell imaging to be a highly selective fluorescence turn-on probe for real-time and continuous tracking and monitoring of rG4 structural dynamics in live cells. It was also applied in the visualization of rG4s unwinding by helicase [143]. Nonetheless, the fluorescence intensity of this ligand decreases in the presence of other competing G4s ligands. The interaction between QUMA-1 and rG4 was demonstrated to be caused by the rotational constraint experienced by the ligand at higher energy levels because of a conformational rearrangement [143].

Laguerre et al. [144] reported another multifunctional G4 smart probe (ligand and fluorescence turn-on probe) developed using the template-assembled synthetic G-quartets (TASQ) method. They used TASQ to develop pyrene template-assembled synthetic G-quartets (PyroTASQ) as both a smart G4 ligand and a fluorescence probe. This ligand and probe were demonstrated to recognize and bind to both DNA and RNA G4s and it was shown to occur through an interesting approach, in which the ligand causes a 'quadruplex-promoted conformational switch' that leads to the assembling of four guanines into a G-quartet. Subsequently, the pyrene's fluorescence is released [144]. However, the application of PyroTASQ to detect G4s in live cells proved difficult as it aggregates in the cells [108]. To address this issue, the same group demonstrated another multitasking G4 probe synthesized in an approach similar to that of PyroTASQ but replacing the pyrene group with naphthalene to form a Naptho-TASQ (N-TASQ) [108]. The authors were able to visualize RNA G4s in live cells using the multi-photon microscopy method [108] and both RNA and DNA imaging using confocal microscopy [145]. The interaction occurs through an approach similar to that of PyroTASQ [108]. However, no binding competition with other G4 ligands was shown.

Table 1. Representative fluorescent turn-on G4 ligands and their corresponding characteristics and applications

Class	Ligand and Commercial Availability (CAS no.)	Structure and Fluorescence Properties	Representative Applications	Advantages and Limitations	Ref.
	N-methyl mesoporphyrin IX (NMM), Yes (142234-85-3)	$\lambda_{ex. max}, \lambda_{em. max}$ (393 nm, 610 nm)	— Highly specific parallel telomeric G4s binding, stabilization, and structural rearrangement. — Specific inhibitor of G4 unwinding by helicase (of *Saccharomyces cerevisiae* and human BM1). In the presence of NMM the helicase gets trapped on the NMM-G4 complex. — Real time specific G4 based fluorescence assay for RNase sensing and inhibition. — A label free sensor for sensing iodide and melamine. Based on thymine-melamine-thymine (T-M-T)/thymine-Hg²⁺-thymine (T-Hg²⁺-T) and G4-NMM complex. — Highly sensitive microbial pathogen sensor based on quaternized magnetic nanoparticle exonuclease III assisted DNA amplification assays. Based on conformational transition from hairpin to G4 (assisted by Exo III nuclease) and subsequent specific interaction (of the G4) with NMM.	— Asymmetric anionic porphyrin — Inhibitors of different enzymes — Easy to develop label free sensors — Selective and sensitive G4 ligand — Allow real time study of G4 — Specific binding to parallel telomeric G4 — Microbial pathogen sensing — In live cell imaging, a Stokes shift and a red-shift emission were observed when applied, both of which were higher than the emissions seen with a different class of ligand, thioflavin T (ThT) — Not shown to provide visual discrimination of various G4s	[75,76,79,84, 146,147]
Porphyrin	5,10,15,20-tetra-[4-[2-(1-methyl-1-piperidinyl)ethoxy]phenyl] porphyrin (TMPipEOPP), No	$\lambda_{ex. max}, \lambda_{em. max}$ (422 nm, 660 nm)	— G4s specific probe that allow visual discrimination between G4s, duplexes, and single stranded DNAs.	— Cationic porphyrin — Aid visual differentiation of various G4s — Not shown to have enzymatic potentials	[86]
	Pyridinium, 4,4',4'',4'''-(21*H*,23*H*-porphine-5, 10,15,20-tetrayl)tetrakis[1-methyl-, 4-methylbenzenesulfonate (1:4) (TMPyP4), Yes (36951-72-1)	$\lambda_{ex. max}, \lambda_{em. max}$ (425 nm, 650 nm)	— A ligand specific metabolic regulation of nitrate assimilation in *Paracoccus denitrificans* (a Gram-negative soil bacterium), based on stabilization of G4.	— Cationic porphyrin — Metabolic regulator nitrate assimilation — Not shown to provide visual discrimination of various G4s. — Not shown to have inhibitory potentials	[85]

Table 1. *Cont.*

Class	Ligand and Commercial Availability (CAS no.)	Structure and Fluorescence Properties	Representative Applications	Advantages and Limitations	Ref.
Benzothiazole	3,6-dimethyl-2-(4-dimethylaminophenyl) benzothiazolium cation Thioflavin T (ThT), Yes (2390-54-7)	$\lambda_{ex, max}$, $\lambda_{em, max}$ (425 nm, 490 nm)	— Sensitive and efficient G4 fluorescence sensor for human telomeric DNA. — Fluorescence sensor for the determination of cysteine and glutathione. Also, shown to detects biothiols in blood samples. Based on ThT ability to induced conformational specific G4. — Highly sensitive sensor for thrombin detection using Förster resonance energy transfer (FRET). Based on ThT ability to induce G4 and used as an acceptor with a conjugated polymer as the donor. — Specific fluorescence probe for G4 formation. Based on direct interaction between ThT and the target. — Aptasensor for Adenosine deaminase activity and inhibition. — Fluorescence probe for the detection of G4s in *Chlamydomonas reinhardtii*. — Fluorescence probe for the detection of G4s in zika virus. — Fluorescence probe for the detection of G4s in papillomaviruses.	— Has low background fluorescence intensity, which translates to a high signal-to-noise ratio — Highly sensitive probe for the detection of G4s in different species and in different samples — Induced conformational specific G4 — Shown to have enzymatic activity and inhibition — An ethyl substituted ThT allows naked-eye visualization of G4 in solution under ultraviolet light — Highly specific to parallel G4s — In live cells imaging, it produces less emissions compared to what was observed with a different class of ligand, NMM — In live cell imaging, its green fluorescence can easily coincide with the intrinsic fluorescence of the cell's other components — ThT induced G4s can potentially cause topological changes — Produces false positive and false negative results — It binds tightly to non-G4 G–A-rich containing sequences and dimerizes them into a parallel double-stranded mode — Difficult to use for effective monitoring of G4s in the chromatin of live cells because of its inability to stain the nuclei	[72,74,97,99, 104–106,110, 148]
	N-Isopropyl-2-(4-N, N-dimethylanilino)-6-methylbenzothiazole (IMT), No	$\lambda_{ex, max}$, $\lambda_{em, max}$ (415 nm, 500 nm)	— Real time fluorescence probe for monitoring the formation of G4 in live cells and its response to chemical treatment demonstrated.	— Live cell monitoring of G4 formation in real time — Selectively bind G4s in a cell's chromatin (with negligible cytotoxicity) — Toxicity analysis only performed using single method instead of using two different methods in parallel	[51]
	ThT-NE, No	$\lambda_{ex, max}$, $\lambda_{em, max}$ (459 nm, 493 nm)	— Cell permeable and highly specific G4 based fluorescence turn-on probe for real time imaging of native viral RNA genome in hepatitis C virus (HCV). This method was shown to allow subcellular monitoring and continuous live-cell monitoring of infected cells.	— Allows real time subcellular and continuous live-cell monitoring of native viral RNA genome — Toxicity effect to cells not shown/reported	[107]

174

Table 1. *Cont.*

Class	Ligand and Commercial Availability (CAS no.)	Structure and Fluorescence Properties	Representative Applications	Advantages and Limitations	Ref.
Triphenylmethane (TPM)	Crystal Violet (CV), Yes (548-62-9)	$\lambda_{ex. max}$, $\lambda_{em. max}$ (540 nm, 640 nm)	— Label free fluorescence aptasensor for specific detection of CV based on G4 interaction with CV. — A label-free G4 based fluorescence turn-on probe for the selective detection of ATP in aqueous medium. This is based on the ability of CV to specifically binds to G4. — Live cells visualization of G4 role in alternative splicing via RNA-binding protein hnRNPF. — G4-based fluorescence aptasensor for the selective detection of thrombin protein. Based on CV-G4 fluorescence. — Fluorescence probe for monitoring G4 structural differences (as a function of cation) and sensing of K^+. — Fluorescence probe for homogenous detection of K^+ based on the fluorescence intensity changes of CV-G4 complex.	— Distinguishes intramolecular from intermolecular G4s — Distinguishes single DNA strands from duplex DNAs — Widely employed in biosensing — Distinguishes between parallel and anti-parallel G4 topologies (preferentially binds to anti-parallel G4s)	[73,116–120]
	Malachite Green (MG), Yes (569-64-2)	$\lambda_{ex. max}$, $\lambda_{em. max}$ (617 nm, 650 nm)	— Fluorescence G4 based aptasensor for binding recognition to MG ligand.	— Widely employed in (bio)sending — Not shown to allow naked eye visualization of G4s in solution	[146]
Triangulenium	Morpholino containing bis-substituted triangulenium (DAOTA-M2), **No**	$\lambda_{ex. max}$, $\lambda_{em. max}$ (501 nm, 539 nm)	— Fluorescence probe for G4 visualization in live cells, based fluorescence lifetime imaging microscopy. This probe was demonstrated to be cell permeable, have low toxicity, and be localized in the nucleus.	— Allows live cell visualization of G4 — High cell permeability — Low cytotoxicity — Can localize in the nucleus — One-to-one G4-specific sensor — Allows the visualization of interactions between ligands and G4s by fluorescence lifetime microscopy	[52]

Table 1. *Cont.*

Class	Ligand and Commercial Availability (CAS no.)	Structure and Fluorescence Properties	Representative Applications	Advantages and Limitations	Ref.
	Ethyl 2-(6-(4-(4-((4-(4-methylpiperazin-1-yl)phenyl)-1H-imidazol-2-yl)phenoxy)methyl)-1H-1,2,3-triazol-1-yl)butoxy)-3-oxo-3H-xanthen-9-yl)benzoate (IZFL-2), No	$\lambda_{ex\ max}$, $\lambda_{em\ max}$ (450 nm, 520 nm)	— A tunable fluorescence activation probe for the specific detection of c-Myc G4. This was demonstrated to differentiate between wild-type c-Myc G4 and other G4s.	— Its fluorescence can be tuned — Distinctive smart sensor specific only for c-Myc G4s — Not yet demonstrated in live cells	[139]
Imidazole	2,4,5-triaryl-substituted imidazole (IZCM-1), No	$\lambda_{ex\ max}$, $\lambda_{em\ max}$ (450 nm, 525 nm)	— Fluorescence turn-on probe for the specific detection of parallel G4 without affecting their topology and thermal stability.	— Effectively and specifically binds to parallel G4s	[137]
	[2-(4-(4,5-bis(4-(4-methylpiperazin-1-yl)phenyl)-1H-imidazol-2-yl)phenyl)-6-(4-methylpiperazin-1-yl)-1H-benzo[de]isoquinoline-1,3(2H)-dione] (IZNP-1), No	$\lambda_{ex\ max}$, $\lambda_{em\ max}$ (400 nm, 540 nm)	— Fluorescence turn-on probe for the specific targeting of telomeric multimeric G4 structures, shown to occur via intercalation into the pocket between two G-quartet units.	— Can discriminate between telomeric multimeric G4s and monomeric G4s— Induce apoptosis and senescence in cancer cells	[138]
Acridine	3,6,9-trisubstituted Acridine; cyanine dye 1, No	$\lambda_{ex\ max}$, $\lambda_{em\ max}$ (400 nm, 475 nm)	— Water soluble dual function probe for G4 specific binding; pH sensitive and fluorescence probe for G4 stabilization and detection that operate by a push–pull mechanism.	— Highly water soluble — pH sensitive — Application not demonstrated in vivo	[133]

Table 1. *Cont.*

Class	Ligand and Commercial Availability (CAS no.)	Structure and Fluorescence Properties	Representative Applications	Advantages and Limitations	Ref.
	(E)-3-((7-(diethylamino)-2-oxo-2H-chromen-3-yl)methylene)-6,7-difluoro-4-methyl-9-oxo-1,2,3,9-tetrahydropyrrolo[2,1-b]quinazolin-4-ium iodide (ISCH-1), No	$\lambda_{ex, max}, \lambda_{em, max}$ (570 nm, 652 nm)	— Multifunctional (colorimetric and red-emitting fluorescence) turn-on probe for specific G4 detection. This method is ideal for reliability and diverse applications.	— Multifunctional (colorimetric and fluorescence) — Reliable and potential for numerous applications — Not shown to allow specific targeting of G4s in a given region (such as the 5′-UTR)	[141]
Alkaloid	(E)-3-((7-(diethylamino)-2-oxo-2H-chromen-3-yl)methylene)-7-fluoro-4-methyl-9-oxo-6-(prop-2-yn-1-yloxy)-1,2,3,9-tetrahydropyrrolo[2,1-b]quinazolin-4-ium iodide (ISCH-oa1), No	$\lambda_{ex, max}, \lambda_{em, max}$ (630 nm, 650 nm)	— G-quadruplex-triggered fluorogenic hybridization (GTFH) probe, that selectively allows the visualization of the G-quadruplexes that form in a particular region interest (NRAS mRNA 5′-UTR region was demonstrated) both in vitro and in cells. The ligand consists of two segments, which are a fluorescent light-up fluorophore and oligonucleotide sequence that can hybridize with the sequence adjacent to the guanine rich sequence in the NRAS mRNA 5′-UTR or other regions of interest.	— Allows specific targeting of G4s in a particular region such as 5′-UTR — Can be use both in vivo and in vitro — Cannot detect the in situ spots of a given RNA in single cell — Requires RNAs to be transfected into cells to increase their concentration	[142]
	(E)-2-(2-(7-(diethylamino)-2-oxo-2H-chromen-3-yl)vinyl)-6-fluoro-1-methyl-7-(4-methylpiperazin-1-yl)quinolin-1-ium iodide (QUMA-1), No	$\lambda_{ex, max}, \lambda_{em, max}$ (555 nm, 660 nm)	— Highly selective fluorescence turn-on probe for real time and continuous tracking and monitoring of rG4 structural dynamics in live cells, this application has been demonstrated in through live cell imaging. Also, applied in visualization of rG4s unwinding by helicase.	— Allows live cell monitoring and tracking of rG4s — Allows the imaging of rG4 unwinding — Fluorescence intensity decreases in the presence of competing G4s ligands	[143]
Acetone	Bis(4-aminobenzylidene)acetone derivative referred to as GD3, No	$\lambda_{ex, max}, \lambda_{em, max}$ (450 nm, 600 nm)	— An effective red emitting fluorescence turn-on ligand for parallel G4s structures. Its biological application was demonstrated in fixed cells and shown to allow the visualization and monitoring of G4s structures. It was also shown to occur based on dipole moment created in the microenvironment of the ligand and restriction of the fluorophore resulting in altered charge transfer in the system, hence an enhanced light-up observed	— Red emitting ligand — Specific for parallel G4s — Allows monitoring of G4s in fixed cells	[136]

Table 1. *Cont.*

Class	Ligand and Commercial Availability (CAS no.)	Structure and Fluorescence Properties	Representative Applications	Advantages and Limitations	Ref.
Pyrene	Pyrene template-assembled synthetic G-quartet (PyroTASQ), No	$\lambda_{ex.\ max}$, $\lambda_{em.\ max}$ (420 nm, 450 nm)	— Multitasking G4s smart probe (stabilizing ligand and fluorescence turn-on probe). This ligand and probe were demonstrated to recognize and bind to both DNA and RNA G4s, and shown to occur through an interesting approach; in which the ligand causes a 'quadruplex-promoted conformational switch' that leads to assembling of four guanines into a G-quartet, and subsequently the pyrene's fluorescence is release	— Multifunctional (stabilization and fluorescence turn-on) — Can bind to both DNA and RNA G4s — Failed for in vivo studies as it forms aggregates in cells	[144]
Naphthalene	Naptho-template-assembled synthetic G-quartet (N-TASQ), No	$\lambda_{ex.\ max}$, $\lambda_{em.\ max}$ (286 nm, 400 nm)	— Multitasking G4s smart probe stabilizing ligand and fluorescence turn-on probe for live cell visualization of RNA G4s using multi-photon microscopy technique, while both RNA and DNA G4s were visualized using confocal microscopy. The interaction occurs through similar approach with Pyro-TASQ.	— Multifunctional (stabilization and fluorescence turn-on) — Can bind to both DNA and RNA G4s — G4 visualization in live cells using the multi-photon microscopy — Allows both RNA and DNA G4 imaging using confocal microscopy — No binding competition with other G4 ligands shown	[108,145]

2.5. Future Perspectives of the Development and Applications of Fluorescent Turn-On Ligands

As seen from above sections, most ligands have different binding modes, and G4 and other nucleic acid structural motifs can sometimes significantly influence the ligand's fluorescence enhancement [122]. This raises some concerns that need to be addressed: is the ligand-binding mechanism to G4s dependent on the loop length, bulge, inter versus intra-molecular G4s, parallel versus antiparallel G4 topologies, or number of G-quartets? Understanding the binding modes between the ligands and G4s, as well as the dimensions of the G4s grooves, is critical to understanding the mechanism of interactions between the ligands and G4s. Also, future high-resolution 3D structures with bound ligands will potentially allow a better picture of the ligand binding modes for future ligand design and G4 targeting.

Also, some of these ligands showed a decreased fluorescent enhancement in presence of other competing ligands, as such, ligand competition studies with other ligands are needed to fully ascertain the selectivity of the ligands of interest, this will allow the design and development of ligands with better fluorescent properties and this could prevent the off-target effects of some of these ligands (that leads to cell cytotoxicity) [87], and can also address the false positive and false negative results [97] produced by some of the ligands as a result of their abilities to induce topological changes [101]. More so, as mentioned earlier, only few of these ligands can effectively penetrate the cells [107] and reach their desired target [108]. Therefore, permeability, affinity, and selectivity are critical factors that need to be further improved when designing and developing advance novel fluorescence G4 probes.

Lastly, application-wise, many of these ligands are not yet applied in vivo [133] and can only allow monitoring of G4s in fixed cells [136], while others still requires RNAs to be transfected into cells to increase their concentration and thus signal [142]. Therefore, more advanced ligands are required with an improved property to reach their targets in cells and across different species, as well as increase their potential for real-time monitoring and single G4 detection application. We anticipate that, by addressing these issues, we could shed lights into the better understanding of the folding status, dynamics, and localization of G4s in cells and their biological roles in different cellular processes.

3. G-Quadruplex-Containing Nucleic Acid Aptamers

While biologically-relevant G4 targets can be detected and visualized by fluorescent turn-on ligands in vitro and in cells as described above, another exciting and emerging field of research is the identification and development of G4-containing aptamers, which may serve as molecular tools for diverse chemical and biological applications. Aptamers are single-stranded DNA or RNA sequences that are able to recognize natural and synthetic targets ranging from metal ions, small molecules, dyes, proteins, toxins, microbes, and cells [149]. The most well-established screening method for nucleic acid aptamers is the iterative SELEX process, which selects aptamers for targets of interest from a library of random sequences [150]. Aptamers are proposed to function as alternatives to other affinity reagents (e.g., protein-based antibodies) owing to several key advantages, such as simple synthesis and modification, design flexibility, high target specificity, and good stability. These properties can be successfully exploited in drug delivery, molecular imaging, clinical diagnosis, and biochemical research [151,152].

Aptamers can adopt various structural arrangements, which enable their recognition functionality. Among several architectures, the G4 structures are commonly found in aptamers [153]. One possible reason is that G4s involve sophisticated tertiary folding and display remarkable structure polymorphism and tunable conformation depending on the oligonucleotide sequences and different conditions of cations, ligands, or pH level [48,154], which give them strong structural discriminatory ability and contribute to their affinity and specificity for target binding. In addition, the high negative charge density of G4 gives them an advantage in the selection process for binding to positively charged surfaces of targets, such as proteins with positively charged amino acids (e.g., arginine, lysine, histidine) and metal ions via electrostatic interactions [153]. The first reported G4-containing aptamer was a 15-nucleotide thrombin-binding DNA aptamer, with the sequence of d(GGTTGGTGTGGTTGG) (Table 2), first selected using SELEX to bind thrombin [155]. The aptamer structure was later determined in NMR study to consist of two G-quartets [156]. Other G4-containing DNA aptamers have since been reported against targets including proteins and small molecules (Table 2). RNA is also equipped to form aptamers owing to its great structural flexibility that recognize small molecules, as exemplified in naturally occurring riboswitches [157,158]. A list of representative G4s-containing DNA and RNA aptamers is shown in Table 2.

The existence of G4 structures in aptamers ideally combines the superior properties of G4 and the intrinsic binding capabilities of aptamers. These features favor the application of G4-containing aptamers in biosensing, bioimaging, and therapeutics, as described below (Figure 3).

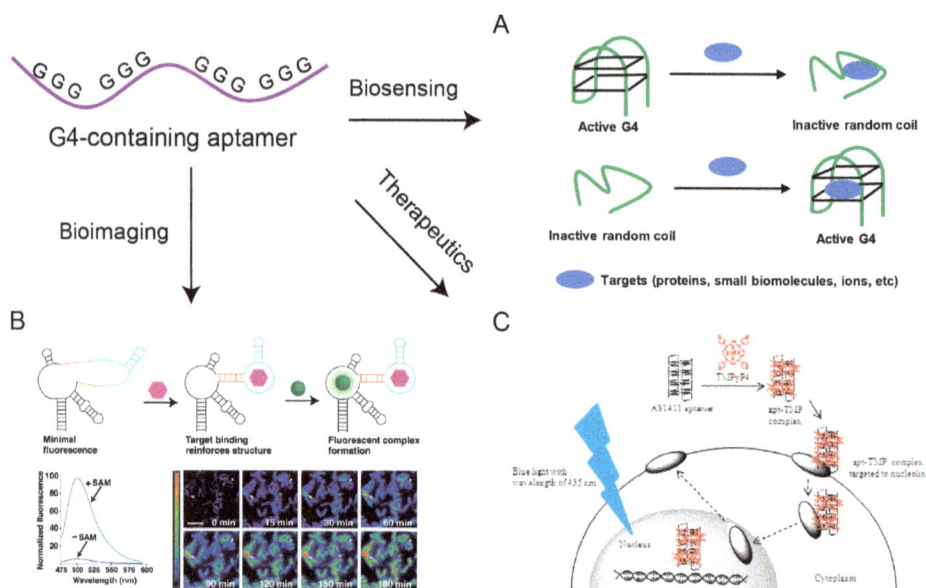

Figure 3. Representative applications of G-quadruplex-containing aptamers in biosensing, bioimaging and therapeutics. (**A**) Biosensors based on the conformational change of G-quadruplex-containing aptamers. Targets binding can destabilize/stabilize the G4 structure of aptamers and this conformational change is designed to cause signal change in the system. (**B**) Imaging metabolite (e.g., SAM) in living cells with fluorogenic RNA [159]. Reprinted with permission from [159]. Copyright 2012 American Association for the Advancement of Science. (**C**) Proposed mechanism of a photodynamic therapy strategy by using AS1411 as drug carrier to target cancer cells [160]. Reprinted with permission from [160].Copyright 2010 American Chemical Society.

3.1. Biosensing Applications of G-Quadruplex-Containing Aptamers

Biomolecules are of great importance in regulating various biochemical reactions and cellular metabolic processes. Aptamer-based biosensors have been widely used for biomolecule detection and for understanding their biological functions [151,161]. In addition, by using disease-related biomolecules as analytes, aptamer-based biosensors have become powerful diagnostic tools [162]. Various sensing strategies and signal readout techniques are used to develop sensing systems for a variety of targets [151]. Here, we summarize the fluorometric biomolecule aptasensors that utilize the G4 structure of aptamers in strategic design. Most aptasensors are based on the conformational switching of aptamers. Target binding can cause distortion on aptamers and stabilize or destabilize the G4 structure (Figure 3A). This conformational switch can be effectively monitored by several fluorescence signal output methods, such as nanomaterials [163,164], molecular beacons [165] and organic dyes, especially G4-selective fluorogenic ligands [99,117,166–169], which can give a fluorescence response upon target binding. Examples of the use of fluorometric G4 aptamer-based biosensors include the detection of proteins, small biomolecules and cations.

Regarding protein detection, thrombin has been employed as an analyte in some aptasensors. Li et al. [163] developed a FRET aptasensor for thrombin in both buffer and blood serum based on a fluorescein amidite (FAM)-labelled aptamer and graphene. A single-stranded thrombin aptamer was absorbed onto the surface of graphene due to noncovalent assembly and the fluorescence of FAM was quenched because of the FRET effect. With the addition of thrombin, it interacted with the aptamer and formed a G4-thrombin complex, which had weak affinity to the graphene and thus dissociated from the graphene, resulting in fluorescence recovery. A similar aptasensor was developed by Chu and coworkers using MoS$_2$ nanosheets and an FAM-labelled thrombin aptamer [164]. In some other assays, nucleic acid-interacting dyes are used to avoid labelling of aptamers. Zhou et al. [166] designed a thrombin aptasensor based on a four-branched pyrazine derivative (TASPI). The thrombin aptamer can eliminate the fluorescence of TASPI, whereas in the presence of thrombin, its aptamer specifically bound to thrombin and folded into a G4 structure, releasing TASPI molecules. Liu et al. [99] reported a FRET-based aptasensor for thrombin by using ThT as an energy acceptor and a water-soluble conjugated polymer (CP) as an energy donor. In this approach, ThT was bound to a thrombin aptamer (TBA) first, which induced TBA to fold into a G4 structure, forming a fluorescent ThT–TBA complex. The electrostatic attractions between the ThT–TBA complex and CP resulted in a high FRET signal. While in the presence of thrombin, TBA formed a G4-thrombin complex first, resulting in a longer distance between ThT and CP, which led to a low FRET signal. This method can also be used for human serum thrombin detection.

Regarding G4 aptamer-based fluorometric biosensors for small biomolecules, ATP has been used as a target in many assays because of its biological significance. In these assays, G4-selective fluorescent ligands were widely used to transduce the target binding into a fluorescence signal change. For example, Ji et al. [167] developed an ATP detection method using an ATP aptamer and ThT. The G4 structure of the ATP aptamer allowed the intercalation of ThT to produce strong fluorescence. However, upon ATP binding to its aptamer, a conformation change occurred in the aptamer. ThT was released into the solution, causing drastic suppression of the fluorescence intensity. This method was capable of detecting ATP in human serum and cell extracts. Other methods adopting similar principles have also been reported for ATP detection by using other G4 selective fluorescent ligands, such as CV [117], zinc(II)-protoporphyrin IX [168], and berberine [169]. An alternative approach to detecting ATP was based on a molecular beacon as the signal output. Willner et al. [165] assembled ATP aptamers into hairpin DNA, which was modified with a fluorescent dye (FAM) as a fluorophore at its 5′ terminus and a black hole quencher (BHQ1) at its 3′ terminus. In the absence of ATP, FAM, and BHQ1 were in close proximity, resulting in fluorescence quenching of FAM due to the FRET effect. However, in the presence of ATP, the hairpin DNA switched to a G4 structure and was bound to ATP. The re-organized G4 hairpin structure allowed Exo III to hydrolytically digest the 3′-end strand, and thus BHQ1 was released into solution and the fluorescence of FAM was recovered.

Pei et al. [170] used G4 aptamer-based fluorometric biosensors for cation detection. They proposed a sensing strategy for Pb^{2+} based on target-induced G4 formation and found a G-rich sequence (AGRO100) that works as a Pb^{2+} aptamer and forms a G4 conformation induced by Pb^{2+}. The G4-Pb^{2+} complex binds to NMM, giving a turn-on fluorescence response to Pb^{2+}. Another interesting work reported by the Wei group achieved the in vivo detection of K$^+$ in living organisms (brains and tumors) [171]. They selected a G-rich DNA probe that was selectively induced to form a parallel G4 by K$^+$. The G4-K$^+$ complex can enhance the fluorescence of PPIX. Thus, the concentration of K$^+$ could be detected by modulating the fluorescence of the system. A similar study was reported by Tan et al. [172] for human blood K$^+$ detection using a G4 aptamer of K$^+$ and a G4-binding ligand (EBMVC-B). This was the first attempt to exploit G4 aptamer-based fluorescent sensing for direct assay of blood targets. This concept also holds great potential for other ions' detection by selecting their corresponding G4-containing aptamers.

3.2. Bioimaging Applications of G-Quadruplex-Containing Aptamers

Monitoring the distribution and tracking of intracellular biomolecules contributes to the understanding of their cellular location, dynamics, and functions, which is vital for gene regulation, disease diagnosis, and drug discovery [173]. Fluorescence imaging is a major technique for identifying the expression and spatial and temporal dynamics of biomolecules [174]. A few G4-containing aptamer-based strategies have been reported for bioimaging applications.

A particular example of this application is RNA Spinach, which is a 98nt SELEX-identified RNA aptamer that can fold into a G4 structure and switch on the fluorescence of 3,5-difluoro-4-hydroxybenzylidene imidazolinone (DFHBI) [175]. RNA Spinach has been demonstrated to be a powerful bioimaging tool because of its strong resistance to photo-bleaching [175]. Spinach was successfully implemented for RNA imaging in living mammalian cells [175] and bacteria [176], as well for cellular metabolite [159] and protein [177] imaging in bacteria. The common strategy of Spinach-based bioimaging is to express 'fusion RNAs' that comprise Spinach and an additional RNA tag that can recognize targets and give a fluorescence response. For example, Jaffrey and coworkers [159] established a strategy to image cellular metabolites in *E. coli* based on Spinach (Figure 3B). They fused the target-binding aptamer to RNA Spinach via a transducer stem and destroyed the G4 motif of Spinach. Target binding to the aptamer promoted stabilization of the transducer stem, enabling Spinach to fold and activating DFHBI fluorescence. They also adapted this approach to monitor protein levels in *E. coli* [177]. In addition to the original Spinach, other versions of Spinach, like Spinach-mini [175], Spinach1.2 [178], Spinach2 [178], Spinach2-mini [179] and Baby Spinach [180], all adopt a G4 structure. A compelling alternative to RNA Spinach has been identified by in vitro selection, termed as Mango. Mango has a more rigid G4 structure, which activates the fluorescence of thiazole orange derivatives [109]. RNA Mango has also been used to bioimaging systems. For example, Jepsen et al. [181] developed a FRET sensing system by using RNA origami scaffolds consisting of Spinach and Mango. The fluorescent aptamers Spinach and Mango were placed in close proximity to obtain FRET and a new fluorophore was synthesized to increase the spectral overlap. The FRET-based constructs were finally expressed in *E. coli*. These bioimaging applications reveal the fact that G4-containing aptamers can provide promising platform for efficient intracellular monitoring of biomolecules in living cells and organisms.

3.3. Therapeutic Applications of G-Quadruplex-Containing Aptamers

For therapeutic functions, several G-quartet-containing oligonucleotides have been demonstrated to have potential as drugs, such as HIV inhibitors [182,183]. DNA sequences (termed 93del and 112del) adopting the G4 folding topology have been reported to exhibit anti-HIV1 integrase activity in a nanomolar range [182,183]. Another DNA aptamer (T30695) with a sequence similar to that of 93del and 112del but with a rather different G4 folding topology has also been identified as an HIV1 integrase inhibitor [182]. Despite the existence of quite a few anti-HIV1 integrase aptamers, delivering them to intracellular targets is still a challenge. Jing et al. [184] developed a system to deliver an HIV1 integrase inhibitor (T40214) into the target cell nuclei, which successfully decreased HIV1 replication, thus demonstrating the possible use of G4-containing nucleic acid aptamers as anti-HIV drugs.

The AS1411 aptamer is a 26nt G-rich DNA sequence that can fold into a G4 structures and bind to nucleolin with strong affinity and specificity [185]. AS1411 has been widely employed to target higher nucleolin-expressing cancer cells. For example, Shieh et al. [160] developed an aptamer-based photodynamic therapy strategy by using AS1411 as a drug carrier to target cancer cells (Figure 3C). Willner and co-workers [186] also designed a drug delivery method based on AS1411-functionalized metal–organic framework nanoparticles loaded with anti-cancer drugs. AS141 was used to target the cancer cells, and VEGF in the target cells can trigger the release of the anti-cancer drug. This concept could be adapted to other diseases that involve cellular biomarkers and their aptamers as gating units.

3.4. Current Challenges and Future Perspectives of the Development and Applications of G4-Containing Aptamers

Since the thrombin-binding aptamer (TBA, Table 2) was first identified as a G4-containing aptamer, G4 structure has been reported in a number of DNA and RNA aptamers towards various targets (Table 2). The potential applications of these G4-containing aptamers have been illustrated in different areas as discussed earlier. Nonetheless, the development and applications are still in the early stages and suffer from several challenges.

Firstly, high-resolution structures of targets with and without aptamer bound are necessary to reveal the structural basis of these complexes, which will allow development and optimization of aptamer's sequence and structure, and provide insights to further enhance the aptamer's properties for desired applications. So far, only a few G4-containing aptamers have been structurally determined (TBA, Spinach, Mango, etc.) [156,187,188], whereas the structures of other G4-containing aptamers are still poorly understood, making it challenging to improve the design and properties of those G4-containing aptamers. In addition, as the number of G4-containing aptamer is still limited, identifying novel G4-containing aptamers against new targets will broaden the scope of this research area.

Secondly, the folding of G4-containing aptamers should be experimentally investigated to ensure their specificity both in vitro and vivo, as the aptamer structure might re-fold in cellular environment. The selected aptamers' folding can be inhibited by cell machinery and physiochemical environment when used in cells/in vivo, which decrease the aptamer's ability to bind to targets. Therefore, more tests in different conditions are required to ensure the aptamer specificity. In addition, new experimental structure mapping techniques [32,48] and cell imaging have been developed to examine G4 folding, allowing us to verify the formation of G4 structure in the G4-containing aptamer in both in vitro and in vivo settings.

Thirdly, most of the G4-containing aptamer-based systems are still proof-of-concept studies, which were performed in vitro or in cells. The application of them from bench to diagnosis and therapy are still elusive and need to be fully investigated. One main obstacle for therapeutic applications is the biological barrier existing during the drug delivery process [161], such as cell membrane internalization. In addition, the nucleases present in biological system also pose another key issue. To solve these, more efforts should be made to develop G4-containing aptamer-based systems that can penetrate across the biological barrier, such as the use of other biocompatible species like nanomaterials to facilitate intracellular delivery of the therapeutic G4-containing aptamers [189]. To resist nuclease digestion and increase G4-containing aptamer's lifetime in cells/in vivo, unnatural nucleotide base modifications can be used, such as 2'O-methylation, lock nucleic acids, and phosphothioate. Further improvement in this area will facilitate the better G4-containing aptamer stability and delivery in complex system. Taken together, with these challenges to be addressed, G4-containing aptamers will likely achieve their diagnostic and therapeutic potential, leading to a new chapter in the application of G4-containing aptamer research.

Table 2. Representative list of G-quadruplex-containing nucleic acid aptamers.

Aptamer	Target	Sequence (5'-3')	Length	Ref.
		DNA G-quadruplex-containing aptamers		
TBA	Thrombin	d(GGTTGGTGTGGTTGG)	15	[156]
AS1411	Nucleolin	d(GGTGGTGGTGGTTGTGGTGGTGGTGG)	26	[85]
T40214	Stat3 [a]	d(GGGCGGGCGGGCGGGGC)	16	[190]
T40231	Stat3	d(GGTGGTGTGGTGGG)	14	[190]
22AG	Human TEBPs [b]	d(AGGGTTAGGGTTAGGGTTAGGG)	22	[95]
N.A.	Ciliate TEBPs	d(TTTTGGGGTTTTGGGG)	16	[191]
ISIS5320	HIV-1 gp120	d(TTGGGGTT)	8	[192]
93del	HIV-1 integrase	d(GGGGTGGGAGGAGGGT)	16	[82]
112del	HIV-1 integrase	d(CGGGCTGGGTGGGTGT)	16	[183]
T30695	HIV-1 integrase	d(GGGTGGGTGCGTGGGT)	16	[82]
RT5	HIV-1 reverse transcriptase	d(CAGGCGCCCGGGGGGGGTGGAATACAGTGATCAGCG)	35	[41]
RT6	HIV-1 reverse transcriptase	d(CAGGCGTTAGGGAAGGGCGTCGAAAGCAGGGTGGG)	35	[41]
RT47	HIV-1 reverse transcriptase	d(CAGGCCTTGGCGGGCCGGACAATGGAGAGATTT)	35	[41]
ODN93	HIV-1 reverse transcriptase	d(GGGGGTGGGAGGAGGGTAGGCCTTAGGTTTCTGA)	34	[193]
r10/43.	HCV RdRp [c]	d(GGGCGTGCGTGGGTGGGGTACTAATAATGTGCGTTTG)	36	[194]
G5	SARS Coronavirus Helicase	d(AGCGGGCCATATGCTGTGTGGGTGTATGGTC)	30	[195]
N.A.	Insulin	d(GGTGTGCGGGGGGGTTGGTAGGGTGTCTTC)	30	[196]
N.A.	Hematoporphyrin IX	d(ATGGGGTCGGCGCGGGCCGGGTGTC)	24	[197]
PS2M	Hemin	d(GTGGGTAGGGCGGGTTGG)	18	[198]
ABA	ATP	d(ACCTGGGGGAGTATTGCGGAGGAAGGT)	27	[67]
		RNA G-quadruplex-containing aptamers		
Spinach	DFHBI [d]	r(GACGCAACUGAAUGAAAUGGUGAAGGACGGUCCAGGUGUGCCUGCUUCGGCCAGUGCAGCUUGUUGAGUAGAGUGUGAGCGUCCUGCUGUAACUAGUCCGCGUC)	98	[175]
Spinach mini	DFHBI	r(GACGCGACCGAAAUGGUGAAGGACGGUCCAGUGCUUCGGCACUGUUGAGUAGAGUGUGAGCUCCGUAACUGGUCCGCGUC)	80	[175]
Spinach1.2	DFHBI	r(GACGCGACCGAAUGAAAUGGUGAAGGACGGUCCAGCCGGCUUCGGCCGGCUCCGUAACUGGUCCGCGUC)	95	[178]
Spinach2	DFHBI	r(GAUGUAACUGAAUGAAAUGGUGAAGGACGGUCCAGGUGUGGCUUCGGCCAGCCUACUUGUUGAGUAGAGUGUGAGCUCCGUAACUAGUUACAUC)	95	[178]
Spinach2 mini	DFHBI	r(GAUGUAACUGAAAUGGUGAAGGACGGUCCAGUGCUUCGGCACUGUUGAGAGUGUGAGCUCCGUAACUAGUUACAUC)	80	[179]
Baby Spinach	DFHBI	r(GGUGAAGGACGGUCCAGUAGUCCGUACUGUUGAGAGUGUGAGCUCC)	51	[180]
Broccoli	DFHBI	r(GAGACGGUCGGGUCCAGAUAUUCGUAUCUGUCGAGUAGAGUGUGGGCUC)	49	[199]

Table 2. *Cont.*

Aptamer	Target	Sequence (5'-3')	Length	Ref.
Corn	DFHO[e]	r(CGAGGAAGGAGGUCUGAGGAGGUCACUG)	28	[200]
Mango	Thiazole orange-biotin	r(GGCACGUACGAAGGGACCGUGCCGAGGACGAGAGUACGUG)	39	[109]
Mango-II	Thiazole orange-biotin	r(GCCUACGAAGGAGGAGGAAGGAGGAGAGUACGC)	36	[201]
Mango-III	Thiazole orange-biotin	r(GCUACGAAGGAAGGAAUUCGUAUGUGGUAUAUUCGUAGC)	38	[202]
ApT4-A	Thyroxine hormone	r(GUGGAGGGGGACGUGCUGCAUCCGCAGUGCGUCUUGGGUUGUG)	44	[203]
N.A.	Human receptor activator of NF-*k*B	r(ACGGAUUCGUAUGGGUGGGAUCGGAAGGGCUACGAACACCGU)	43	[204]
N.A.	HIV-1 integrase	r(GGAGGGGAGGGGAU) or r(GGAGUUAGGGGCU)	13	[205]
N.A.	Prion protein rPrP23-231	r(CACUGCUACCUUAGAGUAGAGCGGGACGAGGGUUGUUGGGACGUGGGUAUGAUCC AUACAUUAGGAAGCUGGUGAGCUGGCACC)	86	[206]
N2	Trypanosome	r(AAGAAGCGCGCGAGGCACGACGCAGGCAGUGAGCGCUGUCCGA)	43	[207]

[a], Signal transducer and activator of transcription 3; [b], Telomere end-binding proteins; [c], RNA-dependent RNA polymerase; [d], 3,5-difluoro-4-hydroxybenzylidene imidazolinone; [e], 3,5-difluoro-4-hydroxybenzylidene-imidazolinone-2-oxime.

4. Conclusions

Over the years, impressive progress has been made in the G4 field with respect to G4 fluorescent turn-on ligands and G4-containing aptamers. Remarkable discoveries and applications have been reported in these two promising fields, including the interaction mechanism and applications of several classes of G4 fluorescent turn-on ligands (Table 1), as well as the G4-containing aptamers (Table 2) and their uses in biosensing, bioimaging, and therapy. With such developments achieved in the investigation and applications of G4s, the study of G4 fluorescent turn-on ligands and G4-containing aptamers is expected to open new perspectives towards wider biological understanding and applications of G4s both in vitro and in cells.

Author Contributions: Writing—original draft preparation, M.I.U., D.J., C.-Y.C., and C.K.K.; Writing—review and editing, M.I.U., D.J., C.-Y.C., and C.K.K.; Funding acquisition, C.K.K. and M.I.U.

Funding: The Kwok laboratory is funded by the Research Grants Council of the Hong Kong SAR, China (project nos. CityU 21302317, CityU 11100218, N_CityUI110/17), the Croucher Foundation (project no. 9500030), and City University of Hong Kong (project no. 9680261). M.I.U. received some support from the Petroleum Technology Development Fund from the Nigerian government.

Acknowledgments: We thank the Kwok lab members for discussion. We apologize to colleagues whose works are not cited due to space limitations.

Conflicts of Interest: The authors declare no conflict of interest.

References

1. Davis, J.T. G-quartets 40 years later: From 5′-GMP to molecular biology and supramolecular chemistry. *Angew. Chem.* **2004**, *43*, 668–698. [CrossRef] [PubMed]
2. The Role of Cations in Determining Quadruplex Structure and Stability. In *Quadruplex Nucleic Acids*; Neidle, S.; Balasubramanian, S. (Eds.) The Royal Society of Chemistry: London, UK, 2006; pp. 100–130.
3. Huppert, J.L.; Balasubramanian, S. Prevalence of quadruplexes in the human genome. *Nucleic Acids Res.* **2005**, *33*, 2908–2916. [CrossRef] [PubMed]
4. Hazel, P.; Huppert, J.; Balasubramanian, S.; Neidle, S. Loop-Length-Dependent Folding of G-Quadruplexes. *J. Am. Chem. Soc.* **2004**, *126*, 16405–16415. [CrossRef] [PubMed]
5. Guedin, A.; Gros, J.; Alberti, P.; Mergny, J.L. How long is too long? Effects of loop size on G-quadruplex stability. *Nucleic Acids Res.* **2010**, *38*, 7858–7868. [CrossRef] [PubMed]
6. Varizhuk, A.; Ischenko, D.; Tsvetkov, V.; Novikov, R.; Kulemin, N.; Kaluzhny, D.; Vlasenok, M.; Naumov, V.; Smirnov, I.; Pozmogova, G. The expanding repertoire of G4 DNA structures. *Biochimie* **2017**, *135*, 54–62. [CrossRef] [PubMed]
7. Mukundan, V.T.; Phan, A.T. Bulges in G-quadruplexes: Broadening the definition of G-quadruplex-forming sequences. *J. Am. Chem. Soc.* **2013**, *135*, 5017–5028. [CrossRef] [PubMed]
8. Das, K.; Srivastava, M.; Raghavan, S.C. GNG Motifs Can Replace a GGG Stretch during G-Quadruplex Formation in a Context Dependent Manner. *PLoS ONE* **2016**, *11*, e0158794. [CrossRef] [PubMed]
9. Qin, M.; Chen, Z.; Luo, Q.; Wen, Y.; Zhang, N.; Jiang, H.; Yang, H. Two-quartet G-quadruplexes formed by DNA sequences containing four contiguous GG runs. *J. Phys. Chem. B* **2015**, *119*, 3706–3713. [CrossRef]
10. Li, X.M.; Zheng, K.W.; Zhang, J.Y.; Liu, H.H.; He, Y.D.; Yuan, B.F.; Hao, Y.H.; Tan, Z. Guanine-vacancy-bearing G-quadruplexes responsive to guanine derivatives. *Proc. Natl. Acad. Sci. USA* **2015**, *112*, 14581–14586. [CrossRef]
11. Heddi, B.; Martin-Pintado, N.; Serimbetov, Z.; Kari, T.M.; Phan, A.T. G-quadruplexes with (4n-1) guanines in the G-tetrad core: Formation of a G-triad.water complex and implication for small-molecule binding. *Nucleic Acids Res.* **2016**, *44*, 910–916. [CrossRef]
12. Lim, K.W.; Phan, A.T. Structural basis of DNA quadruplex-duplex junction formation. *Angew. Chem.* **2013**, *52*, 8566–8569. [CrossRef] [PubMed]
13. Bing, T.; Zheng, W.; Zhang, X.; Shen, L.; Liu, X.; Wang, F.; Cui, J.; Cao, Z.; Shangguan, D. Triplex-quadruplex structural scaffold: A new binding structure of aptamer. *Sci. Rep.* **2017**, *7*, 15467. [CrossRef] [PubMed]
14. Zhang, S.; Wu, Y.; Zhang, W. G-quadruplex structures and their interaction diversity with ligands. *ChemMedChem* **2014**, *9*, 899–911. [CrossRef] [PubMed]

15. Dvorkin, S.A.; Karsisiotis, A.I.; Webba da Silva, M. Encoding canonical DNA quadruplex structure. *Sci. Adv.* **2018**, *4*, eaat3007. [CrossRef] [PubMed]
16. Rhodes, D.; Lipps, H.J. G-quadruplexes and their regulatory roles in biology. *Nucleic Acids Res.* **2015**, *43*, 8627–8637. [CrossRef] [PubMed]
17. Fay, M.M.; Lyons, S.M.; Ivanov, P. RNA G-Quadruplexes in Biology: Principles and Molecular Mechanisms. *J. Mol. Biol.* **2017**, *429*, 2127–2147. [CrossRef] [PubMed]
18. Hansel-Hertsch, R.; Di Antonio, M.; Balasubramanian, S. DNA G-quadruplexes in the human genome: Detection, functions and therapeutic potential. *Nat. Rev. Mol. Cell Biol.* **2017**, *18*, 279–284. [CrossRef]
19. Harris, L.M.; Merrick, C.J. G-quadruplexes in pathogens: A common route to virulence control? *PLoS Pathog.* **2015**, *11*, e1004562. [CrossRef]
20. Kikin, O.; D'Antonio, L.; Bagga, P.S. QGRS Mapper: A web-based server for predicting G-quadruplexes in nucleotide sequences. *Nucleic Acids Res.* **2006**, *34*, W676–W682. [CrossRef]
21. Bedrat, A.; Lacroix, L.; Mergny, J.-L. Re-evaluation of G-quadruplex propensity with G4Hunter. *Nucleic Acids Res.* **2016**, *44*, 1746–1759. [CrossRef]
22. Garant, J.M.; Perreault, J.P.; Scott, M.S. Motif independent identification of potential RNA G-quadruplexes by G4RNA screener. *Bioinformatics (Oxf. Engl.)* **2017**, *33*, 3532–3537. [CrossRef] [PubMed]
23. Sahakyan, A.B.; Chambers, V.S.; Marsico, G.; Santner, T.; Di Antonio, M.; Balasubramanian, S. Machine learning model for sequence-driven DNA G-quadruplex formation. *Sci. Rep.* **2017**, *7*, 14535. [CrossRef] [PubMed]
24. del Villar-Guerra, R.; Trent, J.O.; Chaires, J.B. G-Quadruplex Secondary Structure Obtained from Circular Dichroism Spectroscopy. *Angew. Chem. Int. Ed. Engl.* **2018**, *57*, 7171–7175. [CrossRef] [PubMed]
25. Mergny, J.-L.; Phan, A.-T.; Lacroix, L. Following G-quartet formation by UV-spectroscopy. *FEBS Lett.* **1998**, *435*, 74–78. [CrossRef]
26. Scalabrin, M.; Palumbo, M.; Richter, S.N. Highly Improved Electrospray Ionization-Mass Spectrometry Detection of G-Quadruplex-Folded Oligonucleotides and Their Complexes with Small Molecules. *Anal. Chem.* **2017**, *89*, 8632–8637. [CrossRef]
27. Webba da Silva, M. NMR methods for studying quadruplex nucleic acids. *Methods (San Diego Calif.)* **2007**, *43*, 264–277. [CrossRef] [PubMed]
28. Mendez, M.A.; Szalai, V.A. Fluorescence of unmodified oligonucleotides: A tool to probe G-quadruplex DNA structure. *Biopolymers* **2009**, *91*, 841–850. [CrossRef]
29. Han, H.; Hurley, L.H.; Salazar, M. A DNA polymerase stop assay for G-quadruplex-interactive compounds. *Nucleic Acids Res.* **1999**, *27*, 537–542. [CrossRef]
30. Williamson, J.R.; Raghuraman, M.K.; Cech, T.R. Monovalent cation-induced structure of telomeric DNA: The G-quartet model. *Cell* **1989**, *59*, 871–880. [CrossRef]
31. Kwok, C.K.; Balasubramanian, S. Targeted Detection of G-Quadruplexes in Cellular RNAs. *Angew. Chem. Int. Ed. Engl.* **2015**, *54*, 6751–6754. [CrossRef]
32. Kwok, C.K.; Sahakyan, A.B.; Balasubramanian, S. Structural Analysis using SHALiPE to Reveal RNA G-Quadruplex Formation in Human Precursor MicroRNA. *Angew. Chem. Int. Ed.* **2016**, *55*, 8958–8961. [CrossRef] [PubMed]
33. Chambers, V.S.; Marsico, G.; Boutell, J.M.; Di Antonio, M.; Smith, G.P.; Balasubramanian, S. High-throughput sequencing of DNA G-quadruplex structures in the human genome. *Nat. Biotechnol.* **2015**, *33*, 877–881. [CrossRef] [PubMed]
34. Hänsel-Hertsch, R.; Beraldi, D.; Lensing, S.V.; Marsico, G.; Zyner, K.; Parry, A.; Di Antonio, M.; Pike, J.; Kimura, H.; Narita, M.; et al. G-quadruplex structures mark human regulatory chromatin. *Nat. Genet.* **2016**, *48*, 1267. [CrossRef] [PubMed]
35. Kwok, C.K.; Marsico, G.; Sahakyan, A.B. rG4-seq reveals widespread formation of G-quadruplex structures in the human transcriptome. *Nat. Methods* **2016**, *13*, 841–844. [CrossRef] [PubMed]
36. Guo, J.U.; Bartel, D.P. RNA G-quadruplexes are globally unfolded in eukaryotic cells and depleted in bacteria. *Science (N.Y.)* **2016**, *353*, aaf5371. [CrossRef] [PubMed]
37. Yang, S.Y.; Lejault, P.; Chevrier, S.; Boidot, R.; Robertson, A.G.; Wong, J.M.Y.; Monchaud, D. Transcriptome-wide identification of transient RNA G-quadruplexes in human cells. *Nat. Commun.* **2018**, *9*, 4730. [CrossRef] [PubMed]

38. Collie, G.W.; Parkinson, G.N. The application of DNA and RNA G-quadruplexes to therapeutic medicines. *Chem. Soc. Rev.* **2011**, *40*, 5867–5892. [CrossRef] [PubMed]

39. Tian, T.; Xiao, H.; Zhou, X. A Review: G-Quadruplex's Applications in Biological Target Detection and Drug Delivery. *Curr. Top. Med. Chem.* **2015**, *15*, 1988–2001. [CrossRef]

40. Platella, C.; Riccardi, C.; Montesarchio, D.; Roviello, G.N.; Musumeci, D. G-quadruplex-based aptamers against protein targets in therapy and diagnostics. *Biochim. Biophys. Acta Gener. Subj.* **2017**, *1861*, 1429–1447. [CrossRef]

41. Michalowski, D.; Chitima-Matsiga, R.; Held, D.M.; Burke, D.H. Novel bimodular DNA aptamers with guanosine quadruplexes inhibit phylogenetically diverse HIV-1 reverse transcriptases. *Nucleic Acids Res.* **2008**, *36*, 7124–7135. [CrossRef]

42. Andreola, M.-L.; Pileur, F.; Calmels, C.; Ventura, M.; Tarrago-Litvak, L.; Toulmé, J.-J.; Litvak, S. DNA Aptamers Selected against the HIV-1 RNase H Display in Vitro Antiviral Activity. *Biochemistry* **2001**, *40*, 10087–10094. [CrossRef] [PubMed]

43. Mashima, T.; Matsugami, A.; Nishikawa, F.; Nishikawa, S.; Katahira, M. Unique quadruplex structure and interaction of an RNA aptamer against bovine prion protein. *Nucleic Acids Res.* **2009**, *37*, 6249–6258. [CrossRef] [PubMed]

44. Rosenberg, J.E.; Bambury, R.M.; Van Allen, E.M.; Drabkin, H.A.; Lara, P.N., Jr.; Harzstark, A.L.; Wagle, N.; Figlin, R.A.; Smith, G.W.; Garraway, L.A.; et al. A phase II trial of AS1411 (a novel nucleolin-targeted DNA aptamer) in metastatic renal cell carcinoma. *Investig. New Drugs* **2014**, *32*, 178–187. [CrossRef] [PubMed]

45. Weerasinghe, P.; Li, Y.; Guan, Y.; Zhang, R.; Tweardy, D.J.; Jing, N. T40214/PEI complex: A potent therapeutics for prostate cancer that targets STAT3 signaling. *Prostate* **2008**, *68*, 1430–1442. [CrossRef] [PubMed]

46. Kwok, C.K.; Tang, Y.; Assmann, S.M.; Bevilacqua, P.C. The RNA structurome: Transcriptome-wide structure probing with next-generation sequencing. *Trends Biochem. Sci.* **2015**, *40*, 221–232. [CrossRef] [PubMed]

47. Kwok, C.K.; Marsico, G.; Balasubramanian, S. Detecting RNA G-Quadruplexes (rG4s) in the Transcriptome. *Cold Spring Harb. Perspect. Biol.* **2018**, *10*. [CrossRef]

48. Kwok, C.K.; Merrick, C.J. G-Quadruplexes: Prediction, Characterization, and Biological Application. *Trends Biotechnol.* **2017**, *35*, 997–1013. [CrossRef]

49. Chan, K.L.; Peng, B.; Umar, M.I.; Chan, C.Y.; Sahakyan, A.B.; Le, M.T.N.; Kwok, C.K. Structural analysis reveals the formation and role of RNA G-quadruplex structures in human mature microRNAs. *Chem. Commun.* **2018**, *54*, 10878–10881. [CrossRef]

50. Neidle, S.; Balasubramanian, S. *Quadruplex Nucleic Acids*; The Royal Society of Chemistry: London, UK, 2006.

51. Zhang, S.; Sun, H.; Wang, L.; Liu, Y.; Chen, H.; Li, Q.; Guan, A.; Liu, M.; Tang, Y. Real-time monitoring of DNA G-quadruplexes in living cells with a small-molecule fluorescent probe. *Nucleic Acids Res.* **2018**, *46*, 7522–7532. [CrossRef]

52. Shivalingam, A.; Izquierdo, M.A.; Le Marois, A.; Vysniauskas, A.; Suhling, K.; Kuimova, M.K.; Vilar, R. The interactions between a small molecule and G-quadruplexes are visualized by fluorescence lifetime imaging microscopy. *Nat. Commun.* **2015**, *6*, 8178. [CrossRef]

53. Ma, D.L.; Dong, Z.Z.; Vellaisamy, K.; Cheung, K.M.; Yang, G.; Leung, C.H. Luminescent Strategies for Label-Free G-Quadruplex-Based Enzyme Activity Sensing. *Chem. Rec.* **2017**, *17*, 1135–1145. [CrossRef] [PubMed]

54. Ma, D.L.; Zhang, Z.; Wang, M.; Lu, L.; Zhong, H.J.; Leung, C.H. Recent Developments in G-Quadruplex Probes. *Chem. Biol.* **2015**, *22*, 812–828. [CrossRef] [PubMed]

55. Ma, D.L.; Wang, M.; Lin, S.; Han, Q.B.; Leung, C.H. Recent Development of G-Quadruplex Probes for Cellular Imaging. *Curr. Top. Med. Chem.* **2015**, *15*, 1957–1963. [PubMed]

56. Vummidi, B.R.; Alzeer, J.; Luedtke, N.W. Fluorescent probes for G-quadruplex structures. *ChemBioChem Eur. J. Chem. Biol.* **2013**, *14*, 540–558. [CrossRef] [PubMed]

57. Leung, K.H.; He, H.Z.; Ma, V.P.; Chan, D.S.; Leung, C.H.; Ma, D.L. A luminescent G-quadruplex switch-on probe for the highly selective and tunable detection of cysteine and glutathione. *Chem. Commun.* **2013**, *49*, 771–773. [CrossRef] [PubMed]

58. Dong, Z.-Z.; Lu, L.; Wang, W.; Li, G.; Kang, T.-S.; Han, Q.; Leung, C.-H.; Ma, D.-L. Luminescent detection of nicking endonuclease Nb.BsmI activity by using a G-quadruplex-selective iridium(III) complex in aqueous solution. *Sens. Actuators B Chem.* **2017**, *246*, 826–832. [CrossRef]

59. Lin, S.; Lu, L.; Liu, J.B.; Liu, C.; Kang, T.S.; Yang, C.; Leung, C.H.; Ma, D.L. A G-quadruplex-selective luminescent iridium(III) complex and its application by long lifetime. *Biochim. Biophys. Acta. Gener. Subj.* **2017**, *1861*, 1448–1454. [CrossRef]

60. Lin, S.; Kang, T.S.; Lu, L.; Wang, W.; Ma, D.L.; Leung, C.H. A G-quadruplex-selective luminescent probe with an anchor tail for the switch-on detection of thymine DNA glycosylase activity. *Biosens. Bioelectron.* **2016**, *86*, 849–857. [CrossRef]

61. Lin, S.; Lu, L.; Kang, T.S.; Mergny, J.L.; Leung, C.H.; Ma, D.L. Interaction of an Iridium(III) Complex with G-Quadruplex DNA and Its Application in Luminescent Switch-On Detection of Siglec-5. *Anal. Chem.* **2016**, *88*, 10290–10295. [CrossRef]

62. Lu, L.; Wang, W.; Yang, C.; Kang, T.-S.; Leung, C.-H.; Ma, D.-L. Iridium(iii) complexes with 1,10-phenanthroline-based N^N ligands as highly selective luminescent G-quadruplex probes and application for switch-on ribonuclease H detection. *J. Mater. Chem. B* **2016**, *4*, 6791–6796. [CrossRef]

63. Ma, D.-L.; Che, C.-M.; Yan, S.-C. Platinum(II) Complexes with Dipyridophenazine Ligands as Human Telomerase Inhibitors and Luminescent Probes for G-Quadruplex DNA. *J. Am. Chem. Soc.* **2009**, *131*, 12. [CrossRef] [PubMed]

64. Yat-Wah Man, B.; Shiu-Hin Chan, D.; Yang, H.; Ang, S.-W.; Yang, F.; Yan, S.-C.; Ho, C.-M.; Wu, P.; Che, C.-M.; Leungy, C.-H.; et al. A selective G-quadruplex-based luminescent switch-on probe for the detection of nanomolar silver(I) ions in aqueous solutionw. *Chem. Commun.* **2010**, *46*, 3. [CrossRef]

65. Wang, P.; Leung, C.-H.; Ma, D.-L.; Yan, S.C.; Che, C.M. Structure-based design of platinum(II) complexes as c-myc oncogene down-regulators and luminescent probes for G-quadruplex DNA. *Chemistry* **2010**, *16*, 6900–6911. [CrossRef] [PubMed]

66. Suntharalingam, K.; White, A.J.; Vilar, R. Synthesis, structural characterization, and quadruplex DNA binding studies of platinum(II)-terpyridine complexes. *Inorg. Chem.* **2009**, *48*, 9427–9435. [CrossRef] [PubMed]

67. Naud-Martin, D.; Landras-Guetta, C.; Verga, D.; Ghosh, D.; Achelle, S.; Mahuteau-Betzer, F.; Bombard, S.; Teulade-Fichou, M.P. Selectivity of Terpyridine Platinum Anticancer Drugs for G-quadruplex DNA. *Molecules* **2019**, *24*, 404.

68. Piraux, G.; Bar, L.; Abraham, M.; Lavergne, T.; Jamet, H.; Dejeu, J.; Marcelis, L.; Defrancq, E.; Elias, B. New Ruthenium-Based Probes for Selective G-Quadruplex Targeting. *Chemistry* **2017**, *23*, 11872–11880. [CrossRef] [PubMed]

69. Wachter, E.; Howerton, B.S.; Hall, E.C.; Parkin, S.; Glazer, E.C. A new type of DNA "light-switch": A dual photochemical sensor and metalating agent for duplex and G-quadruplex DNA. *Chem. Commun.* **2014**, *50*, 311–313. [CrossRef]

70. Wachter, E.; Moya, D.; Parkin, S.; Glazer, E.C. Ruthenium Complex "Light Switches" that are Selective for Different G-Quadruplex Structures. *Chemistry* **2016**, *22*, 550–559. [CrossRef]

71. Gama, S.; Rodrigues, I.; Mendes, F.; Santos, I.C.; Gabano, E.; Klejevskaja, B.; Gonzalez-Garcia, J.; Ravera, M.; Vilar, R.; Paulo, A. Anthracene-terpyridine metal complexes as new G-quadruplex DNA binders. *J. Inorg. Biochem.* **2016**, *160*, 275–286. [CrossRef]

72. Tong, L.L.; Li, L.; Chen, Z.; Wang, Q.; Tang, B. Stable label-free fluorescent sensing of biothiols based on ThT direct inducing conformation-specific G-quadruplex. *Biosens. Bioelectron.* **2013**, *49*, 420–425. [CrossRef]

73. Huang, H.; Zhang, J.; Harvey, S.E.; Hu, X.; Cheng, C. RNA G-quadruplex secondary structure promotes alternative splicing via the RNA-binding protein hnRNPF. *Genes Dev.* **2017**, *31*, 2296–2309. [CrossRef] [PubMed]

74. Tang, X.; Wu, K.; Zhao, H.; Chen, M.; Ma, C. A Label-Free Fluorescent Assay for the Rapid and Sensitive Detection of Adenosine Deaminase Activity and Inhibition. *Sensors* **2018**, *18*, 2441. [CrossRef] [PubMed]

75. Huber, M.D.; Lee, D.C.; Maizels, N. G4 DNA unwinding by BLM and Sgs1p: Substrate specificity and substrate-specific inhibition. *Nucleic Acids Res.* **2002**, *30*, 3954–3961. [CrossRef] [PubMed]

76. Hu, D.; Pu, F.; Huang, Z.; Ren, J.; Qu, X. A quadruplex-based, label-free, and real-time fluorescence assay for RNase H activity and inhibition. *Chemistry* **2010**, *16*, 2605–2610. [CrossRef] [PubMed]

77. Yingfu Li, C.R.G.; Sen, D. Recognition of Anionic Porphyrins by DNA Aptamers. *Biochemistry* **1996**, *35*, 12. [CrossRef]

78. Haribabu Arthanari, S.B.; Kawano, T.L.; Bolton, P.H. Fluorescent dyes specific for quadruplex DNA. *Nucleic Acids Res.* **1998**, *26*, 5. [CrossRef]

79. Nicoludis, J.M.; Barrett, S.P.; Mergny, J.L.; Yatsunyk, L.A. Interaction of human telomeric DNA with N-methyl mesoporphyrin IX. *Nucleic Acids Res.* **2012**, *40*, 5432–5447. [CrossRef]

80. Tippana, R.; Xiao, W.; Myong, S. G-quadruplex conformation and dynamics are determined by loop length and sequence. *Nucleic Acids Res.* **2014**, *42*, 8106–8114. [CrossRef]

81. Sabharwal, N.C.; Savikhin, V.; Turek-Herman, J.R.; Nicoludis, J.M.; Szalai, V.A.; Yatsunyk, L.A. N-methylmesoporphyrin IX fluorescence as a reporter of strand orientation in guanine quadruplexes. *FEBS J.* **2014**, *281*, 1726–1737. [CrossRef]

82. Ren, J.; Qin, H.; Wang, J.; Luedtke, N.W.; Wang, E.; Wang, J. Label-free detection of nucleic acids by turn-on and turn-off G-quadruplex-mediated fluorescence. *Ana. Bioanal. Chem.* **2011**, *399*, 2763–2770. [CrossRef]

83. Li, M.; Zhao, A.; Ren, J.; Qu, X. N-Methyl Mesoporphyrin IX as an Effective Probe for Monitoring Alzheimer's Disease beta-Amyloid Aggregation in Living Cells. *ACS Chem. Neurosci.* **2017**, *8*, 1299–1304. [CrossRef] [PubMed]

84. Sun, Y.; Zhao, C.; Yan, Z.; Ren, J.; Qu, X. Simple and sensitive microbial pathogen detection using a label-free DNA amplification assay. *Chem. Commun.* **2016**, *52*, 5. [CrossRef] [PubMed]

85. Waller, Z.A.; Pinchbeck, B.J.; Buguth, B.S.; Meadows, T.G.; Richardson, D.J.; Gates, A.J. Control of bacterial nitrate assimilation by stabilization of G-quadruplex DNA. *Chem. Commun.* **2016**, *52*, 13511–13514. [CrossRef] [PubMed]

86. Zhu, L.N.; Zhao, S.J.; Wu, B.; Li, X.Z.; Kong, D.M. A new cationic porphyrin derivative (TMPipEOPP) with large side arm substituents: A highly selective G-quadruplex optical probe. *PLoS ONE* **2012**, *7*, e35586. [CrossRef] [PubMed]

87. Gabelica, V.; Maeda, R.; Fujimoto, T.; Yaku, H.; Murashima, T.; Sugimoto, N.; Miyoshi, D. Multiple and cooperative binding of fluorescence light-up probe thioflavin T with human telomere DNA G-quadruplex. *Biochemistry* **2013**, *52*, 5620–5628. [CrossRef] [PubMed]

88. Paramasivan, S.; Bolton, P.H. Mix and measure fluorescence screening for selective quadruplex binders. *Nucleic Acids Res.* **2008**, *36*, e106. [CrossRef] [PubMed]

89. Hu, D.; Huang, Z.; Pu, F.; Ren, J.; Qu, X. A label-free, quadruplex-based functional molecular beacon (LFG4-MB) for fluorescence turn-on detection of DNA and nuclease. *Chemistry* **2011**, *17*, 1635–1641. [CrossRef]

90. Zhao, C.; Wu, L.; Ren, J.; Qu, X. A label-free fluorescent turn-on enzymatic amplification assay for DNA detection using ligand-responsive G-quadruplex formation. *Chem. Commun.* **2011**, *47*, 5461–5463. [CrossRef]

91. Yao, X.; Song, D.; Qin, T.; Yang, C.; Yu, Z.; Li, X.; Liu, K.; Su, H. Interaction between G-Quadruplex and Zinc Cationic Porphyrin: The Role of the Axial Water. *Sci. Rep.* **2017**, *7*, 10951. [CrossRef]

92. Wheelhouse, R.T.; Sun, D.; Han, H.; Han, F.X.; Hurley, L.H. Cationic Porphyrins as Telomerase Inhibitors: The Interaction of Tetra-(N-methyl-4-pyridyl)porphine with Quadruplex DNA. *J. Am. Chem. Soc.* **1998**, *120*, 2. [CrossRef]

93. Biancalana, M.; Koide, S. Molecular mechanism of Thioflavin-T binding to amyloid fibrils. *Biochim. Biophysi. Acta* **2010**, *1804*, 1405–1412. [CrossRef] [PubMed]

94. Inbar, P.; Li, C.Q.; Takayama, S.A.; Bautista, M.R.; Yang, J. Oligo(ethylene glycol) derivatives of thioflavin T as inhibitors of protein-amyloid interactions. *ChemBioChem Eur. J. Chem. Biol.* **2006**, *7*, 1563–1566. [CrossRef]

95. Mohanty, J.; Barooah, N.; Dhamodharan, V.; Harikrishna, S.; Pradeepkumar, P.I.; Bhasikuttan, A.C. Thioflavin T as an efficient inducer and selective fluorescent sensor for the human telomeric G-quadruplex DNA. *J. Am. Chem. Soc.* **2013**, *135*, 367–376. [CrossRef] [PubMed]

96. Liu, S.; Peng, P.; Wang, H.; Shi, L.; Li, T. Thioflavin T binds dimeric parallel-stranded GA-containing non-G-quadruplex DNAs: A general approach to lighting up double-stranded scaffolds. *Nucleic Acids Res.* **2017**, *45*, 12080–12089. [CrossRef]

97. Renaud de la Faverie, A.; Guedin, A.; Bedrat, A.; Yatsunyk, L.A.; Mergny, J.L. Thioflavin T as a fluorescence light-up probe for G4 formation. *Nucleic Acids Res.* **2014**, *42*, e65. [CrossRef] [PubMed]

98. Lee, I.J.; Patil, S.P.; Fhayli, K.; Alsaiari, S.; Khashab, N.M. Probing structural changes of self assembled i-motif DNA. *Chem. Commun.* **2015**, *51*, 3747–3749. [CrossRef] [PubMed]

99. Liu, X.; Hua, X.; Fan, Q.; Chao, J.; Su, S.; Huang, Y.Q.; Wang, L.; Huang, W. Thioflavin T as an Efficient G-Quadruplex Inducer for the Highly Sensitive Detection of Thrombin Using a New Foster Resonance Energy Transfer System. *ACS Appl. Mater. Interfaces* **2015**, *7*, 16458–16465. [CrossRef]

100. Zeng, H.; Zhu, Y.; Ma, L.; Xia, X.; Li, Y.; Ren, Y.; Zhao, W.; Yang, H.; Deng, R. G-quadruplex specific dye-based ratiometric FRET aptasensor for robust and ultrafast detection of toxin. *Dyes Pigments* **2019**, *164*, 35–42. [CrossRef]

101. Yuka Kataoka, H.F.; Kasahara, Y.; Yoshihara, T.; Tobita, S.; Kuwahara, M. Minimal Thioflavin T Modifications Improve Visual Discrimination of Guanine-Quadruplex Topologies and Alter Compound-induced Topological Structures. *Anal. Chem.* **2014**, *86*, 12078–12084. [CrossRef] [PubMed]

102. Zhang, S.; Sun, H.; Chen, H.; Li, Q.; Guan, A.; Wang, L.; Shi, Y.; Xu, S.; Liu, M.; Tang, Y. Direct visualization of nucleolar G-quadruplexes in live cells by using a fluorescent light-up probe. *Biochim. Biophys. Acta Gener. Subj.* **2018**, *1862*, 1101–1106. [CrossRef]

103. Guan, A.J.; Zhang, X.F.; Sun, X.; Li, Q.; Xiang, J.F.; Wang, L.X.; Lan, L.; Yang, F.M.; Xu, S.J.; Guo, X.M.; et al. Ethyl-substitutive Thioflavin T as a highly-specific fluorescence probe for detecting G-quadruplex structure. *Sci. Rep.* **2018**, *8*, 2666. [CrossRef] [PubMed]

104. Fleming, A.M.; Ding, Y.; Alenko, A.; Burrows, C.J. Zika Virus Genomic RNA Possesses Conserved G-Quadruplexes Characteristic of the Flaviviridae Family. *ACS Infect. Dis.* **2016**, *2*, 674–681. [CrossRef] [PubMed]

105. Vinyard, W.A.; Fleming, A.M.; Ma, J.; Burrows, C.J. Characterization of G-Quadruplexes in Chlamydomonas reinhardtii and the Effects of Polyamine and Magnesium Cations on Structure and Stability. *Biochemistry* **2018**, *57*, 6551–6561. [CrossRef]

106. Zahin, M.; Dean, W.L.; Ghim, S.J.; Joh, J.; Gray, R.D.; Khanal, S.; Bossart, G.D.; Mignucci-Giannoni, A.A.; Rouchka, E.C.; Jenson, A.B.; et al. Identification of G-quadruplex forming sequences in three manatee papillomaviruses. *PLoS ONE* **2018**, *13*, 23. [CrossRef] [PubMed]

107. Luo, X.; Xue, B.; Feng, G.; Zhang, J.; Lin, B.; Zeng, P.; Li, H.; Yi, H.; Zhang, X.L.; Zhu, H.; et al. Lighting up the Native Viral RNA Genome with a Fluorogenic Probe for the Live-Cell Visualization of Virus Infection. *J. Am. Chem. Soc.* **2019**, *141*, 5182–5191. [CrossRef]

108. Laguerre, A.; Hukezalie, K.; Winckler, P.; Katranji, F.; Chanteloup, G.; Pirrotta, M.; Perrier-Cornet, J.M.; Wong, J.M.; Monchaud, D. Visualization of RNA-Quadruplexes in Live Cells. *J. Am. Chem. Soc.* **2015**, *137*, 8521–8525. [CrossRef]

109. Jeng, S.C.; Chan, H.H.; Booy, E.P.; McKenna, S.A.; Unrau, P.J. Fluorophore ligand binding and complex stabilization of the RNA Mango and RNA Spinach aptamers. *RNA* **2016**, *22*, 1884–1892. [CrossRef]

110. Xu, S.; Li, Q.; Xiang, J.; Yang, Q.; Sun, H.; Guan, A.; Wang, L.; Liu, Y.; Yu, L.; Shi, Y.; et al. Thioflavin T as an efficient fluorescence sensor for selective recognition of RNA G-quadruplexes. *Sci. Rep.* **2016**, *6*, 24793. [CrossRef] [PubMed]

111. Guo, J.H.; Zhu, L.N.; Kong, D.M.; Shen, H.X. Triphenylmethane dyes as fluorescent probes for G-quadruplex recognition. *Talanta* **2009**, *80*, 607–613. [CrossRef] [PubMed]

112. Stanoeva, T.; Neshchadin, D.; Gescheidt, G.; Ludvik, J.; Lajoie, B.; Batchelor, S.N. An Investigation into the Initial Degradation Steps of Four Major Dye Chromophores: Study of Their One-Electron Oxidation and Reduction by EPR, ENDOR, Cyclic Voltammetry, and Theoretical Calculations. *J. Phys. Chem. A* **2005**, *109*, 7. [CrossRef]

113. Kong, D.M.; Ma, Y.E.; Wu, J.; Shen, H.X. Discrimination of G-quadruplexes from duplex and single-stranded DNAs with fluorescence and energy-transfer fluorescence spectra of crystal violet. *Chemistry* **2009**, *15*, 901–909. [CrossRef] [PubMed]

114. Li, F.; Feng, Y.; Zhao, C.; Tang, B. Crystal violet as a G-quadruplex-selective probe for sensitive amperometric sensing of lead. *Chem. Commun.* **2011**, *47*, 11909–11911. [CrossRef]

115. Song, J.; Wu, F.-Y.; Wan, Y.-Q.; Ma, L.-H. Ultrasensitive turn-on fluorescent detection of trace thiocyanate based on fluorescence resonance energy transfer. *Talanta* **2015**, *132*, 619–624. [CrossRef] [PubMed]

116. Chen, Y.; Wang, J.; Zhang, Y.; Xu, L.; Gao, T.; Wang, B.; Pei, R. Selection and characterization of a DNA aptamer to crystal violet. *Photochem. Photobiol. Sci.* **2018**, *17*, 800–806. [CrossRef] [PubMed]

117. He, H.Z.; Ma, V.P.; Leung, K.H.; Chan, D.S.; Yang, H.; Cheng, Z.; Leung, C.H.; Ma, D.L. A label-free G-quadruplex-based switch-on fluorescence assay for the selective detection of ATP. *Analyst* **2012**, *137*, 1538–1540. [CrossRef]

118. De-Ming, K.; Ma, Y.-E.; Guo, J.-H.; Yang, W.; Shen, H.-X. Fluorescent Sensor for Monitoring Structural Changes of G-Quadruplexes and Detection of Potassium Ion. *Anal. Chem.* **2009**, *81*, 7. [CrossRef]

119. Jin, Y.; Bai, J.; Li, H. Label-free protein recognition using aptamer-based fluorescence assay. *Analyst* **2010**, *135*, 1731–1735. [CrossRef] [PubMed]

120. Kong, D.M.; Guo, J.H.; Yang, W.; Ma, Y.E.; Shen, H.X. Crystal violet-G-quadruplex complexes as fluorescent sensors for homogeneous detection of potassium ion. *Biosens. Bioelectron.* **2009**, *25*, 88–93. [CrossRef] [PubMed]

121. Zheng, B.; Cheng, S.; Dong, H.; Liang, H.; Liu, J.; Lam, M.H.-W. Label Free Determination of Potassium Ions Using Crystal Violet and Thrombin-Binding Aptamer. *Anal. Lett.* **2014**, *47*, 1726–1736. [CrossRef]

122. Ivancic, V.A.; Ekanayake, O.; Lazo, N.D. Binding Modes of Thioflavin T on the Surface of Amyloid Fibrils Studied by NMR. *ChemPhysChem* **2016**, *17*, 2461–2464. [CrossRef] [PubMed]

123. Zhang, X.Y.; Luo, H.Q.; Li, N.B. Crystal violet as an i-motif structure probe for reversible and label-free pH-driven electrochemical switch. *Anal. Biochem.* **2014**, *455*, 55–59. [CrossRef] [PubMed]

124. Introduction: Quadruplexes and their Biology. In *Therapeutic Applications of Quadruplex Nucleic Acids*; Neidle, S. (Ed.) Science Elsevier: London, UK, 2012; pp. 1–20.

125. Gunaratnam, M.; Greciano, O.; Martins, C.; Reszka, A.P.; Schultes, C.M.; Morjani, H.; Riou, J.F.; Neidle, S. Mechanism of acridine-based telomerase inhibition and telomere shortening. *Biochem. Pharmacol.* **2007**, *74*, 679–689. [CrossRef] [PubMed]

126. Perrone, R.; Nadai, M.; Frasson, I.; Poe, J.A.; Butovskaya, E.; Smithgall, T.E.; Palumbo, M.; Palu, G.; Richter, S.N. A dynamic G-quadruplex region regulates the HIV-1 long terminal repeat promoter. *J. Med. Chem.* **2013**, *56*, 6521–6530. [CrossRef] [PubMed]

127. Le, D.D.; di Antonio, M.; Chan, L.K.M.; Balasubramanian, S. G-quadruplex ligands exhibit differential G-tetrad selectivity. *Chem. Commun.* **2015**, *51*. [CrossRef] [PubMed]

128. Koirala, D.; Dhakal, S.; Ashbridge, B.; Sannohe, Y.; Rodriguez, R.; Sugiyama, H.; Balasubramanian, S.; Mao, H. A single-molecule platform for investigation of interactions between G-quadruplexes and small-molecule ligands. *Nat. Chem.* **2011**, *3*, 782–787. [CrossRef] [PubMed]

129. Muller, S.; Kumari, S.; Rodriguez, R.; Balasubramanian, S. Small-molecule-mediated G-quadruplex isolation from human cells. *Nat. Chem.* **2010**, *2*, 1095–1098. [CrossRef] [PubMed]

130. Muller, S.; Sanders, D.A.; Di Antonio, M.; Matsis, S.; Riou, J.F.; Rodriguez, R.; Balasubramanian, S. Pyridostatin analogues promote telomere dysfunction and long-term growth inhibition in human cancer cells. *Org. Biomol. Chem.* **2012**, *10*, 6537–6546. [CrossRef] [PubMed]

131. Rodriguez, R.; Miller, K.M.; Forment, J.V.; Bradshaw, C.R.; Nikan, M.; Britton, S.; Oelschlaegel, T.; Xhemalce, B.; Balasubramanian, S.; Jackson, S.P. Small-molecule-induced DNA damage identifies alternative DNA structures in human genes. *Nat. Chem. Biol.* **2012**, *8*, 301–310. [CrossRef]

132. Mahmood, T.; Paul, A.; Ladame, S. Synthesis and spectroscopic and DNA-binding properties of fluorogenic acridine-containing cyanine dyes. *J. Org. Chem.* **2010**, *75*, 204–207. [CrossRef]

133. Percivalle, C.; Mahmood, T.; Ladame, S. Two-in-one: A pH-sensitive, acridine-based, fluorescent probe binds G-quadruplexes in oncogene promoters. *Med. Chem. Commun.* **2013**, *4*, 211–215. [CrossRef]

134. Machireddy, B.; Kalra, G.; Jonnalagadda, S.; Ramanujachary, K.; Wu, C. Probing the Binding Pathway of BRACO19 to a Parallel-Stranded Human Telomeric G-Quadruplex Using Molecular Dynamics Binding Simulation with AMBER DNA OL15 and Ligand GAFF2 Force Fields. *J. Chem. Inf. Model.* **2017**, *57*, 2846–2864. [CrossRef] [PubMed]

135. Jin, B.; Zhang, X.; Zheng, W.; Liu, X.; Qi, C.; Wang, F.; Shangguan, D. Fluorescence light-up probe for parallel G-quadruplexes. *Anal. Chem.* **2014**, *86*, 943–952. [CrossRef] [PubMed]

136. Yang, C.; Hu, R.; Li, Q.; Li, S.; Xiang, J.; Guo, X.; Wang, S.; Zeng, Y.; Li, Y.; Yang, G. Visualization of Parallel G-Quadruplexes in Cells with a Series of New Developed Bis(4-aminobenzylidene)acetone Derivatives. *ACS Omega* **2018**, *3*, 10487–10492. [CrossRef]

137. Chen, S.-B.; Wu, W.-B.; Hu, M.-H.; Ou, T.-M.; Gu, L.-Q.; Tan, J.-H.; Huang, Z.-S. Discovery of a New Fluorescent Light-Up Probe Specific to Parallel G-Quadruplexes. *Chem. Commun.* **2014**, *50*. [CrossRef] [PubMed]

138. Hu, M.H.; Chen, S.B.; Wang, B.; Ou, T.M.; Gu, L.Q.; Tan, J.H.; Huang, Z.S. Specific targeting of telomeric multimeric G-quadruplexes by a new triaryl-substituted imidazole. *Nucleic Acids Res.* **2017**, *45*, 1606–1618. [CrossRef]

139. Hu, M.H.; Zhou, J.; Luo, W.H.; Chen, S.B.; Huang, Z.S.; Wu, R.; Tan, J.H. Development of a Smart Fluorescent Sensor that Specifically Recognizes the c-MYC G-Quadruplex. *Anal. Chem.* **2019**. [CrossRef] [PubMed]

140. Kotar, A.; Wang, B.; Shivalingam, A.; Gonzalez-Garcia, J.; Vilar, R.; Plavec, J. NMR Structure of a Triangulenium-Based Long-Lived Fluorescence Probe Bound to a G-Quadruplex. *Angew. Chem.* **2016**, *55*, 12508–12511. [CrossRef]

141. Yan, J.W.; Chen, S.B.; Liu, H.Y.; Ye, W.J.; Ou, T.M.; Tan, J.H.; Li, D.; Gu, L.Q.; Huang, Z.S. Development of a new colorimetric and red-emitting fluorescent dual probe for G-quadruplex nucleic acids. *Chem. Commun.* **2014**, *50*, 6927–6930. [CrossRef]

142. Chen, S.B.; Hu, M.H.; Liu, G.C.; Wang, J.; Ou, T.M.; Gu, L.Q.; Huang, Z.S.; Tan, J.H. Visualization of NRAS RNA G-Quadruplex Structures in Cells with an Engineered Fluorogenic Hybridization Probe. *J. Am. Chem. Soc.* **2016**, *138*, 10382–10385. [CrossRef]

143. Chen, X.C.; Chen, S.B.; Dai, J.; Yuan, J.H.; Ou, T.M.; Huang, Z.S.; Tan, J.H. Tracking the Dynamic Folding and Unfolding of RNA G-Quadruplexes in Live Cells. *Angew. Chem.* **2018**. [CrossRef]

144. Laguerre, A.; Stefan, L.; Larrouy, M.; Genest, D.; Novotna, J.; Pirrotta, M.; Monchaud, D. A twice-as-smart synthetic G-quartet: PyroTASQ is both a smart quadruplex ligand and a smart fluorescent probe. *J. Am. Chem. Soc.* **2014**, *136*, 12406–12414. [CrossRef] [PubMed]

145. Laguerre, A.; Wong, J.M.; Monchaud, D. Direct visualization of both DNA and RNA quadruplexes in human cells via an uncommon spectroscopic method. *Sci. Rep.* **2016**, *6*, 32141. [CrossRef]

146. Flinders, J.; DeFina, S.C.; Brackett, D.M.; Baugh, C.; Wilson, C.; Dieckmann, T. Recognition of planar and nonplanar ligands in the malachite green-RNA aptamer complex. *ChemBioChem Eur. J. Chem. Biol.* **2004**, *5*, 62–72. [CrossRef] [PubMed]

147. Dai, R.; Wang, X.; Wang, Z.; Mu, S.; Liao, J.; Wen, Y.; Lv, J.; Huang, K.; Xiong, X. A sensitive and label-free sensor for melamine and iodide by target-regulating the formation of G-quadruplex. *Microchem. J.* **2019**, *146*, 592–599. [CrossRef]

148. Hsu, J.C.; Chen, E.H.; Snoeberger, R.C., 3rd.; Luh, F.Y.; Lim, T.S.; Hsu, C.P.; Chen, R.P. Thioflavin T and its photoirradiative derivatives: Exploring their spectroscopic properties in the absence and presence of amyloid fibrils. *J. Phys. Chem. B* **2013**, *117*, 3459–3468. [CrossRef]

149. Iliuk, A.B.; Hu, L.; Tao, W.A. Aptamer in bioanalytical applications. *Anal. Chem.* **2011**, *83*, 4440–4452. [CrossRef]

150. Tuerk, C.; Gold, L. Systematic Evolution of Ligands by Exponential Enrichment: RNA Ligands to Bacteriophage T4 DNA Polymerase. *Science* **1990**, *249*, 505–510. [CrossRef]

151. Song, S.; Wang, L.; Li, J.; Fan, C.; Zhao, J. Aptamer-based biosensors. *Trends Anal. Chem.* **2008**, *27*, 108–117. [CrossRef]

152. Li, F.; Zhang, H.; Wang, Z.; Newbigging, A.M.; Reid, M.S.; Li, X.-F.; Le, X.C. Aptamers Facilitating Amplified Detection of Biomolecules. *Anal. Chem.* **2014**, *87*, 274–292. [CrossRef]

153. Gatto, B.; Palumbo, M.; Sissi, C. Nucleic Acid Aptamers Based on the G-Quadruplex Structure: Therapeutic and Diagnostic Potential. *Curr. Med. Chem.* **2009**, *16*, 1248–1265. [CrossRef] [PubMed]

154. Phan, A.T. Human telomeric G-quadruplex: Structures of DNA and RNA sequences. *FEBS J.* **2010**, *277*, 1107–1117. [CrossRef] [PubMed]

155. Bock, L.C.; Griffin, L.C.; Latham, J.A.; Vermaas, E.H.; Toole, J.J. Selection of single-stranded DNA molecules that bind and inhibit human thrombin. *Nature* **1992**, *355*, 564–566. [CrossRef]

156. Macaya, R.F.; Schultiz, P.; Smith, F.W.; Roe, J.A.; Feigon, J. Thrombin-binding DNA aptamer forms a unimolecular quadruplex structure in solution. *Proc. Natl. Acad. Sci. USA* **1993**, *90*, 3745–3749. [CrossRef] [PubMed]

157. Jasinski, D.; Haque, F.; Binzel, D.W.; Guo, P. Advancement of the Emerging Field of RNA Nanotechnology. *ACS Nano* **2017**, *11*, 1142–1164. [CrossRef] [PubMed]

158. Xia, Y.; Zhang, R.; Wang, Z.; Tian, J.; Chen, X. Recent advances in high-performance fluorescent and bioluminescent RNA imaging probes. *Chem. Soc. Rev.* **2017**, *46*, 2824–2843. [CrossRef]

159. Paige, J.S.; Nguyen-Duc, T.; Song, W.; Jaffrey, S.R. Fluorescence imaging of cellular metabolites with RNA. *Science* **2012**, *335*, 1194. [CrossRef]

160. Shieh, Y.A.; Yang, S.J.; Wei, M.F.; Shieh, M.J. Aptamer-based tumor-targeted drug delivery for photodynamic therapy. *ACS Nano* **2010**, *4*, 1433–1442. [CrossRef] [PubMed]

161. Meng, H.; Liu, H.; Kuai, H.; Peng, R.; Mo, L.; Zhang, X. Aptamer-integrated DNA nanostructures for biosensing, bioimaging and cancer therapy. *Chem. Soc. Rev.* **2016**, *45*, 2583–2602. [CrossRef] [PubMed]

162. Dhiman, A.; Kalra, P.; Bansal, V.; Bruno, J.G.; Sharma, T.K. Aptamer-based point-of-care diagnostic platforms. *Sens. Actuators B Chem.* **2017**, *246*, 535–553. [CrossRef]
163. Chang, H.; Tang, L.; Wang, Y.; Jiang, J.; Li, J. Graphene fluorescence resonance energy transfer aptasensor for the thrombin detection. *Anal. Chem.* **2010**, *82*, 2341–2346. [CrossRef]
164. Ge, J.; Ou, E.-C.; Yu, R.-Q.; Chu, X. A novel aptameric nanobiosensor based on the self-assembled DNA-MoS2 nanosheet architecture for biomolecule detection. *J. Mater. Chem. B* **2014**, *2*, 625–628. [CrossRef]
165. Liu, X.; Freeman, R.; Willner, I. Amplified fluorescence aptamer-based sensors using exonuclease III for the regeneration of the analyte. *Chemistry* **2012**, *18*, 2207–2211. [CrossRef] [PubMed]
166. Yan, S.; Huang, R.; Zhou, Y.; Zhang, M.; Deng, M.; Wang, X.; Weng, X.; Zhou, X. Aptamer-based turn-on fluorescent four-branched quaternary ammonium pyrazine probe for selective thrombin detection. *Chem. Commun.* **2011**, *47*, 1273–1275. [CrossRef] [PubMed]
167. Ji, D.; Wang, H.; Ge, J.; Zhang, L.; Li, J.; Bai, D.; Chen, J.; Li, Z. Label-free and rapid detection of ATP based on structure switching of aptamers. *Anal. Biochem.* **2017**, *526*, 22–28. [CrossRef] [PubMed]
168. Zhang, Z.; Sharon, E.; Freeman, R.; Liu, X.; Willner, I. Fluorescence detection of DNA, adenosine-5′-triphosphate (ATP), and telomerase activity by zinc(II)-protoporphyrin IX/G-quadruplex labels. *Anal. Chem.* **2012**, *84*, 4789–4797. [CrossRef] [PubMed]
169. Wei, Y.; Chen, Y.; Li, H.; Shuang, S.; Dong, C.; Wang, G. An exonuclease I-based label-free fluorometric aptasensor for adenosine triphosphate (ATP) detection with a wide concentration range. *Biosens. Bioelectron.* **2015**, *63*, 311–316. [CrossRef]
170. Xu, L.; Shen, X.; Hong, S.; Wang, J.; Zhang, Y.; Wang, H.; Zhang, J.; Pei, R. Turn-on and label-free fluorescence detection of lead ions based on target-induced G-quadruplex formation. *Chem. Commun.* **2015**, *51*, 8165–8168. [CrossRef] [PubMed]
171. Cheng, H.; Qiu, X.; Zhao, X.; Meng, W.; Huo, D.; Wei, H. Functional Nucleic Acid Probe for Parallel Monitoring K(+) and Protoporphyrin IX in Living Organisms. *Anal. Chem.* **2016**, *88*, 2937–2943. [CrossRef]
172. Yang, L.; Qing, Z.; Liu, C.; Tang, Q.; Li, J.; Yang, S.; Zheng, J.; Yang, R.; Tan, W. Direct Fluorescent Detection of Blood Potassium by Ion-selective Formation of Intermolecular G-quadruplex and Ligand Binding. *Anal. Chem.* **2016**. [CrossRef]
173. Lord, S.J.; Lee, H.L.; Moerner, W.E. Single-molecule spectroscopy and imaging of biomolecules in living cells. *Anal. Chem.* **2010**, *82*, 2192–2203. [CrossRef]
174. Johnsson, N.; Johnsson, K. Chemical tools for biomolecular imaging. *ACS Chem. Biol.* **2007**, *2*, 31–38. [CrossRef] [PubMed]
175. Paige, J.S.; Wu, K.Y.; Jaffrey, S.R. RNA mimics of green fluorescent protein. *Science* **2011**, *333*, 642–646. [CrossRef] [PubMed]
176. Han, K.Y.; Leslie, B.J.; Fei, J.; Zhang, J.; Ha, T. Understanding the photophysics of the Spinach-DFHBI RNA aptamer-fluorogen complex to improve live-cell RNA imaging. *J. Am. Chem. Soc.* **2013**, *135*, 19033–19038. [CrossRef] [PubMed]
177. Song, W.; Strack, R.L.; Jaffrey, S.R. Imaging bacterial protein expression using genetically encoded RNA sensors. *Nat. Methods* **2013**, *10*, 873–875. [CrossRef] [PubMed]
178. Strack, R.L.; Disney, M.D.; Jaffrey, S.R. A superfolding Spinach2 reveals the dynamic nature of trinucleotide repeat-containing RNA. *Nat. Methods* **2013**, *10*, 1219–1224. [CrossRef] [PubMed]
179. Okuda, M.; Fourmy, D.; Yoshizawa, S. Use of Baby Spinach and Broccoli for imaging of structured cellular RNAs. *Nucleic Acids Res.* **2017**, *45*, 1404–1415. [CrossRef] [PubMed]
180. Warner, K.D.; Chen, M.C.; Song, W.; Strack, R.L.; Thorn, A.; Jaffrey, S.R.; Ferre-D'Amare, A.R. Structural basis for activity of highly efficient RNA mimics of green fluorescent protein. *Nat. Struct. Mol. Biol.* **2014**, *21*, 658–663. [CrossRef]
181. Jepsen, M.D.E.; Sparvath, S.M.; Nielsen, T.B.; Langvad, A.H.; Grossi, G.; Gothelf, K.V.; Andersen, E.S. Development of a genetically encodable FRET system using fluorescent RNA aptamers. *Nat. Commun.* **2018**, *9*, 18. [CrossRef]
182. Chou, S.H.; Chin, K.H.; Wang, A.H. DNA aptamers as potential anti-HIV agents. *Trends Biochem. Sci.* **2005**, *30*, 231–234. [CrossRef]
183. de Soultrait, V.R.; Lozach, P.-Y.; Altmeyer, R.; Tarrago-Litvak, L.; Litvak, S.; Andréola, M.L. DNA Aptamers Derived from HIV-1 RNase H Inhibitors are Strong Anti-integrase Agents. *J. Mol. Biol.* **2002**, *324*, 195–203. [CrossRef]

184. Jing, N.; Xiong, W.; Guan, Y.; Pallansch, L.; Wang, S. Potassium-dependent folding: A key to intracellular delivery of G-quartet oligonucleotides as HIV inhibitors. *Biochemistry* **2002**, *41*, 5397–5403. [CrossRef] [PubMed]

185. Li, T.; Shi, L.; Wang, E.; Dong, S. Multifunctional G-quadruplex aptamers and their application to protein detection. *Chemistry* **2009**, *15*, 1036–1042. [CrossRef] [PubMed]

186. Chen, W.H.; Yang Sung, S.; Fadeev, M.; Cecconello, A.; Nechushtai, R.; Willner, I. Targeted VEGF-triggered release of an anti-cancer drug from aptamer-functionalized metal–organic framework nanoparticles. *Nanoscale* **2018**, *10*, 4650–4657. [CrossRef] [PubMed]

187. Huang, H.; Suslov, N.B.; Li, N.S.; Shelke, S.A.; Evans, M.E.; Koldobskaya, Y.; Rice, P.A.; Piccirilli, J.A. A G-quadruplex-containing RNA activates fluorescence in a GFP-like fluorophore. *Nat. Chem. Biol.* **2014**, *10*, 686–691. [CrossRef] [PubMed]

188. Trachman, R.J., 3rd.; Demeshkina, N.A.; Lau, M.W.L.; Panchapakesan, S.S.S.; Jeng, S.C.Y.; Unrau, P.J.; Ferre-D'Amare, A.R. Structural basis for high-affinity fluorophore binding and activation by RNA Mango. *Nat. Chem. Biol.* **2017**, *13*, 807–813. [CrossRef] [PubMed]

189. Singh, R.; Lillard, J.W., Jr. Nanoparticle-based targeted drug delivery. *Exp. Mol. Pathol.* **2009**, *86*, 215–223. [CrossRef]

190. Weerasinghe, P.; Garcia, G.E.; Zhu, Q.; Yuan, P.; Feng, L.; Mao, L.; Jing, N. Inhibition of Stat3 activation and tumor growth suppression of non-small cell lung cancer by G-quartet oligonucleotides. *Int. J. Oncol.* **2007**, *31*, 129–136. [CrossRef]

191. Paeschke, K.; Simonsson, T.; Postberg, J.; Rhodes, D.; Lipps, H.J. Telomere end-binding proteins control the formation of G-quadruplex DNA structures in vivo. *Nat. Struct. Mol. Biol.* **2005**, *12*, 847–854. [CrossRef]

192. Stoddart, C.A.; Rabin, L.; Hincenbergs, M.; Moreno, M.E.; Steppes, V.L.; Leeds, J.M.; Truong, L.A.; Wyatt, J.R.; Ecker, D.J.; Mccune, J.M. Inhibition of human immunodeficiency virus type 1 infection in SCID-hu Thy/Liv mice by the G-Quartet-forming oligonucleotide, ISIS 5320. *Antimicrob. Agents Chemother.* **1998**, *42*, 2113–2115. [CrossRef]

193. Pileur, F.; Andreola, M.-L.; Dausse, E.; Michel, J.; Moreau, S.; Yamada, H.; Gaidamakov, S.A.; Crouch, R.J.; Toulmé, J.-J.; Cazenave, C. Selective inhibitory DNA aptamers of the human RNase H1. *Nucleic Acids Res.* **2003**, *31*, 5776–5788. [CrossRef]

194. Jones, L.A.; Clancy, L.E.; Rawlinson, W.D.; White, P.A. High-affinity aptamers to subtype 3a hepatitis C virus polymerase display genotypic specificity. *Antimicrob. Agents Chemother.* **2006**, *50*, 3019–3027. [CrossRef] [PubMed]

195. Shum, K.T.; Tanner, J.A. Differential inhibitory activities and stabilisation of DNA aptamers against the SARS coronavirus helicase. *ChemBioChem Eur. J. Chem. Biol.* **2008**, *9*, 3037–3045. [CrossRef] [PubMed]

196. Yoshida, W.; Mochizuki, E.; Takase, M.; Hasegawa, H.; Morita, Y.; Yamazaki, H.; Sode, K.; Ikebukuro, K. Selection of DNA aptamers against insulin and construction of an aptameric enzyme subunit for insulin sensing. *Biosens. Bioelectron.* **2009**, *24*, 1116–1120. [CrossRef] [PubMed]

197. Okazawa, A.; Maeda, H.; Fukusaki, E.; Katakura, Y.; Kobayashi, A. In vitro selection of Hematoporphyrin binding DNA aptamers. *Bioorg. Med. Chem. Lett.* **2000**, *10*, 2653–2656. [CrossRef]

198. Li, T.; Dong, S.; Wang, E. G-quadruplex aptamers with peroxidase-like DNAzyme functions: Which is the best and how does it work? *Chem. Asian J.* **2009**, *4*, 918–922. [CrossRef] [PubMed]

199. Filonov, G.S.; Moon, J.D.; Svensen, N.; Jaffrey, S.R. Broccoli: Rapid selection of an RNA mimic of green fluorescent protein by fluorescence-based selection and directed evolution. *J. Am. Chem. Soc.* **2014**, *136*, 16299–16308. [CrossRef]

200. Warner, K.D.; Sjekloca, L.; Song, W.; Filonov, G.S.; Jaffrey, S.R.; Ferre-D'Amare, A.R. A homodimer interface without base pairs in an RNA mimic of red fluorescent protein. *Nat. Chem. Biol.* **2017**, *13*, 1195–1201. [CrossRef]

201. Trachman, R.J., 3rd.; Abdolahzadeh, A.; Andreoni, A.; Cojocaru, R.; Knutson, J.R.; Ryckelynck, M.; Unrau, P.J.; Ferre-D'Amare, A.R. Crystal Structures of the Mango-II RNA Aptamer Reveal Heterogeneous Fluorophore Binding and Guide Engineering of Variants with Improved Selectivity and Brightness. *Biochemistry* **2018**, *57*, 3544–3548. [CrossRef]

202. Trachman, R.J., 3rd.; Autour, A.; Jeng, S.C.Y.; Abdolahzadeh, A.; Andreoni, A.; Cojocaru, R.; Garipov, R.; Dolgosheina, E.V.; Knutson, J.R.; Ryckelynck, M.; et al. Structure and functional reselection of the Mango-III fluorogenic RNA aptamer. *Nat. Chem. Biol.* **2019**, *15*, 472–479. [CrossRef]

203. Levesque, D.; Beaudoin, J.D.; Roy, S.; Perreault, J.P. In vitro selection and characterization of RNA aptamers binding thyroxine hormone. *Biochem. J.* **2007**, *403*, 129–138. [CrossRef]

204. Mori, T.; Oguro, A.; Ohtsu, T.; Nakamura, Y. RNA aptamers selected against the receptor activator of NF-kappaB acquire general affinity to proteins of the tumor necrosis factor receptor family. *Nucleic Acids Res.* **2004**, *32*, 6120–6128. [CrossRef] [PubMed]

205. Liu, Y.; Zhang, Y.; Ye, G.; Yang, Z.; Zhang, L.; Zhang, L. In vitro selection of G-rich RNA aptamers that target HIV-1 integrase. *Sci. China Series B Chem.* **2008**, *51*, 401–413. [CrossRef]

206. Weiss, S.; Proske, D.; Neumann, M.; Groschup, M.H.; Kretzschmar, H.A.; Famulok, M.; Winnacker, E.-L. RNA aptamers specifically interact with the prion protein PrP. *J. Virol.* **1997**, *71*, 8790–8797. [PubMed]

207. Homann, M.; Lorger, M.; Engstler, M.; Zacharias, M.; Göringer, H.U. Serum-stable RNA aptamers to an invariant surface domain of live african trypanosomes. *Comb. Chem. High Throughput Screen.* **2006**, *9*, 491–499. [PubMed]

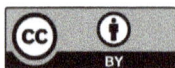

MDPI

St. Alban-Anlage 66

4052 Basel

Switzerland

Tel. +41 61 683 77 34

Fax +41 61 302 89 18

www.mdpi.com

Molecules Editorial Office

E-mail: molecules@mdpi.com

www.mdpi.com/journal/molecules